Biochemistry

For Churchill Livingstone

Publisher: Michael Parkinson
Project Editor: Barbara Simmons
Project Controller: Frances Affleck
Design Direction: Erik Bigland

Churchill's Mastery of Medicine

Biochemistry

Alexander C. Brownie

PhD DSc FRSE
Teaching and Research Fellow,
Consultant in Biochemistry,
University of Dundee, UK;
Distinguished Teaching Professor Emeritus,
University at Buffalo, NY, USA

John C. Kernohan

MA PhD
Senior Lecturer, Department of Biochemistry,
University of Dundee, UK

Illustrations by
**Jane Templeman and
Chartwell Illustrators**

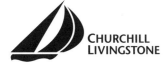
CHURCHILL
LIVINGSTONE

EDINBURGH, LONDON, NEW YORK, PHILADELPHIA, ST LOUIS,
SYDNEY, TORONTO 1999

CHURCHILL LIVINGSTONE
A Division of Harcourt Publishers Limited

Churchill Livingstone, 1–3 Baxter's Place, Leith Walk, Edinburgh
EH1 3AF

© Harcourt Publishers Limited 1999

 is a registered trade mark of Harcourt Publishers Limited

The right of Professor Alexander Brownie and Dr John Kernohan
to be identified as authors of this book has been asserted by them
in accordance with the Copyright, Designs and Patents Act 1988.

ISBN 0443 056935

British Library of Cataloguing in Publication Data
A catalogue record for this book is available from the British
Library.

Library of Congress Cataloging in Publication Data
A catalog record for this book is available from the Library of
Congress.

Medical knowledge is constantly changing. As information
becomes available, changes in treatment, procedures, equipment
and the use of drugs become necessary. The author and publisher
have, as far as it is possible, taken care to ensure that the
information given in the text is accurate and up-to-date. However,
readers are strongly advised to confirm that the information,
especially with regard to drug usage, complies with current
legislation and standards of practice.

The
publisher's
policy is to use
**paper manufactured
from sustainable forests**

Printed in China

Acknowledgements

Both authors have been teaching general biochemistry to medical, dental and science students for many years. During this time we have had many colleagues whose input to jointly taught courses have impacted on our teaching and therefore this text. ACB wishes to express his extreme indebtedness to the late Dr John F. Moran, with whom he taught metabolism at the University at Buffalo School of Medicine and Biomedical Sciences. Jack Moran and ACB developed many of the course notes that have served as a guide for much of the material on normal function contained in Chapters 7, 8, 9, 10, 11 and 12. Also, Dr Steven M. Simasko, College of Veterinary Medicine, Pullman, Washington State, with whom ACB taught in Buffalo, has influenced the treatment of the endocrine system presented in Chapter 18. We thank Dr Josephine Alfano, University at Buffalo, who reviewed and edited Chapter 18.

The authors thank their colleagues at the University of Dundee who reviewed most of the chapters. Professor Michael J. Rennie provided the diagrams in Chapter 9 on protein turnover and reviewed that chapter as well as the nutritional biochemistry presented in Chapter 19. Dr Michael Stark, University of Dundee provided material incorporated into Chapter 21 on biochemical genetics and reviewed that chapter. Dr Roger Booth reviewed all of the metabolism chapters plus Chapters 2, 3, 4, 5 and 6.

We thank Michael Parkinson and Barbara Simmons at Churchill Livingstone as well as Dr Jane Ward who, as copy-editor, helped clarify our text.

Lastly, we acknowledge the support of our wives, Willy Brownie-Bakhuizen and Kathy Kernohan, who tolerated our commitment to many hours of work on the text.

Contents

Using this book

Philosophy of the book

Both the General Medical Council in Great Britain and the Licensing Committee on Medical Education in the United States have recommended significant changes in the medical curriculum. Phase 1 of such a new curriculum emphasises integration, a systems approach and the presentation of core knowledge. The teaching of a core biochemistry course to Medical (or Dental) students represents a major challenge. The problem that we face in designing biochemistry courses for first year students is that it is difficult to identify *anything* that is not core. This applies especially in the rapidly developing area of molecular biology and the fact-rich area of metabolism. We are writing this core text as part of the Churchill Livingstone series stimulated by the multiple requests from our students for a text that they can use to guide them in Phase 1 of the new curriculum. It is also designed to be of use to first year BDS students.

Within a text of this length we cannot cover the entire breadth of medical biochemistry knowledge that will be discussed throughout the medical course. Rather, we have focussed upon knowledge that will allow students to survive the first year in medical school. Based upon that core material we expect students will want to expand their knowledge and consult several biochemistry texts that cover the discipline in a comprehensive fashion.

Layout of the book

This book covers General and Applied Biochemistry. Some of our colleagues who teach in the first year medical curriculum have provided us with the learning objectives for their lectures and we have designed the book to conform with these. Since this is a text primarily directed at medical students we have included brief 'clinical notes' in order to demonstrate the applications of core biochemistry knowledge to clinical practice.

We recognise that self-assessment by our students is the key to them dealing with the intensity of the medical curriculum and have prepared many exercises that complement the various chapters in this core text.

Studying biochemistry

The field of biochemistry has changed enormously since the Second World War and the pace of advances is increasing. Core knowledge essential for students in the life sciences has not become easier, but because of the application of tools of modern molecular biology we now can describe the systems in a clearer fashion. How should students deal with the knowledge explosion in a core course? Our advice is as follows.

- Make the most of basic courses in chemistry, biology, mathematics and physics
- Read the appropriate section of this core text *before* attending lectures. If detailed lecture hand-outs are part of the course, read them in advance as well. If necessary, read relevant material in one of the many excellent comprehensive texts available.
- Try to be honest and admit when there are areas or points that you find confusing. The key is not to delay in filling in these gaps in your understanding. Often you can clear up problems by talking to a colleague but, failing that, talk to the teacher or teaching assistant. Students who fail miserably and who have not asked for help do not impress anyone!
- You will find that many new terms will be introduced in your biochemistry course. Be consistent in listing those terms that you do not know with certainty. Prepare a *glossary* by making use of this text and the other texts. Writing down definitions and descriptions will help fix the information in your memory.
- During the course, prepare a list of headings of the various sub-sections of the material well spaced out on sheets of paper. Closer to exam time take these sheets and fill in as much of the gaps as you can. Comparison with your notes will establish two things: (a) what you know well and (b) what you need to study once more. In this way you avoid reading through your entire course notes or course book again and again.
- Your aim should be to arrive at the examination hall knowing what you know. You are there simply to let the teachers know what you know. To accomplish this simplistic aim you will need to indulge in regular and extensive *self-assessment*. Each chapter in this textbook ends with a series of self-assessment questions. Try them after you have reviewed the material in the chapter. Get a colleague to grade you if you want to feel even more confident of your knowledge. Make sure you use any self-assessment exercises that your teachers have prepared; they may be easy to access through your university computer network.

Examination techniques

There is a lot of variation in the exam formats used in the different universities. Since medical classes are usually large, easily-scored multiple choice questions are frequently used, but it is also useful to develop skills in answering short-essay questions. Here are some hints.

- Multiple choice questions need particular attention since a single word can change the answer dramatically. **Read the stem more than once**. Although this is not obvious at first glance, every choice in a MCQ is between **true** or **false**. If there is a customised key to the MCQ you can then examine your answers in the context of that customised key and make an appropriate choice. If you are given no guidance as to the number of true and false statements in a MCQ, in most cases you get credit for all correct answers selected but you lose points for incorrect ones (negative marking). Be cautious but definitely attempt each MCQ and give each your best shot! Too much caution rarely succeeds. Watch out for traps! It is advisable to find out in advance whether your teachers are using negative marking since this can influence the strategy you employ. Know if the exam guidelines allow for challenges!

- Words in the stem such as 'direct' and 'indirect' can make terrific differences to the answers. Words such as 'only' and 'never' are often giveaways that the choice is false but there is no hard and fast rule.

- If you are taking exams with short answers or essays, make sure to start by sketching out the major points you will cover: ask for scrap paper! This helps to organise your answer and will be appreciated by the examiner. Do not fail to take opportunities to illustrate your answers with well-conceived, clear diagrams. Do not drift from the point of the question; examiners get tired and angry reading through a mass of irrelevancy! Ration your time since it is advisable to write *all* of the required essays. Practise writing answers to questions that appeared in previous years' exams; they are usually provided but if not, ask for them! Find out if the teacher is willing to give you an opinion on your practice efforts.

- If your teachers provide you with computer banks of questions that cover the learning objectives of your course, try them. Integrated exams in Phase 1 can be taken by students at a computer terminal and students who practise with the computer bank of sample questions improve their chances of success in the degree exams.

Biochemistry and medicine

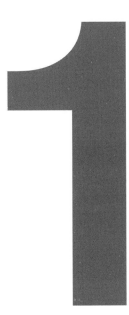

Most biochemists will tell you that the enormous strides which have been made in advancing medical knowledge have been largely the result of development of methods that allow us to examine physiological and pathological processes at the molecular level. In fact, almost every branch of clinical medicine research is carried out using the latest molecular biology techniques. The fact that the newspapers report these advances on an almost daily basis and terms such as 'recombinant DNA' and 'cloning' are printed without explanation is surely reason enough why medical graduates must be better informed than the lay public.

Surely the parents of a child with a metabolic disorder (diabetes affects millions in the UK alone!) should expect their general practitioner to know enough about intermediary metabolism that they can explain the diagnostic techniques available and the biochemical basis of treatment regimens.

You need to understand the background to the screening of newborn infants for inborn errors of metabolism, which are carried out routinely in most technically advanced countries. Interpretation of the data requires a knowledge of basic aspects of metabolism and biochemical genetics.

Given the major role that (bad) diet plays in the extraordinarily high incidence of coronary heart disease in the UK (the rate is not low in North America or in Northern Europe), it is surely unacceptable for medical students not to understand basic aspects of lipoprotein metabolism. Similarly, it is imperative that our medical graduates appreciate the mechanisms that are involved in the beneficial actions of vitamins in important periods of life such as pregnancy and growth and development.

If you have a patient who may have had a heart attack, you need to know about the enzyme assays that support the diagnosis and when you may need to request more specific tests.

Table 1 is a (incomplete) list of clinical biochemical studies carried out on patients in hospital and on out-

Table 1 Some clinical biochemical studies and the related biochemistry

Clinical biochemistry	Core biochemistry
Blood glucose	Carbohydrate metabolism and its control
Blood urea	Amino acid catabolism The urea cycle Liver function
Serum cholesterol	Lipid and lipoprotein metabolism
Serum fatty acids	Lipid and lipoprotein metabolism
Serum albumin	Protein synthesis; liver function; nutrition
Prothrombin time	Blood coagulation, protein synthesis
Lactate dehydrogenase	Enzyme kinetics; electrophoresis; enzyme assay
Creatine kinase	Enzyme kinetics; electrophoresis
DNA analysis	DNA structure and DNA replication
Serum thyroxine and TSH	Endocrine system
Phenylalanine	Amino acid catabolism; inheritance of disease
Ketone bodies	Ketogenesis; starvation; diabetes mellitus
Serum uric acid	Purine nucleotide metabolism
Serum calcium	Control of calcium metabolism; parathyroid hormone; vitamin D and calcium
Serum bilirubin	Haem degradation; liver function
Liver function tests (LFTs)	Enzyme assays; liver metabolism
Plasma and urinary creatinine	One-carbon metabolism; muscle creatine metabolism
Haemoglobin A_{lc}	Glucose homeostasis; diabetes mellitus

patients and the core biochemistry related to these tests.

The fact that a biochemistry laboratory of high or moderate sophistication is present in every hospital reemphasises the importance of this discipline. Now all one need do is get on with the task of studying biochemistry.

Molecules in cells and water

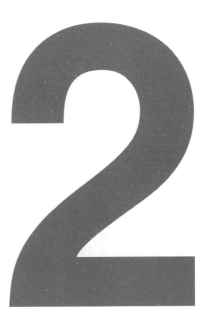

2.1 The nature of biochemistry

Biochemistry is the study of the molecular events that correspond to the phenomenon of life. It is concerned with the relationship between the structure and the function of the molecules that occur in living systems. Biochemists believe that it is possible to give an account of physiological observations, such as muscle contraction, gas exchange in the lung and nerve conduction, in terms of the molecules involved and the laws of physics and chemistry. Most of the processes that interest a biochemist occur, or at least start, in cells, so we begin by asking what kinds of molecule we find in cells.

Molecules in cells

Cells contain a great variety of molecules, ranging from enormous polymers containing millions of atoms to small building block and fuel molecules with less than 100 atoms. Before we start our study of the molecules that are the main subject matter of biochemistry, the proteins, nucleic acids, polysaccharides, lipids and metabolites, we must first consider the most abundant molecule in cells: water.

2.2 The importance of water

Water accounts for about 60% of the body weight of an adult. About 63% of this water is within cells and 37% is in the extracellular fluid, about one quarter of the latter being blood plasma. The importance of water in the body is shown by the precision with which the water content of the body is regulated by physiological mechanisms, including thirst and renal function. Deviations of more than 1 or 2% from the normal have adverse effects on our well-being and performance. Uncontrolled water loss from the body, which can occur in diseases such as cholera and untreated diabetes, is life-threatening.

Water is important in biochemistry not only because of its abundance but also because it influences the behaviour of all other molecules of biochemical interest. All biochemical processes occur in, or in contact with, aqueous solution, so we must consider the properties of water if we are to understand how other molecules interact in cells.

Physical properties of water

The molecular formula for water, H_2O, does not reveal what an unusual substance water is. The molecule contains an oxygen atom making covalent bonds with each of two hydrogen atoms. However, the molecule so formed is highly polar; the 'centre of gravity' of its positive charge does not coincide with its centre of negative charge. This polar nature has a strong

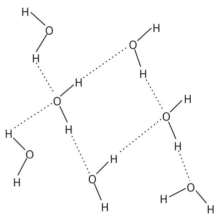

Fig. 1 Cluster of water molecules held together by hydrogen bonds.

influence on its physical properties. Water molecules act as electrostatic dipoles; they attract each other strongly and form clusters (Fig. 1). The clusters formed by water molecules are temporary; molecules are constantly leaving one cluster and joining another. Water in the liquid state is highly mobile and has no regular long-range structure.

Polar interactions and hydrogen bonds make water a liquid at temperatures where all other molecules of a similar size are gases.

Hydrogen bonds

Another important interaction between water molecules that favours cluster formation is the formation of hydrogen bonds. A hydrogen bond is a sharing of two electrons on an oxygen or nitrogen atom with a hydrogen atom carried on another atom, usually oxygen or nitrogen (but not carbon). This bond is weaker and longer than a covalent bond (Fig. 2). The hydrogen bond is about 0.28 nm long compared with a covalent bond length of 0.15 nm. The energy required to break a hydrogen bond is about 20 times lower than that needed to break a covalent bond.

Hydrogen bond formation in water tends to organise water molecules in space. A hydrogen bond is strongest when the hydrogen atom, the oxygen atom to which it is covalently bonded and the other atom forming the hydrogen bond are in line. Ice, or solid water, is an array of water molecules held in place by hydrogen bonds; ice has a regular long-range structure.

Many molecules of biochemical interest are capable of forming hydrogen bonds. Bonds are formed both within and between molecules, but most hydrogen bonds are formed in competition with the bonds that could be formed with water. Water thus provides a medium in which hydrogen bonds can be rapidly formed and broken.

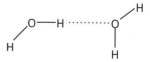

Fig. 2 Hydrogen bond between water molecules.

Although they are weaker than covalent bonds, hydrogen bonds are very important in biochemistry because they are so numerous and because they can be formed and broken so readily. Appropriate spacing of hydrogen bond acceptors and donors provides one mechanism for intermolecular recognition and specific binding.

Solvent and ionising properties of water

Water being polar is an excellent solvent for other polar molecules: molecules such as glucose and the smaller amino acids are polar and are very soluble in water. Water as a consequence of its polar nature has a high dielectric constant. This means that it reduces the electrostatic forces between any charged particles it surrounds. Water is thus an excellent solvent for ionic materials. Sodium and chloride ions in a salt crystal attract each other so strongly that the crystal is a highly stable structure in air or in most solvents. In the presence of water, the ions become hydrated (surrounded by a shell of water molecules) and the attractive forces between the ions are greatly reduced. The hydrated ions can readily separate and enter solution.

An *acid* is a molecule that can dissociate to form a hydrogen ion, H^+, and a *base*. Water can promote the dissociation of hydrogen ions from acids in two ways:

- it acts as an acceptor for the hydrogen ion, which should really be represented not as H^+ but as H_3O^+, and even the H_3O^+ is hydrated; H^+ on its own is unstable so ionisation of acids requires the presence of an ionising solvent such as water
- if the base is negatively charged, water reduces the attractive force between the base and the departing positively charged hydrogen ion.

For example, the dissociation of acetic acid, a typical weak acid, is promoted in water where the H^+ produced can be made more stable by hydration:

$$CH_3COOH + H_2O \rightleftharpoons CH_3COO^- + H_3^+O$$

Hydrogen ions are important in many biochemical processes. They are about 100 times more mobile than any other ions in aqueous solution since water provides a special tunnelling mechanism for their movement. The positive charge representing the hydrogen atom can move along the clusters of water molecules with minimal movement of any atoms (Fig. 3). The concentration of hydrogen ions, $[H^+]$, is always quoted in biochemistry as *pH*, where

$$pH = -\log_{10}[H^+]$$

Strictly speaking, the hydrogen ion activity, not concentration, should be used, but few biochemists make this distinction.

The concentration of hydrogen ions influences many biochemical processes and is controlled in living cells and the fluid surrounding them. Most molecules of biochemical interest have one or more chemical

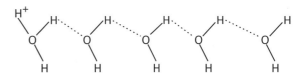

Fig. 3 Mobility of hydrogen ions in water.

groupings that can act as acids or bases: groups which can lose or bind a hydrogen ion. Each hydrogen ion lost decreases the charge on the molecule by one unit and each hydrogen ion gained increases the charge. Since dissociation of acids and binding of hydrogen ions by bases are rapid equilibrium processes, the charge on many biochemical molecules varies with the pH of the medium. This usually influences their properties and functions. Some molecules can have both positive and negative charges, for example amino acids. These molecules are known as *zwitterions*. In most biochemical experiments, pH must be controlled by using buffers.

Water and non-polar molecules

Molecules that are not polar are generally insoluble in water. Water molecules cling to each other, excluding the non-polar molecules, which remain clustered together as solids or immiscible liquids. For example, water is immiscible with liquid hydrocarbons such as hexane and benzene.

Water and amphipathic molecules

Many biochemical molecules cannot be classified as simply polar or non-polar. One part of a molecule may be polar and interact readily with water, and it is said to be *hydrophilic* or 'water-loving', while another part is non-polar and is excluded from water, being *hydrophobic* or 'water-hating'. Such molecules with both a hydrophilic part and a hydrophobic part are said to be amphipathic. Water has a powerful influence on such molecules and can assist in organising them into biochemically important structures such as membranes, folded globular proteins and the double helix of DNA. In all these structures, the hydrophobic parts of the molecules associate with other hydrophobic parts to form a core from which water is excluded. The surface of the structure is composed of the hydrophilic parts of the molecules. The surrounding water molecules stabilise the structure.

Water as a reactant

Biochemical reactions often involve water molecules as a reactant or product. Many reactions in metabolism involve the addition or elimination of a water molecule. The polymerisation of building block molecules to make macromolecules such as proteins or nucleic acids involves the elimination of a water molecule and the formation of a covalent bond between the building blocks. Breakdown of the macromolecules, as in digestion, is by *hydrolysis*, the cleavage of the bond between the building blocks with the introduction of a molecule of water. Because it is present in cells at such a high concentration, water drives hydrolysis reactions. The breakdown of biopolymers in aqueous solution is, therefore, energetically favourable while the synthesis of these polymers from their building blocks requires an input of energy.

Self-assessment: questions

Multiple choice questions

1. The following statements describe water in the body:
   a. Water accounts for more than one half of the mass of the body
   b. Most of the water in the body is inside cells
   c. Most of the extracellular water in the body is in the blood plasma
   d. Water in the body acts as an inert solvent and does not take part in cellular reactions
   e. The water content of the body is so high that changes in its water content are usually well tolerated

2. As a result of the solvent properties of water:
   a. Water is an excellent solvent for non-polar substances like hexane
   b. Water promotes the ionisation of acids such as acetic acid
   c. The amino acids glycine and alanine are very soluble in water since they occur as zwitterions in solution
   d. The attractive electrostatic forces between oppositely charged ions, such as Na^+ and Cl^-, are increased and the repulsive forces between ions having the same charge are decreased
   e. Substances like glucose that have many hydroxyl groups in the molecule are very soluble in water

3. The following statements describe water and hydrogen bonds:
   a. A water molecule can act as a hydrogen bond donor but not as a hydrogen bond acceptor
   b. Hydrogen bonds occur between water molecules in the liquid state but not in ice
   c. Water molecules can form hydrogen bonds with hydrogen atoms attached by covalent bonds to oxygen and carbon atoms but not to those attached to nitrogen
   d. The occurrence of hydrogen bonds between water molecules gives liquid water a regular three-dimensional structure
   e. Hydrogen bonds are important in biochemistry because, although weak, they are numerous and can be made and broken very rapidly

4. Phosphoric acid dissociates in three stages to produce a phosphate ion, according to the following scheme:

$$H_3PO_4 \rightleftharpoons H^+ + H_2PO_4^- \rightleftharpoons H^+ + HPO_4^{2-} \rightleftharpoons H^+ + PO_4^{3-}$$

   a. The species $H_2PO_4^-$ is not an acid because it is not a neutral molecule
   b. The species $H_2PO_4^-$ is an acid because it can dissociate a hydrogen ion
   c. The species $H_2PO_4^-$ is a base because it can accept a hydrogen ion
   d. The species $H_2PO_4^-$ is both an acid and a base
   e. The species H_3PO_4 is a stronger acid than $H_2PO_4^-$ or HPO_4^{2-}

5. The following statements describe water and cellular molecules:
   a. Water has no effect on the structures of macromolecules
   b. Water has no effect on the hydrophobic parts of amphipathic molecules
   c. Water is excluded from cellular membranes so it does not contribute to the stability of their structures
   d. The properties of cellular macromolecules are influenced by changes of pH
   e. The hydrogen ion is hydrated and exists as H_3O^+ in aqueous solution

6. In biochemical reactions:
   a. Water is a reactant in many reactions involved in the digestion of foodstuffs
   b. Water is present in such high concentration that it influences the equilibrium of many cellular reactions
   c. Water is a by-product in the synthesis of many cellular macromolecules
   d. Hydrolysis is the cleavage of a covalent bond with the introduction of the elements of a water molecule
   e. Water is one of the products of the oxidation of foodstuffs

Short essay questions

1. What molecule would you look for first on a planet where you suspected that extraterrestrial life existed? Justify your answer.
2. 'Life is only possible in the presence of liquid water.' Comment on this statement. Also mention any practical applications it might have.

Self-assessment: answers

Multiple choice answers

1. a. **True.** Water accounts for 55 to 65% of the weight of the body.
   b. **True.** About two-thirds of body water is inside cells.
   c. **False.** About one quarter of extracellular water circulates as plasma.
   d. **False.** Far from being an inert solvent, water influences interactions between cellular molecules and takes part in many reactions.
   e. **False.** Although the water content of the body is high, it is also precisely regulated and significant changes in water content can be a serious threat to life.

2. a. **False.** Hexane like all non-polar molecules is insoluble in water.
   b. **True.** Water hydrates H^+ making it more stable. It also promotes dissociation by decreasing the attractive force between H^+ and the acetate ion.
   c. **True.** In water, these amino acids have charged amino and carboxyl groups. Although the molecules have no overall charge they are very polar.
   d. **False.** Water because of its high dielectric constant reduces all electrostatic forces between ions.
   e. **True.** Sucrose is another example.

3. a. **False.** Water can act as both donor and acceptor.
   b. **False.** Ice contains virtually the maximum possible number of hydrogen bonds.
   c. **False.** Hydrogen attached to carbon does not form hydrogen bonds. Hydrogen atoms attached to oxygen and nitrogen generally do.
   d. **False.** Liquid water is composed of temporary irregular clusters of water molecules.
   e. **True.** They are important in most interactions between cellular molecules.

4. a. **False.** Any molecular species from which H^+ can dissociate is an acid.
   b. **True.** Any molecular species from which H^+ can dissociate is an acid.
   c. **True.** Any molecular species to which H^+ can bind is a base.
   d. **True.** $H_2PO_4^-$ can act as an acid or a base; it can dissociate or bind H^+.
   e. **True.** H_3PO_4 dissociates more readily than $H_2PO_4^-$; it has more H atoms and H^+ leaves a neutral molecule more readily than one which has a negative charge.

5. a. **False.** Cellular macromolecules depend on the presence of water for their structures and functions.
   b. **False.** The hydrophobic parts are excluded from the water phase.
   c. **False.** The orientation of amphipathic membrane molecules in the presence of water is a major force for the stability of membrane structure.
   d. **True.** The binding of H^+ to cellular macromolecules, especially proteins, depends on the pH. This changes their charge and the way that they interact with other molecules.
   e. **True.** An unhydrated proton is very unstable.

6. a. **True.** Hydrolysis, the chemical reaction in digestion, requires water.
   b. **True.** The high concentration of water favours hydrolysis.
   c. **True.** The polymerisation reactions by which cellular macromolecules such as proteins and nucleic acids are formed involve the elimination of a water molecule between one building block and the next.
   d. **True.** By definition.
   e. **True.** In catabolism, hydrogen atoms are extracted from foodstuffs, especially fatty acids and sugars, and combine with molecular oxygen to form water. This process is responsible for generating most of the energy required by animal cells.

Short essay answers

1. Water must surely be the first molecule that is looked for. Any form of life that could exist in the absence of water would be so different from life on earth that it would be impossible to predict what molecular form it would take or which of its molecules to look for. The search for ATP on Mars would not make sense unless the NASA scientists already knew that water was present.

2. Most biochemical processes cease or are greatly slowed down in the absence of liquid water. In the complete absence of water or in ice, macromolecules are immobilised and cannot interact at a sufficient rate with smaller molecules such as nutrients, metabolites and building blocks. The biochemical processes, mostly mediated by microorganisms, involved in food spoilage can be controlled by freezing or by desiccation, the removal of water. Biochemicals often spoil at room temperature. In the laboratory they are generally stored in the refrigerator or deep-freeze, or else in freeze-dried form.

Proteins

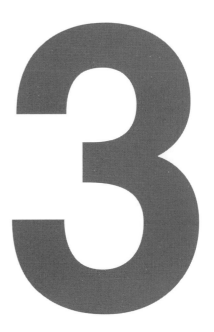

3.1 **Protein function**

Proteins are the first cellular macromolecules to be considered in this book because they are so central to biochemistry. Other macromolecules, while important in some biochemical processes, are generally synthesised, organised, controlled and regulated, packaged and eventually broken down by proteins. It is difficult to think of a biochemical process that does not involve the participation of proteins. The range of protein functions is enormous.

Mechanical functions. Proteins are a major part of the mechanical system of our bodies. Tendons made from collagen, a fibrous protein, are the inelastic ropes that allow our muscles, the protein motors, to move our bones. Bones have some protein content being made from collagen and a calcium phosphate mineral. The bones are held together at our joints by the fibrous elastic protein, elastin.

Energy production. Energy to drive the muscle motors is obtained from metabolic reactions catalysed by enzymes, which are proteins.

Oxygen carriage. Oxygen needed for metabolic reactions that generate energy is carried to our muscles and most other tissues by another protein, haemoglobin.

Regulatory signals. Signal proteins, notably the hormone insulin, regulate the concentrations of fuel molecules circulating to our muscles in our blood. Insulin and many other hormones move in our blood between the glands that secrete them and their target cells where they are detected by protein receptors on the membrane. Once detected, the hormone signal is amplified, combined with other signals and acted upon by further proteins.

Protein synthesis. Proteins are responsible for many aspects of their own synthesis. Nucleic acids, which provide the information for protein synthesis, are synthesised, packaged, regulated and repaired by proteins. Proteins are responsible for catalysis of the actual bond formation needed in protein synthesis and for providing the energy for the process.

Proteins bind other molecules specifically

Considering even this incomplete list of protein functions, it is surprising that a common principle can be discerned in all the biochemical functions of proteins. This common principle is that protein molecules are able to recognise and bind other molecules very specifically and with great affinity. This binding of other molecules occurs very rapidly and is often reversible. Many proteins have multiple binding sites, and the binding of one molecule by a protein often influences its ability to bind others.

The molecules that proteins bind are referred to as *ligands*. A ligand is a small molecule or part of a large molecule that can occupy a binding site. Oxygen is a ligand of haemoglobin, substrates and inhibitors are ligands of enzymes and a hormone molecule is the ligand of the receptor molecule with which it interacts.

Examples of ligand binding in protein function
Proteins involved in forming complex structures assemble by ligand binding. For instance, collagen molecules recognise and bind to other collagen molecules in a regular parallel array to form a fibre and eventually a tendon. Therefore, the ligand for bone collagen molecule is part of another collagen molecule. Collagen molecules that form the matrix of bone have further binding sites where initiation of bone calcification occurs.

Muscle. There are two principal proteins, *myosin* and *actin*, in muscle, which each assemble into filaments: the thick and thin filaments, respectively. These filaments slide over each other as the muscle contracts or relaxes. Further binding sites on the proteins allow the filaments to combine with each other and then separate in a cyclical manner when fuelled by ATP and stimulated by calcium ions. This interaction between the filaments enables the muscle to develop tension and to contract. Myosin, therefore, has binding sites for several different ligands: other myosin molecules, actin filaments, ATP and interaction with calcium ions.

Enzymes. These catalytic proteins bind the molecules that participate in the reactions they catalyse, their substrates. This substrate binding often distorts the substrate making it more reactive. By binding two substrates in an orientation favourable for reaction, the rate of the reaction between them is greatly enhanced. Some enzymes have further binding sites that can be occupied by specific molecules which switch the catalytic activity of the enzyme on or off.

Carriage of oxygen. No molecules composed entirely from amino acids have evolved that are capable of carrying oxygen molecules directly. The haemoglobin which carries oxygen in our blood is formed from a protein, *globin*, which specifically binds an iron-containing organic group, *haem*. Binding of the haem group to globin modifies haem's properties so that it binds oxygen reversibly, a reaction not possible for haem on its own.

Nucleic acid function. The nucleic acids, particularly DNA, carry genetic information: information on the structures of our proteins. Even in this function it needs the participation of protein molecules. Enzymes copy DNA so that after cell division each daughter cell contains an accurate copy of the DNA of the original cell. *Histone* proteins condense the metre length of DNA in each of our cells so that it fits within a cell nucleus with a maximum dimension of perhaps ten millionths of a metre. Other proteins control which parts of the DNA are used to provide information in any particular cell; for example, so that muscle cells make muscle proteins and liver cells make liver proteins. These functions require proteins that can recognise and bind nucleic acids, either to all DNA for

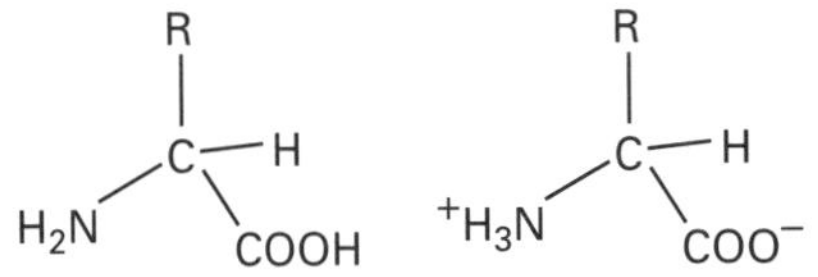

Fig. 4 General structure of an amino acid. Amino acids are often shown as uncharged molecules (left). In solutions with pH near neutrality, as in most physiological situations, the representation with charged amino and carboxyl groups (right) is more accurate.

its replication and packaging or to specific parts of the total DNA when controlling its use to direct protein synthesis.

3.2 Amino acids

If we are to understand how proteins are able to recognise and bind to other molecules we must consider the structure of proteins in some detail. Proteins are polymers of amino acids. The general structure of an amino acid is shown in Figure 4. Four groups are attached by covalent bonds to a single carbon atom, the alpha carbon. Two of these groups, an amino group and an acidic carboxyl group, give their name to this class of compound and are also involved in forming the *peptide bonds* that join the amino acids into long polypeptide chains. The other two groups attached to the alpha carbon are a hydrogen atom, present in all amino acids, and a variable group, the so-called side chain (R). It is the side chain that distinguishes one amino acid from another. All proteins in animals, plants, bacteria and viruses are synthesised from a set of 20 amino acids. The side chains of these 20 amino acids contain a limited range of chemical groups. In the few cases where proteins contain an amino acid that is not a member of this set, the protein is synthesised as a precursor protein. A side chain in the precursor protein is then chemically modified to form the unusual amino acid.

Figure 5 shows the structures of the amino acids. They are arranged in groups with similar amino acids together; noting these structural relationships will help in recognising and distinguishing the amino acids. As the figure shows, the type of side chain alters the character and properties of the amino acids; this results in certain amino acids playing particular roles in protein function; for example, the disulphide bond formed by two cysteine residues is often used to hold a protein in a particular folded configuration.

L-amino acids

All of the amino acids except glycine are optically active, or *chiral*, having four different groups attached to the alpha carbon. Each amino acid can exist in two distinct forms, which are mirror images of each other and are not superimposable. Proteins are composed of amino acids of the so-called L series. Amino acids of the

D series are very rarely found and never in proteins (they do occur in small peptides in some bacterial cell walls). Glycine has two hydrogen atoms attached to its alpha carbon and exists in only one form.

Figure 5 shows two different systems of abbreviated names for amino acids that are in common use: an easily learnt three-letter code and a more concise single letter code, which is used for showing long polypeptide sequences. Only the three-letter code will be used in this book.

The peptide bond

Proteins are composed of amino acids joined by peptide bonds. Peptide bond formation involves the elimination of the elements of water between the alpha carboxyl group of one amino acid and the alpha amino group of another (Fig. 6). The dipeptide that is produced has terminal amino and carboxyl groups that (if free) can participate in further peptide bonds to extend the chain. Side chain carboxyl and amino groups, on those amino acids which possess them, are never involved so polypeptide chains are linear and never branched. The bond formed between the carboxyl carbon and the amino nitrogen is a strong covalent bond that is somewhat shorter than would be expected for a single carbon–nitrogen bond. This is because it has some double bond character (Fig. 7). For this reason, free rotation around the peptide bond is not possible and there are some restrictions on the ways in which a polypeptide chain can be arranged in space.

Another important feature of the peptide bond is the hydrogen-bonding capacity of the atoms around the bond. The oxygen atom attached to the carbon atom of the peptide bond carries a fractional negative charge and is a strong hydrogen bond acceptor. The hydrogen attached to the peptide nitrogen has a fractional positive charge and can form strong hydrogen bonds (Fig. 7). Protein molecules containing many peptide bonds have a great capacity for hydrogen bonding, which must be satisfied. This influences the way in which polypeptide chains fold.

Polypeptide chains typically contain between 50 and 5000 amino acid units. The group of atoms belonging to each amino acid once it is combined in a peptide chain is known as an *amino acid residue*.

N-terminal and C-terminal ends

However long a polypeptide chain becomes it will still have an alpha amino group at one end, known as the N-terminal end, and an alpha carboxyl group at the other, the C-terminal end. Sometimes the N-terminal amino group is not free but is modified by addition of an acetyl or other group. Similarly the C-terminal carboxyl group is sometimes modified to its amide. By convention the sequence of amino acids in a protein is

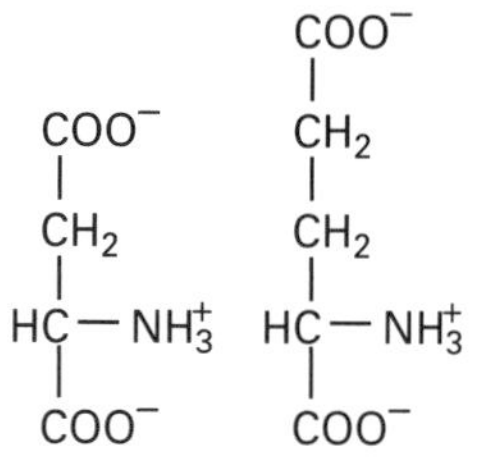

Asp (D)   Glu (E)

Aspartic acid and **glutamic acid** carry acidic carboxyl groups on their side chains.

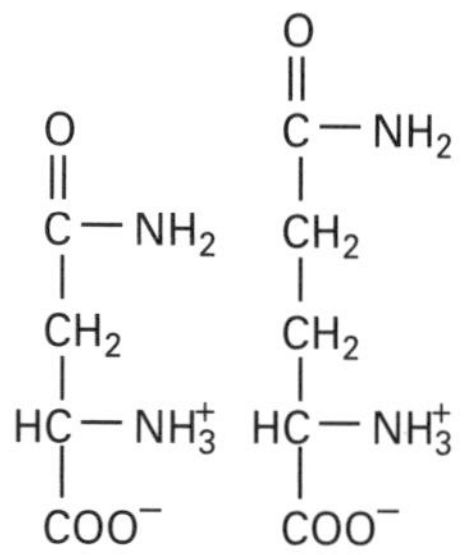

Asn (N)   Gln (Q)

Asparagine and **glutamine** are closely related to aspartic acid and glutamic acid, respectively, the side chain carboxyl groups are modified into uncharged hydrophilic amide groups.

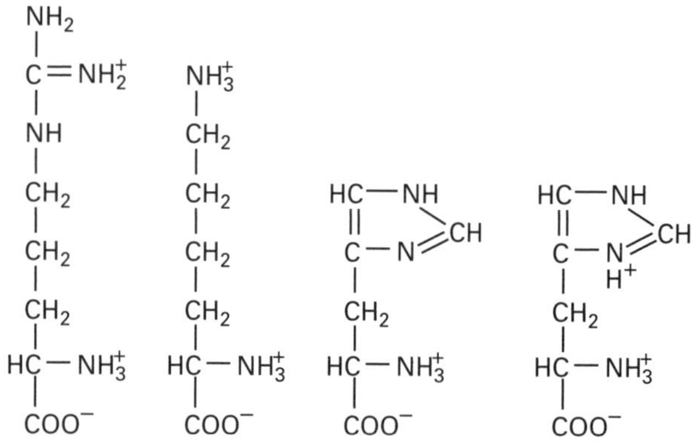

Arg (R)   Lys (K)   His (H)   His (protonated)

Arginine, lysine and histidine carry basic functional groups. Arginine and lysine side chains usually bind protons under physiological conditions and are positively charged. The imidazole group of histidine can exist in either a positively charged form (protonated) or as an uncharged base. Histidine side chains act as buffers at physiological pH.

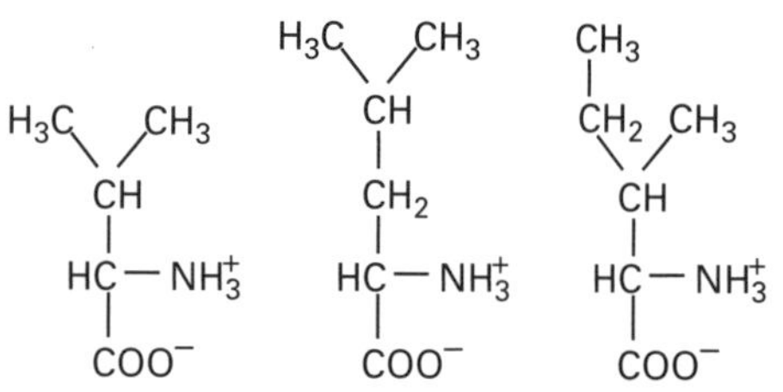

Val (V)   Leu (L)   Ile (I)

Valine, leucine and **isoleucine** have branched aliphatic hydrocarbon side chains, which are very hydrophobic.

Fig. 5 Structure of the amino acids. These are shown with their ionisable groups in their predominant forms found near pH 7.

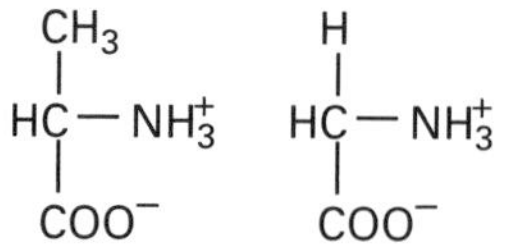

Ala (A)   Gly (G)

Alanine has a methyl group as its side chain; **glycine** has a second hydrogen atom attached to its alpha carbon and can be considered to have no side chain. It is the only amino acid that is not optically active.

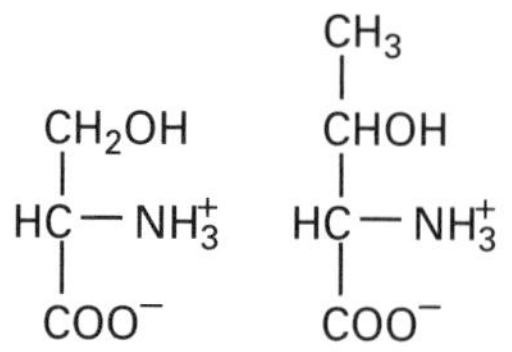

Ser (S)   Thr (T)

Serine and **threonine** have small uncharged side chains containing hydroxyl groups.

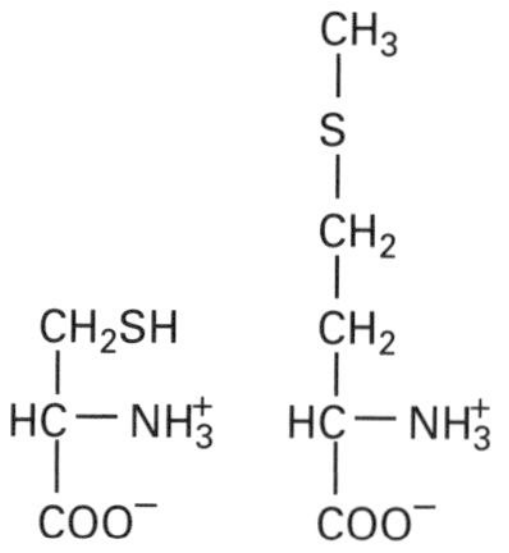

Cys (C)   Met (M)

Cysteine and **methionine** are sulphur-containing amino acids. Cysteine has a thiol or sulphydryl group on its side chain. Two cysteine side chains can react together to form a strong covalent disulphide bond, which is often used to hold different parts of a protein together. Methionine has a methylated sulphur in its side chain.

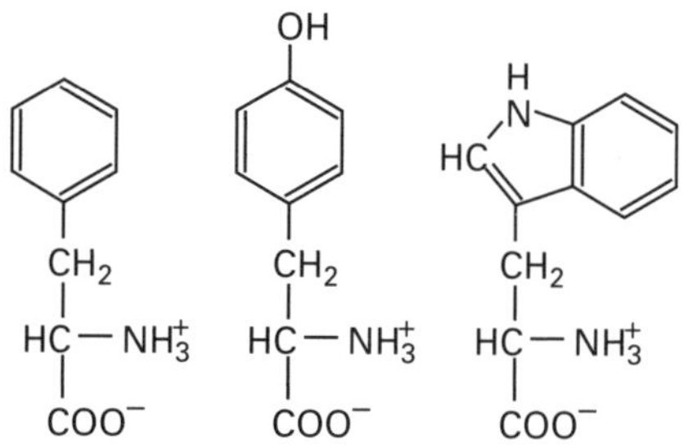

Phe (F)   Tyr (Y)   Trp (W)

Phenylalanine, tyrosine and **tryptophan** all have aromatic side chains. Phenylalanine is very hydrophobic, tyrosine less so since its ring carries a phenolic hydroxyl group. Tryptophan, the largest amino acid, has indole, a double aromatic ring containing a nitrogen atom, as its side chain. It is very hydrophobic.

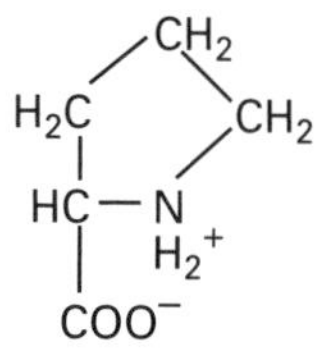

Pro (P)

Proline is the only amino acid to have a secondary amino group, not a primary amino group like all the others. The side chain of proline loops around to make a bond with the amino nitrogen atom, which, therefore, has two covalent bonds to carbon. Strictly speaking proline is an imino acid.

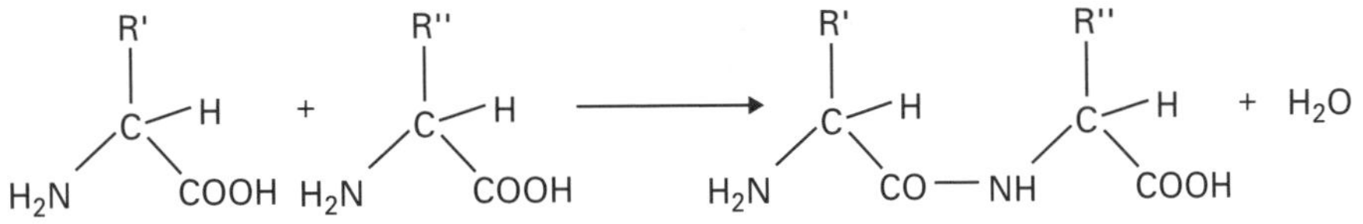

Fig. 6 Peptide bond formation.

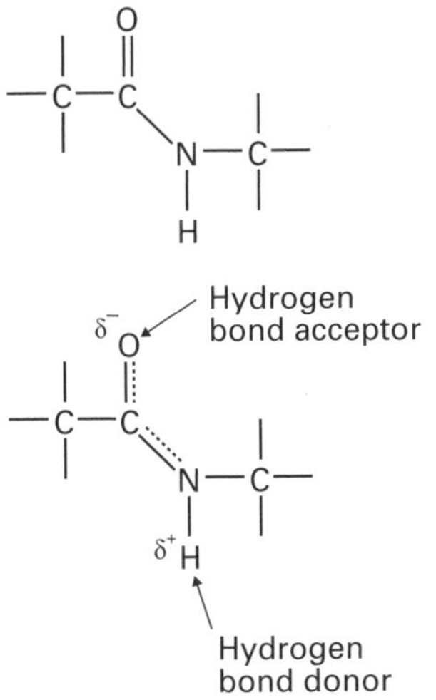

Fig. 7 Nature of the peptide bond. While often shown as the upper form, the properties of the peptide bond show that the lower representation is more accurate. The *trans* configuration shown is adopted by almost all peptide bonds in proteins. All six atoms shown are in a single plane. The carbonyl oxygen and hydrogen on the nitrogen both carry fractional electronic charges and form strong hydrogen bonds. Rotation is allowed around the carbon–carbon bond.

written with the N-terminal on the left. Two amino acids (X and Y) can form two distinct peptides, XY and YX.

3.3 Protein purification and characterisation

Proteins occur mixed with other compounds including proteins so one of the first tasks of a biochemist who wishes to study the relationship between structure and function for a single protein is to purify the protein, to isolate it, separating it from other proteins. Purification is also necessary for proteins used for therapeutic purposes, such as insulin used to treat diabetics and clotting factor VIII used to treat haemophiliacs. Details of the powerful methods that have been developed to purify proteins are beyond the scope of this book but the principles will be mentioned in outline. The methods depend on differences between protein molecules in properties such as

- ligand-binding ability
- size
- solubility
- stability
- electric charge.

Purification of a protein from a complex mixture can rarely be achieved by a one-step process. Usually it is necessary to combine several purification techniques, each of which removes some of the unwanted components of the mixture while retaining the protein to be purified. The success of each stage of the purification process must be monitored by measuring the amount of the protein to be purified and the total protein at the start and finish of each stage. The ratio of the amount of the protein to be purified to the amount of total protein is known as the *specific activity*. The value of this ratio should increase with each successful stage of purification.

Ligand binding

Affinity chromatography is the only method of protein purification that exploits a property related to the function of the protein, ligand-binding ability. The method requires the chemical synthesis of a chromatographic column material that carries a chemical grouping which can be recognised and bound by a ligand-binding site on the required protein. This grouping is generally a chemical analogue of a natural ligand of the protein, for instance a substrate analogue for an enzyme, or a hormone analogue for a hormone receptor protein. The mixture of proteins is poured through the column and protein molecules with an appropriate ligand-binding site will bind to the ligand attached to the column. All other proteins should wash through. The bound protein can then be released from the column by washing with solutions of free ligand. Affinity chromatography can achieve great purification in a single step.

Size

Protein molecules in solution can be separated on the basis of their size by centrifugation or by gel filtration on beads of porous polysaccharide gel, which act as molecular sieves. Measurement of the *sedimentation rates* of protein molecules in the high gravitational fields produced by centrifuges has been used to estimate the molecular size of the molecules. Gel filtration columns can be calibrated with protein molecules of known size and used to obtain estimates of the molecular size of newly discovered proteins.

Solubility

Proteins vary in their solubility, one from another. Their solubility also varies with pH, ionic strength and the presence of solvents other than water. It is often possible to manipulate the physicochemical conditions so that some proteins precipitate while other proteins remain in solution, so allowing separation. Precipitation

Blood donated for transfusion and which has not been used within the few weeks it remains useful is not wasted. The proteins from the plasma are fractionated by precipitation with cold ethanol and the separate fractions are used therapeutically to treat such conditions as low plasma volume following burns and surgery, and to give temporary protection against possible infection.

with soluble salts such as ammonium sulphate or with solvents such as cold ethanol is widely used. Proteins thus precipitated are easily redissolved by dilution of the precipitating agent.

Stability

As will be discussed in more detail later in this chapter, many proteins are readily denatured by exposure to elevated temperatures or to pH values more than two or three units from pH 7. Proteins denatured in this way form insoluble precipitates. If the protein being purified is more resistant to denaturation than other proteins in the mixture, purification can be achieved by exposing the mixture to conditions that selectively denature the unwanted proteins.

Charge

Protein molecules carry electric charge because of their ionised amino acid side chains. The charge depends on the amino acid composition of the protein and also on pH. The charge on each molecule is generally positive at low pH values and falls as the pH increases, reaching zero at a defined pH for each protein, its *isoelectric point*. As the pH rises further beyond the isoelectric point, the charge on the protein becomes increasingly negative. Proteins are separated on the basis of their charge by ion-exchange chromatography. The chromatography material is a porous hydrophilic material, cellulose is often used, modified chemically to carry charged groups. Ion exchangers are available with either fixed positive or fixed negative charges. When a mixture of proteins flows into the chromatographic column, protein molecules opposite in charge to the charge on the column are bound to the column. Other proteins can be washed through. Now changing the pH of the eluting buffer changes the charge on some of the bound proteins and they will elute. If the pH is gradually changed, a series of different proteins will emerge from the column depending on their isoelectric points.

The differences in charge between different proteins is also exploited by the techniques of electrophoresis and isoelectric focussing. *Electrophoresis* is the movement of charged molecules in an electric field. Electrophoresis of proteins is usually carried out in buffer solutions supported by a hydrophobic gel that is

porous enough to allow protein molecules to penetrate. At the end of the electrophoresis procedure, the protein molecules in the gel can be located by a specific or general protein stain. The rate at which proteins move through the gel depends on both their charge and their size. Identical molecules will all move at the same rate so that a sample of purified protein will move as a single band. This makes electrophoresis a valuable tool for establishing how many molecular species of protein a given protein preparation contains. *Isoelectric focussing* is a variant of electrophoresis carried out on a gel that has been set up to contain a gradient of pH. A protein molecule introduced to the gel will move in the electric field to a region where the pH matches its isoelectric point. Here it becomes uncharged and moves no further. Electrophoresis and isoelectric focussing are not often used for protein purification because they must be conducted on a very small scale. Attempts to scale them up must overcome the heating effects of the electric current passing through the electrophoresis buffer.

Choosing a purification method

The methods described above for purifying proteins are used empirically. Methods must be tested experimentally because there is no way of predicting which method will be most successful for any particular protein. The success or otherwise of a particular method cannot usually be related to the biochemical activity of the protein that is being purified.

3.4 Protein structure

Amino acid composition

A count of the number of times each amino acid occurs in a given protein is known as the amino acid composition of the protein. It can be determined by complete hydrolysis of a protein followed by a chromatographic procedure to separate the amino acids. The peptide bond is a strong covalent bond but it can be hydrolysed by prolonged heating in acid or alkali and also by the action of proteolytic enzymes.

The amino acid composition of a protein is often the first information that is available about a protein, but this information, of itself, generally does not reveal much about the relationship between the structure and function of the protein. There are a few exceptions. Haemoglobin contains many more histidine residues than the average protein; the histidine side chains act as a buffer at physiological pH so their presence correlates with the buffering role of haemoglobin in the red cell. One third of the amino acid residues in collagen, the main structural protein of connective tissue, are glycine and one quarter are proline or modified proline. These amino acids have a role in collagen fibre formation. With most proteins there is no obvious relationship between amino acid composition and function.

Proteins have varying levels of structure

Proteins often lose their activity if heated, a few minutes incubation at 60°C to 70°C is sufficient to inactivate many. Exposure to cold dilute acids or bases inactivates the majority of proteins and high concentrations of urea or solvents such as ethanol also inactivate. None of these treatments, which are said to denature the protein, would be expected to cleave peptide bonds or any other covalent bonds involved in protein structure. Some higher level of structure, destroyed by denaturation, must be necessary for protein function. The polypeptide chain must be folded in space to assume its functional form.

The structure of proteins can be considered at varying levels of complexity:

- primary: amino acid sequence established by covalent peptide bonds
- secondary: folding of the chains stabilised by hydrogen bonding between residues that are relatively close together
- tertiary: longer range folding stabilised by interactions between side chains; various bonds including hydrogen bonding and covalent bonds may occur
- quarternary: aggregates of more than one protein chain, folded together and held by various types of bond.

The full three-dimensional structures of many proteins have been determined by X-ray crystallography and nuclear magnetic resonance (NMR) methods. Description of these physical methods is beyond the scope of this book but their results show that the polypeptide chains in proteins are folded specifically. Many relationships between protein structure and function have been revealed.

Primary structure: amino acid sequence

There appears to be no restriction on the order in which amino acids can be joined in a protein, so with 20 possibilities at every position in the sequence, there is clearly an enormous number of possible proteins. Information stored in a nucleic acid base sequence directs the machinery of protein synthesis in a cell to make the proteins appropriate for that cell. The primary structure of a protein, the sequence in which amino acids are joined in a protein, makes that protein distinctive and leads to its further levels of structure, or shape, beyond sequence. Small changes in sequence can lead to large changes in properties and functions. Some inherited diseases are known to be caused by a change involving only one amino acid residue, a change that alters or destroys the function of the protein involved.

The amino acid sequences of many proteins have been determined. The methods used were originally chemical but now physical methods of greater sensitivity are used. Protein amino acid sequences can also be deduced from the base sequences of the nucleic acids that direct their synthesis. Proteins carrying out similar functions and proteins having the same function in different species almost always have closely related primary structures. Primary sequences are stored in data bases. This enables predictions about the structure and function of other proteins, often of medical importance, to be made.

Secondary structure

The folding of the chain of amino acid residues through hydrogen bonding between residues that are close together in the chain is known as the secondary structure of the protein. Folding patterns such as the *alpha helix*, the *beta sheet* and the *triple helix* (occurring in collagen fibres) are examples of secondary structure. Secondary structure can be identified for most proteins, but the best examples of the importance of this level of structure are seen when we consider the structural proteins: the fibrous proteins that make up the structures in our bodies. Fibre formation by these proteins involves formation of regular secondary structures that extend over long distances.

The alpha helix

In the alpha helix, the backbone of the polypeptide chain is folded into a helix (Fig. 8). Folded in this way, the hydrogen-bonding capacity of the back bone peptide bonds can be completely satisfied within the helix and a stable structure results. For each residue,

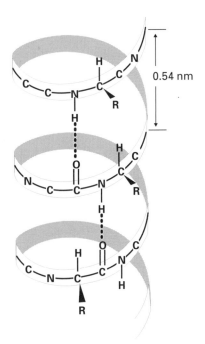

Fig. 8 The alpha helix.

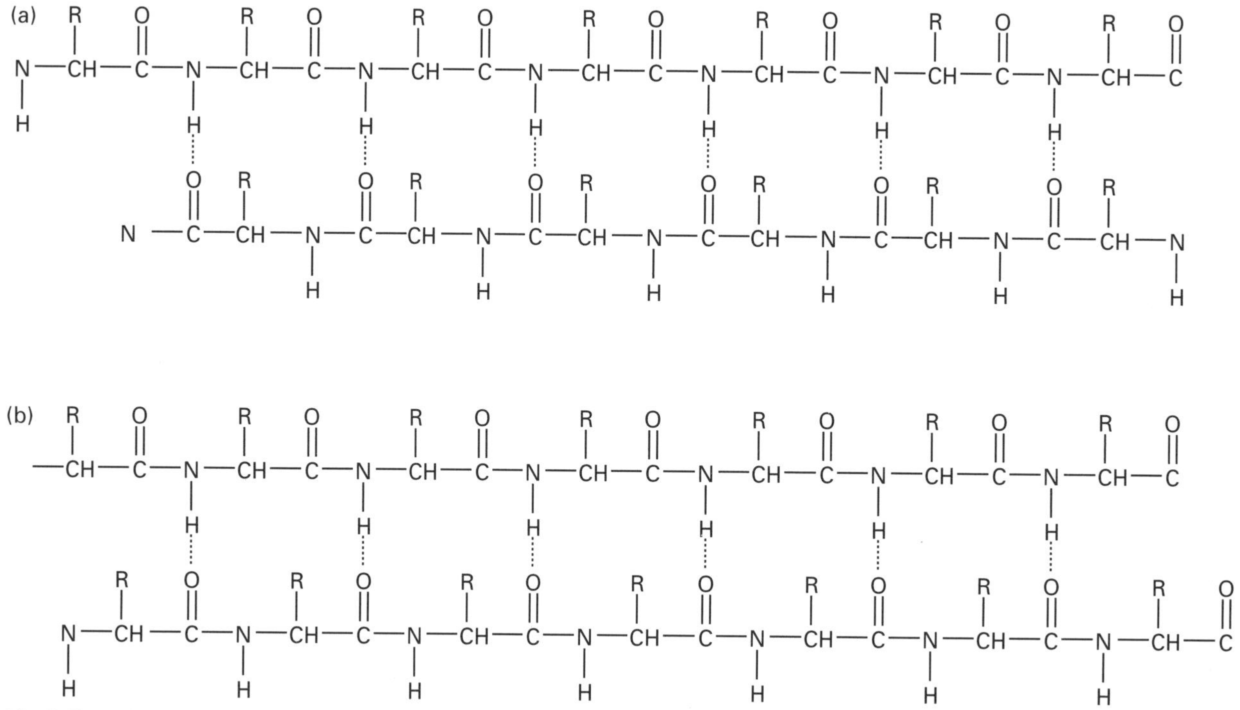

(a)

(Figure 9a: chemical structure of antiparallel beta pleated sheet showing two polypeptide chains with R, O, N, CH, C, H atoms and hydrogen bonds)

(b)

(Figure 9b: chemical structure of parallel beta pleated sheet showing two polypeptide chains with R, O, N, CH, C, H atoms and hydrogen bonds)

Fig. 9 Beta pleated sheets. Sheets comprising antiparallel chains (a) are somewhat more stable than sheets of parallel chains (b).

the amino hydrogen forms a bond to the carbonyl oxygen fourth earlier in the chain and the carbonyl oxygen forms a bond to a later amino hydrogen. Left-handed and right-handed helices are possible but only the latter are found as they are more stable with L-amino acids. In a right-handed helix the chain rises as we move along it to the right. There are 3.6 residues per turn and the pitch of the helix is 0.54 nm, so each residue adds 0.15 nm to the length of the helix. Structural proteins containing the alpha helix have fibres that can be stretched, especially when wet. The alpha helix is the predominant secondary structure of unstretched keratin, the fibrous protein of hair, skin and nails. Many globular proteins contain short sections of alpha helix separated by sequences folded in other ways. The alpha helix does not involve the amino acid side chains which project from the helix.

Beta sheets

In beta sheets, polypeptide chains are almost fully extended and run side by side so that hydrogen bonds can be formed between adjacent chains in the sheet (Fig. 9). Stretched keratin can assume the beta sheet structure. Many globular proteins contain sections of beta sheet or even barrel-like structures formed from a curved sheet.

The triple helix and collagen

The triple helix is found principally in collagen, the protein that makes the strong low-elasticity fibres of connective tissue. Three polypeptide chains that are almost fully extended are wound around each other to

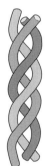

Fig. 10 The collagen triple helix.

form a rope-like structure (Fig. 10). Again much of the stability of the structure results from hydrogen bonds between the backbones of the three chains. For the triple helix to form, it is necessary for each of its component chains to have a glycine residue in every third position in its sequence. Only glycine with a H atom as its side chain can allow the chains to come close enough to form the structure. The individual chains in the helix are in almost fully extended configurations so fibres composed of collagen molecules combine high strength with low elasticity.

Tertiary structure

Consideration of secondary structure can reveal much about the relationship between the structure of fibrous proteins and the physical properties on which the functions of these proteins depend. When we consider globular proteins, we must describe an even higher level of structure, tertiary structure. Physical studies show that many globular proteins have compact struc-

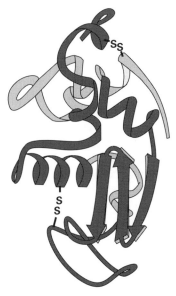

Fig. 11 Tertiary structure of lysozyme. The single polypeptide chain of this small enzyme molecule folds into short sections of alpha helix and a small antiparallel beta pleated sheet as well as into bends and loops where the chain has no recognisable secondary structure. The structure is stabilised by four disulphide bonds, only two of which are visible in the figure. (Based on Wolf, S.L. (1995) *Cell and Molecular Biology*, Wadsworth.)

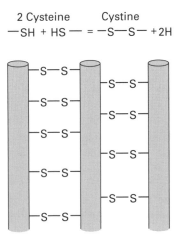

Fig. 12 Disulphide bonds in proteins.

tures, the long polypeptide chains within them must be folded or wound up like a ball of string. Many globular proteins can form crystals: the chains must be folded in the same way in every molecule to give them the identical overall shape needed for them to fit into the crystal. X-ray diffraction studies of protein crystals have led to the determination of the three-dimensional structure of a wide variety of protein molecules. These structures show how the polypeptide chain winds back and forth through the molecule, sometimes in the form of an alpha helix, sometimes forming beta sheets, sometimes in turns and less regular structures (Fig. 11).

Disulphide bonds

Tertiary structures are often stabilised by covalent disulphide bonds. The structures formed by folded polypeptides depend on hydrogen bonds and hydrophobic interactions so they can be fragile and easily disrupted by changes in temperature or pH. Many proteins, especially those that function outside cells, have their folded structures reinforced by disulphide bonds. These bonds can also hold subunits together. Disulphide bonds are formed when the side chains of two cysteine residues that are close together in the folded structure react together, losing the hydrogen atoms of their sulphydryl (also known as thiol) groups in an oxidation reaction (Fig. 12). Disulphide bonds are strong covalent bonds. They are particularly important in keratin, the fibrous structural protein of hair, skin and nails where parallel alpha helices are crosslinked by disulphide bonds. Keratin is chemically very resistant because its structure can maintain its integrity even

after breakage of some peptide or disulphide bonds. It is greatly weakened by reducing agents, which can convert disulphide bonds into free thiol groups. Chemical depilatories (hair removers) exploit this susceptibility of keratin to chemical reduction as do industrial processes to remove the bristles from hides in leather production.

Formation of tertiary structure

The tertiary structure that a protein forms is dependent upon its amino acid sequence. The interpretation of the X-ray studies on protein crystals to discover the three-dimensional structure of a protein depends on knowledge of the primary structure of the protein. Haemoglobin and myoglobin were the first proteins to have their molecular structures described. The relationship between their primary and tertiary structures revealed the general principles of protein tertiary structure. Tertiary structure largely results from the properties of the amino acid side chains. Hydrophobic side chains like those of phenylalanine, valine, leucine and isoleucine are always found on the inside of the structure, out of contact with the water which surrounds the protein molecule, even in the crystal. Charged groups like arginine, lysine, histidine, aspartate and glutamate are almost always on the surface of the molecule. There is no empty space within the molecule; the hydrophobic side chains that form much of the core are close-packed. Groups capable of forming hydrogen bonds, either as donors or acceptors, whether they be on side chains or on the polypeptide backbone, are virtually all in a position to form hydrogen bonds. In myoglobin and in each of the four subunits of haemoglobin, about 75% of the residues are involved in the formation of eight short sections of alpha helix. The remaining residues are situated in the connections between the end of one helix and the start of the next. Myoglobin and haemoglobin are atypical globular proteins in that they have a high content of alpha helix and a complete absence of beta sheet.

Denaturation destroys secondary and tertiary structure

While primary structure depends on covalent bonds, which are strong, secondary and tertiary structures are stabilised by a very large number of weak bonds, principally hydrogen bonds, by hydrophobic forces and by the electrostatic forces between charged groups. A few of these weak bonds can be temporarily disrupted without destroying the tertiary structure. Partners in the broken bonds are still close together in space and the bonds can quickly reform. This dependence of structure on a large number of weak bonds give globular proteins a flexibility and an ability to assume alternative conformations important to their function. However, if too much disruption of the weak stabilising bonds occurs, partners in a broken bond may move too far apart for their bond to be formed again; as a result, the whole structure falls apart.

Primary structure is responsible for specific folding

How do polypeptides achieve the specific folding they need for their function? An important experiment, which showed that polypeptides could acquire their secondary and tertiary structures on their own without the involvement of other agents, was carried out by Anfinsen (Fig. 13). He used a purified enzyme, bovine pancreatic ribonuclease. This is a relatively small enzyme with only 124 amino acid residues in its single polypeptide chain. Like many enzymes secreted into the gut where the physicochemical conditions are not so well controlled as they are within cells, the structure

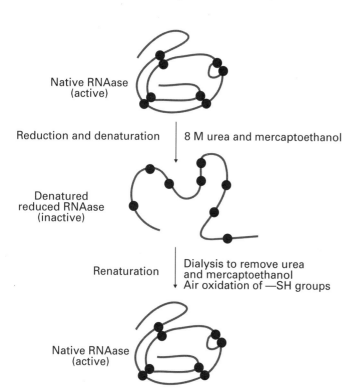

Native RNAase (active)

Reduction and denaturation | 8 M urea and mercaptoethanol

Denatured reduced RNAase (inactive)

Renaturation | Dialysis to remove urea and mercaptoethanol
Air oxidation of —SH groups

Native RNAase (active)

Fig. 13 Anfinsen experiment (see the text for details).

of ribonuclease is reinforced by disulphide bonds. Ribonuclease contains four such bonds. Anfinsen treated the enzyme with a reducing agent to break these bonds and also with a high concentration of urea, a reagent which disrupts hydrogen bonds. This combined treatment completely inactivated the enzyme. He observed that activity could be restored by gradual removal of the reducing agent and urea, if the conditions were mildly oxidising. Restoration of activity was complete. Since no other agent was present that could have brought the partners in the disulphide bonds together, Anfinsen concluded that the polypeptide chain must have refolded as directed by its primary sequence and that once refolded, the original disulphide bonds must have formed again.

While the primary structure of a polypeptide defines the way in which it will fold to form an active protein in the cell, the problem of predicting the actual secondary and tertiary structures of proteins from their amino acid sequences has not been solved. The number of ways in which a chain could fold is so enormous that it is currently beyond the power of even the most powerful computer to predict the stable folding that the majority of proteins appear to achieve within a minute after formation of their primary structure. Limited predictions can be made; some amino acid residues are found more frequently in alpha helixes than in beta sheets and vice versa, so the probable secondary structure of a given section of sequence can often be recognised. Proline cannot be accommodated within an alpha helix and is often found at the junction between one helix and another in globular proteins.

Quaternary structure and subunits

Many proteins contain more than one polypeptide chain. Usually the individual chains fold into subunits that specifically bind to other subunits to make up the complete protein. For example, each molecule of haemoglobin contains four polypeptide chains, each of which is folded to form a subunit that contains a bound haem group. The subunits have complementary binding sites for each other and assemble to form the functional tetramer. The subunits making up a protein are sometimes identical and sometimes not. In the case of the four haemoglobin subunits, there are two alpha chains and two beta chains. Alpha and beta chains have related amino acid sequences and have similar tertiary structures. The related protein myoglobin, which stores oxygen in muscle, exists as a single polypeptide chain with a sequence related to those of the haemoglobin chains. This chain adopts a tertiary structure similar to that of the haemoglobin subunits and binds a haem group but does not assemble into any larger structure.

Multi-subunit proteins are important because they create the possibility of interaction between subunits; the state of one subunit can influence the functioning of another.

The subunits making up a protein are usually held

together by specific but non-covalent forces such as hydrogen bonds, hydrophobic forces and electrostatic attractions. These numerous but weak forces are sometimes reinforced by strong covalent disulphide bonds between the subunits. Immunoglobulin G, a plasma protein that protects the body by recognising antigens, ('non-self' macromolecules in the blood) contains four polypeptide chains, two heavy H chains and two light L chains joined by disulphide bonds (see Fig. 172, p. 253).

Domains

Long polypeptides may contain several folding domains. In some very long polypeptide chains, different parts of the sequence may adopt tertiary structures that are separate from the tertiary structures adopted by other parts of the sequence, forming structures similar to those seen with multiple subunits. These partial structures or domains are tethered to each other by short flexible polypeptide sequences. The heavy H chains of immunoglobulin G each contains four domains while the light L chains each contains two domains.

3.5 **Ligand binding sites**

X-ray crystallography and other physical methods can provide information about the ways in which proteins bind their ligands and the effects ligand binding can have on three-dimensional structure. Proteins achieve specific binding of their ligands by means of forces similar to those they use to achieve specific folding. Achievement of a specific tertiary structure does not involve all the side chains in the amino acid sequence. Other amino acid side chains, usually not near to each other in the primary sequence, can be brought together in space in a specific three-dimensional conformation to form a binding site. This binding site has a structure complementary to the structure of the bound ligand. If the ligand has the potential to form hydrogen bonds, the binding site will have hydrogen bond donor and acceptor groups situated to form bonds with the ligand. If the ligand has a hydrophobic region, hydrophobic side chains in the binding site make close contacts with it. A charged group on the ligand is matched by a group of opposite charge in the binding site. Specificity and affinity of binding are achieved by numerous weak interactions.

Protein function, and hence all of life, depends on the ability of proteins to recognise and bind tightly to their specific ligands even though the ligand molecules may only be present in very small amounts in complex mixtures of similar molecules. For example, the receptor for the protein hormone insulin is present on the surface of many cells. It will recognise, bind and respond to insulin circulating in the blood when blood contains only 10^{-10} moles (6×10^{-7} g) insulin per litre. Insulin is recognised even though blood plasma contains about 60 g per litre or more of total protein, at least a 100 million-fold excess over the amount of insulin present. Other proteins concerned with controlling the expression of our genes can recognise and bind to a section of DNA sequence which represents about one part in 20 billion of the complete DNA sequence in each cell.

Since ligand binding by proteins depends on numerous weak interactions it is reversible and rapid. Ligands do not have to form the ligand–protein complex in one step, they can collide with and occupy part of the binding site and then trigger changes in protein conformation that create other parts of the binding site and hence increase the affinity of binding. Most protein–ligand interactions do not involve covalent bond formation. Ligand binding is important in enzyme function, the subject of the next chapter.

Self-assessment: questions

Multiple choice questions

1. Proteins have a role in the following biochemical processes:
   a. Protein synthesis
   b. Digestion of proteins in the digestive tract
   c. Replication of DNA
   d. Muscle contraction
   e. Transport of glucose across membranes

2. In ligand binding by proteins:
   a. Each globin subunit in haemoglobin has a specific binding site for the haem group
   b. An enzyme can recognise only one ligand, its substrate
   c. Oxygen is a ligand of haemoglobin
   d. In muscle contraction, the muscle proteins actin and myosin bind to each other
   e. Proteins bind specific base sequences in DNA to control synthesis of other proteins

3. Amino acids:
   a. Proteins are made from a set of 20 amino acids and amino acids not in the set are never found in proteins
   b. Amino acids in proteins are distinguished by their different side chains
   c. All amino acids have at least one amino group and at least one carboxyl group
   d. The amino group and a carboxyl group are both attached to the same carbon atom
   e. An alpha amino group and an alpha carboxyl group are involved in the formation of a peptide bond

4. Amino acid side chains:
   a. Aspartic acid and glutamic acid both carry carboxyl groups on their side chains
   b. Cysteine and methionine are the only amino acid side chains that contain sulphur
   c. Phenylalanine and tyrosine have aromatic hydrocarbon rings in their side chains
   d. Lysine, alanine and histidine are the only amino acids with side chains that can carry a positive charge
   e. Glycine is the amino acid with the smallest side chain and proline has a side chain that forms a five-membered ring which includes the amino nitrogen

5. Amino acid residues in proteins:
   a. Serine and threonine both have hydroxyl groups in their side chains.

   b. Glycine is the only amino acid found in proteins which is not an L-amino acid
   c. The most abundant amino acid in collagen is glycine
   d. All the amino acids found in proteins, except proline have a hydrogen atom attached to their alpha carbon
   e. In globular proteins, the side chains of the hydrophobic amino acids valine, leucine and isoleucine are unlikely to be on the surface of the protein

6. The peptide bond:
   a. Joins the alpha carbon of one amino acid with the amino group of the amino acid next in the polypeptide chain
   b. Shows partial double bond character
   c. Is a strong covalent bond
   d. Has an -NH group that can act as a hydrogen bond donor
   e. Has a -CO group that can act as a hydrogen bond acceptor

7. Polypeptide chains:
   a. Are linear and never branched
   b. Rarely show any regularity in the sequence of amino acids they contain
   c. Have an amino acid sequence that is known as the primary structure of a protein
   d. Amino acid sequence, not composition, is what gives each protein its uniqueness
   e. Have two ends that are identical

8. The following techniques for separating proteins from mixtures are commonly used for purifying proteins:
   a. Affinity chromatography
   b. Electrophoresis on polyacrylamide gel
   c. Fractionation by precipitation with ammonium sulphate
   d. Selective denaturation of other proteins in the mixture
   e. Ion exchange chromatography

9. The following techniques for separating proteins depend on properties of proteins directly related to their function:
   a. Affinity chromatography
   b. Electrophoresis on polyacrylamide gel
   c. Fractionation by precipitation with ammonium sulphate
   d. Selective denaturation of other proteins in the mixture
   e. Ion exchange chromatography

10. The following statements describe secondary and tertiary structures of proteins:
    a. The secondary and tertiary structure of a protein depend on its amino acid sequence
    b. The secondary structure of a protein is the three-dimensional configuration of amino acids close together in the sequence
    c. The tertiary structure of a protein is the three-dimensional configuration of all the amino acids in the sequence
    d. The secondary and tertiary structures of a protein are destroyed when the protein is denatured
    e. The secondary and tertiary structures of a protein are stabilised by a large number of weak bonds or forces

11. In protein structures:
    a. The primary structure of a protein is responsible for its tertiary structure
    b. The tertiary structure of a protein can be predicted from its sequence
    c. Anfinsen's experiment showed that peptide chains can only take up their active conformation in the presence of urea
    d. The alpha helix is the predominant secondary structure of unstretched keratin fibres
    e. The alpha helix and the beta pleated sheet are common elements of secondary structure even in globular proteins

12. In denaturation and hydrolysis of proteins:
    a. Peptide bonds are readily hydrolysed by exposure to dilute hydrochloric acid in the cold
    b. Determination of the amino acid composition of a protein involves hydrolysis of all the peptide bonds in the protein and analysis of the amino acids in the hydrolysate
    c. Denaturation alters the primary structure of a protein and destroys its biological activity
    d. Proteins can be denatured by exposure to acids, alkalis and concentrated solutions of urea and by elevated temperatures
    e. Most proteins become less soluble when denatured

13. In protein structures:
    a. Proline residues are never found near the middle of an alpha helix
    b. Lysine and leucine side chains are usually found in the interior of water-soluble globular proteins
    c. Aspartic acid and glutamic acid side chains are usually found on the exterior of water-soluble globular proteins
    d. Pairs of thiol groups from cysteine side chains are often oxidised to form a disulphide bond, which stabilises the tertiary structure of the protein
    e. Polypeptide chains forming a beta pleated sheet are always antiparallel

14. The following statements describe subunits and domains:
    a. The molecules of many proteins contain two or more separate polypeptide chains
    b. Some long polypeptide chains form two or more folding domains separated by flexible sections
    c. Separately folded polypeptide chains within a protein are known as subunits
    d. Subunits in a protein are sometimes identical and sometimes different
    e. Multiple polypeptide chains in a protein are never linked by covalent bonds

Short essay question

'Protein function can be largely explained in terms of specific ligand binding.' Discuss.

Self-assessment: answers

Multiple choice answers

1. a. **True.** Nucleic acids carry information to direct protein synthesis but many proteins are also required, some associated with ribosomes, some enzymes, etc.
   b. **True.** Digestion of dietary protein is carried out by enzymes, which are themselves proteins.
   c. **True.** Several enzymes and DNA-binding proteins are required for DNA replication.
   d. **True.** Actin and myosin are the major proteins involved.
   e. **True.** Proteins that are specific transporters of glucose and other metabolites are found in most cellular membranes.

2. a. **True.** Each globin subunit binds a haem group with high affinity.
   b. **False.** Many enzymes bind other ligands, for example prosthetic groups, second substrates, coenzymes and allosteric effectors.
   c. **True.** By definition: oxygen occupies a binding site on haemoglobin.
   d. **True.** Cyclical binding of myosin to actin filaments is involved in contraction.
   e. **True.** Specific recognition of DNA base sequences by proteins is used by all organisms to control gene expression.

3. a. **False.** Amino acids not in the set of 20 are sometimes found. Some amino acids from the set are incorporated in proteins and modified after incorporation.
   b. **True.** All the other groups around the alpha carbon are identical in all amino acids.
   c. **True.** All have alpha amino groups and alpha carboxyls.
   d. **True.** They are attached to the alpha carbon.
   e. **True.** Some amino acids have second amino groups or carboxyls but these are never involved in peptide bond formation.

4. a. **True.** Aspartic acid and glutamic acid are the only amino acids with second carboxyl groups.
   b. **True.** All the sulphur in proteins is in cysteine and methionine side chains.
   c. **True.** Phenylalanine and tyrosine have similar structures; tyrosine also has a phenolic hydroxyl.
   d. **False.** Lysine, arginine and histidine have basic side chains that can bind an hydrogen ion and carry a positive charge. Alanine has an uncharged methyl side chain.
   e. **True.** Glycine has the smallest possible side chain, a hydrogen atom. The side chain of

proline loops back to form a ring with the alpha nitrogen.

5. a. **True.** Serine and threonine both have hydroxyl groups on the beta carbon.
   b. **True.** Glycine has two hydrogen atoms attached to its alpha carbon so it does not have the asymmetry necessary to be optically active.
   c. **True.** About one third of the residues in collagen are glycine.
   d. **False.** Proline has an alpha hydrogen. It does not have a hydrogen on its nitrogen when it forms a peptide bond.
   e. **True.** Valine, leucine and isoleucine side chains are excluded from solvent water and cluster in the cores of globular proteins.

6. a. **False.** The peptide bond joins the carbonyl carbon of one residue with the amino group of the next.
   b. **True.** It is somewhat shorter than a carbon–nitrogen single bond and longer than the double bond.
   c. **True.** It requires strong reagents or high temperatures to break it.
   d. **True.** The hydrogen atom carries a fractional positive charge.
   e. **True.** The oxygen atom carries a fractional negative charge.

7. a. **True.** Peptide chains are always linear.
   b. **True.** Only a few structural proteins, such as collagen with glycine as every third residue, show any repeating pattern.
   c. **True.** By definition.
   d. **True.** Sequence controls how the chain folds and is essential for biological activity.
   e. **False.** They can be distinguished from each other, one has an amino group not involved in a peptide bond, the other a carboxyl.

8. a. **True.** Much used, it is a very powerful method that can give great purification in a single step.
   b. **False.** Not much used as only minute amounts of proteins can be handled. It is much used as a criterion of purity after separation.
   c. **True.** Much used especially in combination with other methods. It does not give great resolution but can handle large amounts of protein.
   d. **True.** Often useful as a preliminary step.
   e. **True.** Much used especially in combination with other methods. It is capable of great resolution.

9. a. **True.** This method depends on the protein binding a ligand specifically, a property likely to be related to the function of the protein.
    b. **False.** This method depends on the size of the protein and the charge it carries, properties not related to biological function.
    c. **False.** This method depends on solubility of the protein, a property not directly related to biological function.
    d. **False.** This method depends on the stability of the protein, a property not directly related to biological function.
    e. **False.** This method depends on the charge on the protein, a property not related to biological function.

10. a. **True.** The folding of the polypeptide gives the structure minimum energy for its sequence.
    b. **True.** By definition.
    c. **True.** By definition.
    d. **True.** Biological function, which is lost on denaturation, requires specific folding of the polypeptide chain.
    e. **True.** Weak forces such as hydrophobic forces and hydrogen bonds stabilise the folding (covalent disulphide bonds may also occur in tertiary folding).

11. a. **True.** Denatured proteins can often be refolded.
    b. **False.** Prediction needs too many calculations for even modern computers.
    c. **False.** Anfinsen used urea to unfold the protein. It only refolded when he removed the urea.
    d. **True.** Keratin fibres were used in the discovery of the alpha helix.
    e. **True.** About 75% of the residues in haemoglobin are in alpha helical segments. Beta pleated sheets are found in many enzyme molecules.

12. a. **False.** Peptide bonds vary in the ease with which they are hydrolysed but most require heating for hours in strong acid.
    b. **True.** This is how the amino acid composition is determined.
    c. **False.** Denaturation, by definition, destroys biological activity, but it does not alter primary structure.

    d. **True.** These are all common methods of denaturing proteins.
    e. **True.** Coagulation of egg white proteins is the usual example. Insoluble collagen, which when heated converts to soluble gelatin, is the major exception.

13. a. **True.** Proline nitrogen cannot form hydrogen bonds so proline can only occur at the end of a helix.
    b. **False.** Leucine is hydrophobic and is usually in the core of the protein but lysine has a hydrophilic ionised amino group on its side chain that will usually be at the protein surface.
    c. **True.** Aspartic acid and glutamic acid have ionised carboxyl groups in their side chains.
    d. **True.** This is how disulphide bonds are formed.
    e. **False.** Beta pleated sheets having parallel polypeptide chains are found.

14. a. **True.** Haemoglobin with four chains and insulin with two are examples.
    b. **True.** Immunoglobulin G has four chains, two light chains each folded into two domains and two heavy chains each forming four domains.
    c. **True.** By definition.
    d. **True.** For example, the enzyme lactate dehydrogenase is a tetramer of four M-type or H-type subunits and can exist as M_4, M_3H, M_2H_2, MH_3, or H_4.
    e. **False.** For example, the four chains in immunoglobulin G are joined by disulphide bonds and the two chains in insulin have inter and intrachain disulphide bonds.

Short essay answer

Whether protein molecules are functioning as building blocks for structures, as catalysts, as allosteric or controllable catalysts, as transport proteins in blood, as antibodies, as hormone receptors, as packaging for DNA, as pumps or transport mechanisms across membranes, their function always involves recognition and specific binding of other molecules or of parts of other molecules.

Try to think of a protein which has a function that cannot be explained in terms of specific ligand binding!

Enzymes

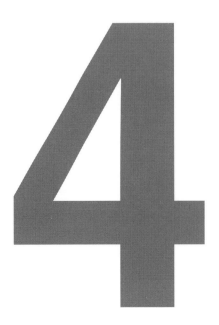

4.1 **Proteins as catalysts**

The living cell is the site of many chemical reactions, most of which require catalysts if they are to proceed at a sufficient rate under physiological conditions for the requirements of the cell. One of the most important functions of proteins is as protein catalysts or enzymes. Enzymes show remarkable properties when compared with the catalysts used by chemists:

* efficiency
* potency
* specificity.

Enzymes are very efficient catalysts

Enzymes do not require elevated temperatures to promote reaction nor do they require that the reactions they catalyse take place in acid, alkali or non-aqueous solution. Enzyme reactions take place at body temperature and, with a few exceptions, take place in aqueous solution near pH 7. No material is wasted in side reactions. The yield from enzyme-catalysed reactions is usually only limited by the equilibrium point of the reaction being catalysed. Enzymes promote reactions that bring chemical systems towards equilibrium but have the ability to couple reactions together so that a 'downhill' (energy-yielding) reaction may appear to drive one that is 'uphill'.

Enzymes are very potent catalysts

Each enzyme molecule is able to promote the conversion of hundreds, thousands or even more substrate molecules to product each second. One molecule of carbonic anhydrase, the enzyme that catalyses the reversible conversion of carbon dioxide and water into bicarbonate and hydrogen ions, can convert about one million molecules of substrate per second.

Enzymes are very specific catalysts

A different enzyme is required for almost every reaction that needs to be catalysed because each enzyme is generally very limited in the range of reactions it can promote. Hexokinase, the enzyme that phosphorylates glucose in preparation for its further metabolism, can also phosphorylate mannose but experiments on the enzyme purified from brain show that it has little or no action on any other monosaccharide. It requires ATP (adenosine triphosphate) as a source of the phosphate group, which it transfers only to the hydroxyl group on carbon-6 of the substrate. Although glucose and mannose have other sites where they could be phosphorylated, the specificity of hexokinase is such that glucose (and mannose) is only phosphorylated at this position (Fig. 14).

Enzymes differ in the degree of specificity that they show. Some enzymes concerned with synthetic reactions are very specific and catalyse only one reaction. Other

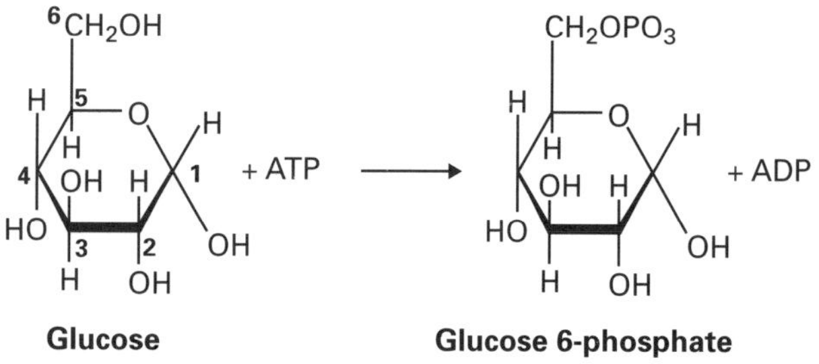

Fig. 14 Specificity of the reaction catalysed by hexokinase: phosphorylation is confined to the hydroxyl group carried by carbon-6.

enzymes, especially those concerned with digestion, can catalyse the hydrolysis of a wide range of similar compounds. For example, *trypsin*, a protein-digesting enzyme that is active in the duodenum, is able to cleave peptide bonds in a large number of proteins and peptides. The structure of most of the substrate molecule does not matter so long as it contains peptide bonds that involve the carboxyl groups of the amino acids arginine and lysine. Trypsin can be considered to be specific for a small part of its substrate. *Chymotrypsin*, a similar enzyme, can only cleave peptide bonds involving the carboxyl group of amino acids with bulky hydrophobic side chains, such as phenylalanine, tryosine and tryptophan. Both of these enzymes can also hydrolyse ester bonds involving these same carboxyl groups, although ester bonds are not found in their natural substrates.

Chemical nature of enzymes

Many enzymes are entirely composed of protein. Others have in addition some non-protein component such as a metal ion or an organic group essential for their catalytic action.

Metalloenzymes

Metalloenzymes have a structure that includes a tightly bound metal ion which is essential for activity. For example, *zinc* is found in carboxypeptidase, carbonic anhydrase and alcohol dehydrogenase, and *copper* is found in many enzymes that use molecular oxygen as a substrate. *Iron, manganese, molybdenum* and *cobalt* have also been found in the structures of some enzymes and are essential for their activity. The metal ion is generally very tightly bound to the enzyme at binding sites that may include cysteine sulphydryl groups, imidazole groups on histidine side chains or other groups on the protein.

Many enzymes have prosthetic groups

Many enzymes contain complex non-protein organic molecules called prosthetic groups that are necessary for their function. These organic molecules provide the enzyme with chemical functional groups that are not available as side chains on amino acids. Some prosthetic groups, such as the haem group found in haemoglobin but also present in many important enzymes, can be completely synthesised in the body. Other prosthetic groups of enzymes cannot be synthesised and are based on *vitamins*: essential organic components of the diet that are required in small amounts (pp. 243–244). For example, flavin adenine dinucleotide, FAD, a prosthetic group found in some enzymes that catalyse oxidation reactions, contains the vitamin *riboflavin*. Cleavage of carbon–carbon bonds to produce carbon dioxide is often catalysed by enzymes having a thiamine pyrophosphate prosthetic group. *Thiamine* is a vitamin. Its deficiency in the diet leads to the disease, beri-beri, which affects many organ systems. A prosthetic group remains bound to its enzyme during the complete catalytic cycle.

Coenzymes are often involved in transfer reactions

Coenzymes are small molecules that are changed in an enzyme-catalysed reaction but will eventually be regenerated; by comparison a substrate usually undergoes further reactions. Many enzyme reactions involve the transfer of a relatively small chemical grouping from one substrate to another: hexokinase transfers a phosphate group from ATP to glucose. ATP is the phosphate donor in many other reactions in which phosphate is transferred. It acts as a common substrate shared by many phosphate-transferring enzymes and is called a coenzyme. Similarly, enzymes catalysing oxidation–reduction reactions usually transfer two hydrogen atoms from a substrate to an acceptor such as NAD$^+$ (nicotinamide adenine dinucleotide), one of the common substrates or coenzymes of hydrogen transfer. Coenzymes also exist for the transfer of acetyl, acyl, glycosyl and other groups. Coenzymes often have a nucleotide unit within their structure, so most of them contain ribose, phosphate and a nitrogenous base such as adenine. Vitamins are required for the synthesis of some but not all coenzymes. *Nicotinamide*, a B vitamin, is required for the synthesis of NAD$^+$ and the related coenzyme NADP$^+$.

Coenzymes differ from prosthetic groups in that they need to move from enzyme to enzyme to carry out their function. For example, ATP is converted to ADP during hexokinase action but another phosphate transfer, catalysed by another enzyme, is required to convert the ADP back to ATP so that it can function again as a phosphate donor.

About fifty years after enzymes were purified sufficiently to demonstrate that they were proteins, RNA molecules with catalytic activity were discovered. Such *ribozymes* appear to have very limited catalytic abilities and to be less efficient than enzymes, which are protein. Ribozymes are involved in the processing of other RNA molecules. They will be mentioned again in Chapter 14.

Enzymes are stereospecific

Molecules that can exist in distinct left-handed and right-handed forms (i.e. their mirror image cannot be exactly superimposed on the 'real' image in any orientation) are said to be optically active or *chiral*. They will rotate a beam of plane-polarised light to the right (+, dextro rotatory) or to the left (–, laevo rotatory). Lactate and all the amino acids except glycine are examples.

Enzymes that act on such molecules or which produce chiral products from non-chiral substrates always show stereospecificity. If the substrate is optically active, only one of the two optical isomers will react. If the product can show optical activity, only one of its isomers will be formed. Lactate dehydrogenase, which is found in many tissues, can only oxidise the L form of lactate to non-chiral pyruvate. It can also catalyse the reduction of pyruvate and produces only L-lactate when it does so.

4.2 Enzyme nomenclature

Enzymes are named after the reactions they catalyse. Their names are generally based on the names of their substrates and indicate the nature of the reaction that is catalysed. They almost always end with the suffix '-ase'. For example, lactate dehydrogenase is the enzyme that oxidises lactate by removing two atoms of hydrogen from it; other *dehydrogenases* will remove hydrogen from other substrates. *Kinases* transfer phosphate groups, often from ATP; thus, hexokinase moves a phosphate group from ATP to the hexoses glucose or mannose. Enzymes that catalyse hydrolytic reactions are often named after their substrates, their class name, *hydrolase*, being assumed. For example, urease hydrolyses urea, sucrase hydrolyses sucrose and maltase hydrolyses maltose. Some digestive enzymes that were discovered before the naming system outlined above came into use have names that do not comply: pepsin, rennin, trypsin, chymotrypsin and thrombin are all *proteases*, which hydrolyse peptide bonds. The names described above are the trivial names, the names used for enzymes in most biochemical writing. An official nomenclature system has been agreed that avoids any ambiguity but it generates very cumbersome names which are useful only for reference. Each enzyme has a full name and an Enzyme Commission (E.C.) number derived from its position in the classification scheme. For instance, *hexokinase* has the full name ATP:D-hexose 6-phosphotransferase and the classification number EC 2.7.1.1. It is a transferase so it is in Group 2; it transfers a phosphate group so it is in subgroup 7; it has an alcohol group as an acceptor so it is in subsubgroup 1 and it is the first such enzyme to be classified. Further description of the classification is beyond the scope of this book.

4.3 Measurement of enzyme activity

The measurement of enzyme activity, or enzyme assay, is a very common operation in biochemical research and medical practice. Assay of enzymes in plasma and other clinical specimens is important for the diagnosis of many diseases. The activity of most enzymes is easy to measure. Even in a sample containing hundreds of enzymes it is possible to measure the activity of an individual enzyme. Enzymes do not have to be purified or separated before they are assayed; indeed enzyme assay is a powerful and essential tool for following the progress of enzyme purification.

Enzymes are assayed by incubating them with their substrates under appropriate conditions and measuring the rate of product formation. Because of enzyme specificity, it is almost always possible to devise conditions where only the enzyme of interest is active. Many other enzymes may be present but they do not interfere because they have no substrates on which to act. Other enzymes that can use the substrate which is provided need not interfere if the substrate is present in excess amount and if they convert this substrate to a different product not measured by the assay.

The aim of an enzyme assay is to measure the initial rate of the enzyme-catalysed reaction. This can be done by producing a graph of the amount of product formed against time. Such a graph is called the *progress curve* of the reaction. The formation of product can be detected by any suitable analytical method. Spectrophotometry, changes in the absorption of visible or ultraviolet light by the sample, is often used. This technique, available in all biochemistry laboratories, combines sensitivity and convenience and will provide a continuous curve (Fig. 15). For even greater sensitivity, radiochemical methods with substrates labelled with radioactive isotopes may be used. In this method, the product of the reaction, which also carries the label, must be separated from excess substrate before its radioactivity is measured. Radiochemical methods are even more sensitive than spectrophotometry but are

more expensive and less convenient. Radiochemical methods are particularly valuable for assaying enzymes that catalyse the synthesis of polymers such as DNA, RNA and glycogen. They make it possible to distinguish newly synthesised polymer from polymer that may be present at the start of the assay as template, primer or contaminant.

Progress curves, however determined, have the same general form; the graph is approximately linear having maximum slope shortly after the start of the reaction (Fig. 15). Later the slope decreases. This decrease in slope can be for a variety of reasons:

- the enzyme may begin to run out of substrate
- conversion of product back into substrate again may become significant as the reaction system approaches equilibrium
- the catalysed reaction may, as it progresses, change a condition such as pH in the assay, leading to lower efficiency for the enzyme
- the enzyme may lose activity as the assay progresses.

The only point on the progress curve where all these factors can be controlled is at the very start of the reaction. Hence during enzyme assay the rate of the enzyme-catalysed reaction is always calculated from the slope of the progress curve as near to the start of the reaction as is feasible. This is known as the *initial rate, v*.

Depending on the analytical method that is used to create the progress curve, the assay can be continuous or point by point.

Continuous assays. The formation of product is followed continuously by the analytical technique. The enzyme lactate dehydrogenase can be assayed continuously by spectrophotometry. As lactate is oxidised to pyruvate, the coenzyme NAD^+ is converted to NADH. NADH absorbs light at a wavelength of 340 nm in the near-ultraviolet while NAD^+ does not. By setting the spectrophotometer wavelength to 340 nm, the amount of NADH in the assay mixture in the cuvette can be measured continuously. If the spectrophotometer is equipped with a pen recorder it will draw the progress curve.

Sampled assay. The enzyme hexokinase cannot be assayed in a direct continuous way. The absorption spectra of its reactants, glucose and ATP, and its products, glucose 6-phosphate and ADP, are so similar that direct spectrophotometric assay cannot be used. Samples of the reaction mixture must be withdrawn and a separate analysis for glucose 6-phosphate formation carried out for each time point. The progress curve must then be constructed from a series of points at different times.

Coupled assay. Another method, which may be used to assay hexokinase, is coupled assay. In this method the product of the enzyme being assayed, in this case glucose 6-phosphate produced by hexokinase, is the substrate of a second enzyme that is more easily

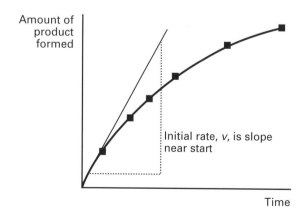

Fig. 15 Progress curve for an enzyme-catalysed reaction.

Amount of product formed

Initial rate, *v*, is slope near start

Time

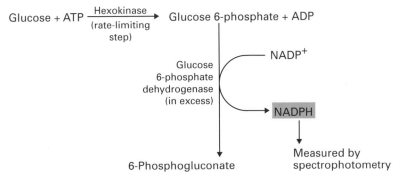

Fig. 16 Reaction scheme for the coupled assay of hexokinase.

assayed (Fig. 16). Glucose 6-phosphate is the substrate of the enzyme glucose 6-phosphate dehydrogenase (G6PDH), which oxidises it using NADP$^+$ as a coenzyme. NADPH absorbs light at 340 nm and its production can be followed by continuous spectro-photometry. If excess purified G6PDH and NADP$^+$ are added to the hexokinase assay, the hexokinase reaction will be the rate-limiting step in the production of NADPH. Coupled assays are used for many other enzymes.

Synthetic substrates. Synthetic substrates that are converted into products easily measured by spectro-photometry are also used to increase the range of enzymes that can be assayed by spectrophotometry. *Phosphatase* enzymes, which catalyse the hydrolysis of many phosphate esters, are easily assayed using nitrophenyl phosphate substrates. These substrates have absorption spectra that are different from the spectra of the free nitrophenol, the product of phosphatase action. Nitrophenol derivatives are used for the assay of a wide range of other hydrolytic enzymes.

Varying enzyme concentration

Since enzyme molecules act independently, the reaction rate measured in an enzyme assay should be proportional to the amount of enzyme present. This proportionality is generally observed and provides a simple test of the validity of the assay method. Any departure from proportionality is almost always an indication of some problem with the assay method.

4.4 Factors influencing enzyme-catalysed reactions

Enzymes are easily inactivated

The catalytic action of an enzyme is influenced by physicochemical conditions, particularly temperature and pH. Changes in these conditions can have irreversible or reversible effects on the enzyme. Enzymes, being proteins, are usually denatured by

BOX 4.1
Clinical note: Enzyme assay in clinical diagnosis

Enzyme assays are performed in hospital labor-atories to further the diagnosis of a wide range of clinical conditions. Many of the assays are performed on blood plasma. Cellular enzymes are usually confined to the cells in which they are synthesised and in which they function. However, if tissue damage occurs during disease, cell membranes may be damaged and enzymes may leak from the cell into the blood where they circulate for several days. Because each cell type has its characteristic complement of enzymes, identification of abnormally high levels of activity of some enzymes in plasma can point to damage of particular tissues. Measurement of the amount of enzyme that has leaked gives a measure of the amount of tissue damage which has occurred. For example, several hours after a coronary blood vessel is blocked, oxygen deprivation damages heart muscle, and *lactate dehydrogenase* and *creatine phosphokinase* activities in the blood rise markedly (Fig. 17). These enzymes leak from the damaged tissue. Their assay can confirm the diagnosis and provides an estimate of how much muscle is involved. The occurrence of isoenzymes, described later in this chapter, can be used to make these clinical tests even more discriminating.

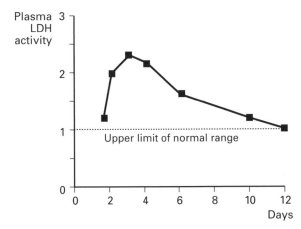

Fig. 17 Use of enzyme assay in clinical diagnosis: lactate dehydrogenase appears in plasma a few hours after heart muscle is damaged (given as a multiple of upper limit of normal range).

high temperatures or by pH values more than a few units away from neutrality. This denaturation is in most cases irreversible. When exploring the effect of changes in temperature and pH on the activity of enzymes, it is best to first define the temperature and pH ranges in which the enzyme is stable. Changes of temperature and pH that do not denature have reversible effects on the enzyme's activity.

Effects of temperature

Enzymes are inactivated by brief exposure to high temperatures. The onset of inactivation occurs over a temperature range of just a few degrees. The actual temperature required for inactivation varies from one enzyme to another but is typically in the range 50–60°C. A few enzymes, notably those from thermophilic microorganisms, can withstand exposure to 100°C. At temperatures below those at which they are inactivated, enzymes show increasing activity with increasing temperature. There is no optimum temperature and enzyme activity measurements should be made at temperatures that are at least a few degrees below the temperature at which the enzyme is inactivated.

Effect of pH

Within the pH range in which they are stable, the activities of enzymes can be strongly influenced by pH. For many enzymes the graph of activity against pH is bell-shaped with a definite optimum (Fig. 18). Enzyme assays should be carried out at the optimum pH. This is generally achieved by adding a buffer of the appropriate pH to the assay. The optimum pH for an enzyme-catalysed reaction does not necessarily coincide with the pH in the compartment of the cell where it is found. This variation of activity with pH results from the ionisation of a limited number of groups on the enzyme or substrate. This is well illustrated by studies on the mechanism of action of lysozyme, described later in this chapter.

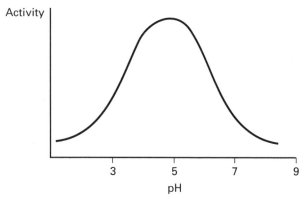

Fig. 18 The effect of pH on the activity of an enzyme, lysozyme. Activity of this enzyme depends on the ionisation state of two carboxyl groups at its active centre; it has a pH optimum of around 5.

BOX 4.2
Clinical note: Therapeutic use of enzymes

Preparations of digestive enzymes from the pancreas are used therapeutically in conditions such as cystic fibrosis where natural secretion is inadequate. Such preparations must be formulated or administered in such a way that they reach the duodenum in an active state and do not become inactivated by exposure to the low pH in the stomach.

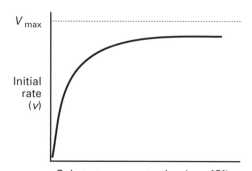

Fig. 19 Effect of varying subtrate concentration on a typical enzyme-catalysed reaction.

Effect of varying substrate concentration

Enzyme kinetics is the investigation of enzyme mechanisms by measuring how the initial rate of reaction is affected by varying experimental conditions, particularly by varying substrate concentrations.

Enzymes show *saturation* with substrate (Fig. 19). At low substrate concentrations, [S], the rate of the enzyme-catalysed reaction is approximately proportional to [S], but as [S] increases further the rate approaches a maximum. This is a consequence of the mechanism of enzymic catalysis.

Most enzyme reactions can be considered to occur in at least three phases. In the first phase the substrate or substrates bind to a specialised binding site on the enzyme, the *active centre*, to form an enzyme–substrate complex. In the second phase, chemical change occurs within this complex to generate the products of the reaction, still bound at the active centre. During this second phase, a transient covalent bond may form between an atom in the substrate and an atom in the enzyme. In the final phase, the products dissociate from the enzyme leaving it free to undergo another catalytic cycle. This mechanism can be represented by the model described by Michaelis and Menten:

$$E + S \leftrightarrow E\text{–}S \rightarrow E\text{–}P \rightarrow E + P$$

where E represents enzyme, S substrate and P product. At high concentrations of substrate, the active centre is fully occupied with substrate and further increases in substrate concentration cannot increase the occupation further. Under these conditions, the rate-limiting step in the catalytic process occurs after substrate has bound. The Michaelis equation, which relates the

(a)

(b)

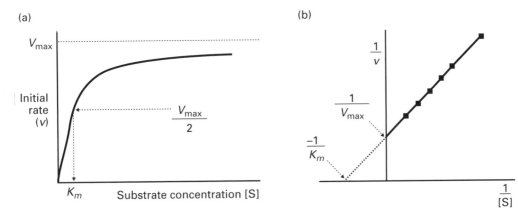

Fig. 20 Estimation of V_{max} and K_m: (a) using a graph of initial rate versus [S] and (b) using a linear plot – the *Lineweaver–Burk* plot – which provides a more accurate estimate.

observed initial rate (v) to the substrate concentration [S], can be derived from this model for enzymic catalysis.

$$v = V_{max} [S]/(K_m + [S])$$

The equation contains two parameters that are characteristic of the rate measurements under the experimental conditions which were used, V_{max}, the maximum reaction rate, and K_m, the *Michaelis constant*. The equation fits the form of the rate versus substrate concentration graph for many enzymes and gives experimental support to the model. V_{max} has the same dimensions as the reaction rate and is the upper limit approached by the reaction rate at high substrate concentrations. The Michaelis constant is the concentration of substrate at which the enzyme gives an observed reaction rate which is one half of V_{max}. V_{max} should be proportional to the amount of enzyme used in the experiments in which it was determined so it is not a characteristic of the enzyme. The value of K_m depends on the relative rates of the reactions involved in the formation of enzyme–substrate complex, its conversion to enzyme–product complex and the dissociation of the enzyme–product complex. It is a characteristic of the enzyme and is a measure of the affinity of the enzyme for its substrate. A low value of K_m indicates that the enzyme has a high affinity for its substrate and a high value that it has a low affinity.

While V_{max} and K_m can be estimated from the graph of v against [S] (Fig. 20a), it is usually more accurate to derive them from a linear transformation of the Michaelis equation, such as the Lineweaver–Burk plot (Fig. 20b). By plotting the reciprocals of rate and [S], a straight line should be obtained. Estimates of V_{max} and K_m can be calculated from the intercepts of this line on the y and x axes. Other statistically more satisfactory methods of estimating V_{max} and K_m from experimental data can also be used. Estimation of its K_m is usually one of the first investigations carried out with any newly discovered enzyme.

The first justification for determining the value of K_m for an enzyme is a very practical one. What concentration of substrate is appropriate for its assay? It is best to assay enzymes using substrate concentrations that are high enough to approach saturation, certainly three or four times the K_m value. In these circumstances, slight departures from the intended substrate concentration will only give small errors in the observed rate. At substrate concentrations below K_m, errors in the substrate concentration will have a more serious effect.

A second reason to determine K_m is to characterise the enzyme and possibly to distinguish it from other enzymes catalysing the same reaction. A single biochemical reaction is often catalysed by a different molecular form of enzyme in different tissues, or even in different compartments of the same cell. These multiple molecular forms of an enzyme are known as *isozymes* or isoenzymes. They can be distinguished in several ways, notably by study of their kinetics and by gel electrophoresis. While they catalyse a single reaction, they often differ from one another in their kinetics and in the ways in which their activity may be controlled. Isoenzymes have K_m values that fit them for their biochemical role. Hexokinase is found in most tissues that rely on blood glucose and has a low K_m for glucose. This means that the rate of glucose phosphorylation is insensitive to the glucose concentration and does not respond to increased glucose concentrations (Fig. 21). Glucose arriving at the cell is

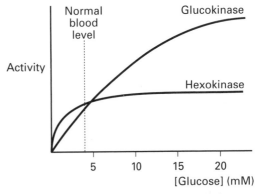

Fig. 21 Hexokinase and glucokinase are isozymes that phosphorylate glucose, the first step in its utilisation. Different K_m values allow hexokinase to supply energy substrates efficiently to cells that rely on blood glucose while glucokinase (in the liver and the pancreas) responds to high glucose levels.

efficiently metabolised. Hexokinase is inhibited by its product and has a low V_{max} so its rate of phosphorylation of glucose does not increase significantly when the blood glucose concentration rises: in effect it is insensitive to blood glucose concentration. *Glucokinase*, an isoenzyme of hexokinase, occurs in liver and in a few other tissues. It has a high K_m and V_{max} and it can respond by increasing the rate of glucose utilisation when large amounts of glucose reach the liver among the products of digestion after a carbohydrate meal. Glucokinase is also the isoenzyme present in the insulin-secreting cells in the pancreas and accounts for the ability of these cells to respond to changing glucose levels in the blood (Fig. 99, p. 139).

The final justification for determining K_m is that it is influenced by certain enzyme inhibitors and reveals their mode of action.

Enzyme inhibitors

Enzymes show diminished catalytic powers or are inhibited in the presence of a wide range of other molecules. Some inhibitors are quite non-specific; they will inhibit many enzymes. Heavy metal ions like mercury, lead and copper usually inhibit enzymes, so even traces of these ions must be removed from water and chemicals to be used in experiments with enzymes. Other inhibitors show more specificity. Specific inhibitors block enzyme action by mimicking the substrate in some way or other; others bind to the enzyme altering its shape and, thus, the configuration of the active site. The inhibitor may bind to and occupy the substrate-binding site forming a specific enzyme–inhibitor complex in which further chemical change does not occur. Other inhibitors get as far as the phase of enzyme action when chemical change occurs. However, instead of forming a transient covalent bond with the enzyme as the substrate does, the inhibitor forms a stable covalent bond so blocking further reaction. Inhibitors can be reversible, bound to the enzyme by non-covalent bonds, and so, in principle at least, able to dissociate from the enzyme again restoring it to activity. Other inhibitors that form a covalent bond

BOX 4.3
Clinical note: Methanol poisoning

There is no sharp dividing line between substrates and competitive inhibitors. The addition of an alternate substrate will decrease the action of an enzyme on a substrate on which it is already acting. This is exploited in the treatment of methanol poisoning. Methanol itself is relatively non-toxic. It is converted into the highly toxic methanal by alcohol dehydrogenase in the liver. Treatment of methanol poisoning is by administration of high concentrations of ethanol. This substrate reduces the rate at which methanol is converted to methanal allowing time for methanol excretion by the kidneys. Methanol poisoning is quite common. Misguided drinkers use it as a substitute for ethanol without appreciating the dangers.

with the enzyme are irreversible in their action. Enzyme inhibition can be described as:

- competitive
- non-competitive
- irreversible.

Competitive inhibitors

One particularly common mode of inhibition is reversible competitive inhibition, where the inhibitor molecule resembles the substrate molecule. The active centre can bind either inhibitor or substrate but not both at once. The amount of enzyme tied up as unproductive enzyme–inhibitor complex depends not only on the concentration of inhibitor but on the concentration of the substrate with which the inhibitor is competing. At high concentrations of substrate, the effects of competitive inhibitors are greatly diminished. (Fig. 22): the effect of the competitive inhibitor is to increase the K_m of the enzyme for its substrate (to K_{mi}): V_{max} remains the same. If the concentration of substrate is increased enough, the active site will be saturated with substrate and the inhibitor excluded. The inhibition of succinate dehydrogenase by malonate is the classic example of competitive inhibition (Fig. 23). The

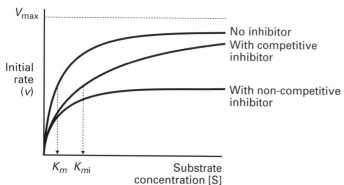

Fig. 22 Competitive and non-competitive inhibitors. A fixed concentration of inhibitor has different effects depending on its mechanism of action.

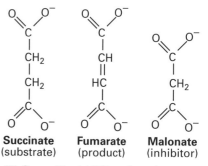

Fig. 23 Competitive inhibition of succinate dehydrogenase by malonate, which has an obvious structural similarity to succinate.

similarity of the succinate and malonate molecules can be easily seen.

Non-competitive inhibitors

Other enzyme inhibitors bind to the enzyme in such a way that the substrate, while it can still bind to the enzyme, cannot undergo reaction or may react more slowly. In this case the extent of inhibition will not be diminished by high substrate concentrations, (Fig. 22) and the inhibition is said to be non-competitive. With a non-competitive inhibitor, V_{max} is lowered but K_m is unaltered. An example is the inhibition of the membrane-bound Na^+/K^+ ATPase by *ouabain*, a toxic glycoside.

Irreversible inhibition: nerve gas inhibitors

Any compound that binds to an enzyme and prevents its catalytic action may irreversibly inhibit the enzyme. One molecule of inhibitor is sufficient to knock out one molecule of enzyme. Serine enzymes are inhibited irreversibly by 'nerve gas' inhibitors such as DIFP, (diisopropyl fluorophosphate). These compounds form stable phosphate esters with the reactive serine side chain and thus block the action of the enzyme. These inhibitors were discovered as very potent and toxic inhibitors of acetylcholinesterase, an enzyme involved in nerve action and which also depends on an activated serine side chain.

4.5 Mechanisms of enzyme action

As we have seen, the catalytic action of enzymes involves the formation of specific complexes between enzymes and their substrates. This accounts for the efficiency, potency and specificity of enzymic catalysis. Many enzymes have had their structures determined both in the absence and presence of competitive inhibitors. These models show how the polypeptide chain is folded and the position of all the amino acid side chains. It is usually impossible to determine

> **BOX 4.4**
> **Clinical note: Enzyme inhibitors are used as drugs**
>
> Many drugs used to control disease inhibit specific enzymes. For instance, in the development of drugs to control the human immunodeficiency virus, HIV, two enzymes involved in replication of the virus have been targeted. *Reverse transcriptase*, the enzyme which makes a DNA copy of the RNA which carries viral genes, is inhibited by AZT and other nucleoside analogues that are currently used as drugs. A specific *protease*, which processes viral proteins, is also the subject of inhibition studies. Since neither of these enzymes is used by the host cell, it should be possible, in principle, to devise drugs that halt viral replication without harming the cells of the host.

enzyme structures in the presence of substrates, but plausible models can be built to represent the structures of enzyme–substrate complexes. The position of the active centre can be deduced from the binding site for competitive inhibitors. Models of substrate molecules can be fitted to the enzyme models, giving an insight into the structure of the enzyme–substrate complex. For each enzyme studied, features of the complex can be identified that promote activation of the substrate and direct its reaction to form a specific product. Table 2 is a list of four of the most studied enzymes and particularly important features which have been identified in the reaction mechanism of each.

The nature of the enzyme–substrate complex

The molecular models show features common to all enzymes. The fit between the substrate and its binding site at the active centre of the enzyme is precise. Charged groups on the substrate are attracted by groups of opposite charge on the enzyme. Hydrogen bond donors and acceptors on the substrate can form bonds with appropriately positioned acceptors and

Table 2 Four much-studied enzymes, the reactions they catalyse and notable features of their reaction mechanisms

Enzyme	Reaction catalysed	Features of reaction mechanism
Carboxypeptidase A	Hydrolyses polar amino acid from C-terminal of peptide	Induced fit: enzyme changes conformation when substrate binds Water molecule on zinc in enzyme made more reactive
Lysozyme	Hydrolyses polysaccharide in cell walls of some bacteria	Monosaccharide unit next to bond that is cleaved is forced into more reactive transition state for reaction Aspartate side chain stabilises carbanion intermediate Glutamate side chain is proton donor for acid catalysis
Chymotrypsin	Hydrolyses peptide bond involving carboxyl group of amino acids with bulky non-polar side chains, e.g. phenylalanine, tyrosine and tryptophan Also hydrolyses ester bonds	Aspartate, histidine and serine side chains interact to enhance serine hydroxyl as a nucleophile Transient covalent intermediate formed and then hydrolysed
Hexokinase	Transfers phosphate group to glucose from ATP	Two substrates, glucose and ATP, are orientated for reaction Water excluded from reaction to prevent hydrolysis, a side reaction

donors on the enzyme. Hydrophobic groups on substrates fit into hydrophobic pockets in the enzyme. At one time it was thought that this fit between the enzyme and its substrate was rigid and could be likened to the fit between a *lock and key*. It is now thought that formation of the enzyme–substrate complex is more dynamic than this. Enzymes can be flexible and many change shape on binding their substrates. Substrates, too, may have to distort and adopt less stable conformations before they fit the binding site on the enzyme. Substrates are forced into a state close to that of the transition state in the reaction they are about to undergo. This concept of enzymes and substrates adapting their structures during complex formation was first described by Koshland and is called *induced fit*.

Proteins can enfold their substrates

Examination of detailed three-dimensional structures determined by X-ray crystallography of enzymes and their complexes with inhibitors or substrates has shown changes in the shape of enzymes when they bind their substrates. These changes in conformation can be used to promote the required reactions and to prevent side reactions. Protein flexibility allows enzymes to enfold their substrates during complex formation, excluding water molecules and thus preventing hydrolysis. Hexokinase shields ATP, its coenzyme substrate, from water while catalysing the transfer of a phosphate group to its other substrate, glucose. ATP hydrolysis is prevented since the only acceptor group accessible to the activated phosphate is on the glucose molecule bound to the enzyme.

Enfolding the substrate can also enhance its reactivity. If a substrate is bound in a region of the enzyme from which bulk solvent water is excluded, electrostatic attractions and repulsions between charged groups on the enzyme and on the substrate are greatly strengthened, increasing the reactivity of the substrate molecule. *Carboxypeptidase*, a zinc-containing protease that hydrolyses an amino acid from the C-terminal end of its peptide substrate, was one of the first enzymes for which clear evidence of a change in conformation on binding of substrate was obtained. A tyrosine side chain in the enzyme swings over the bound substrate, shielding it from solvent water. A single water molecule within the complex has its reactivity enhanced by the zinc atom and cleaves the peptide bond between the C-terminal amino acid and the rest of the substrate.

Bond cleavage

Before we can consider how complex formation can bring about reaction, we need to describe the nature of the chemical reactions important in biochemistry. A covalent bond is the sharing of two electrons by the two atoms involved in the bond. During chemical

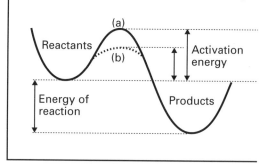

Fig. 24 Energy diagram for a reaction in the absence and presence of an enzyme. The reaction coordinate is a measure of the progress of the reaction. It might, for instance, represent the length of a bond which is being broken.

reaction, a covalent bond is cleaved and a new bond or bonds are formed. In almost all biochemical reactions, both shared electrons remain with one atom after bond cleavage and the other atom takes none. The products of the cleavage are usually unstable and quickly rearrange or form covalent bonds with new partners. Cleavage of a covalent bond is an energetically unfavourable process. If it were otherwise, covalent bonds would not exist. To cleave the bond it is necessary to stretch it until it reaches the *transition state*, the peak on the bond length versus energy graph (Fig. 24). This can be represented in an energy diagram for the reaction. Without a catalyst, the energy for bond stretching must come from thermal collisions with solvent molecules and other molecules in solution. Even if the bond length reaches the critical transition state and cleavage occurs, the molecular fragments produced may recombine producing no net reaction. The presence of an enzyme lowers the energy barrier between reactants and products but has no effect on the overall energy change of the reaction: the rate of reaction is increased but the equilibrium constant remains the same. How can the presence of an enzyme promote the reaction? Two important factors are activation of the substrate and stabilisation of the products.

Activation of the substrate

Several factors seem to be involved in the activation of substrates; the distortion of the substrate towards the transition state, the proximity of chemical groups on the enzyme that can promote reaction, the orientation of the substrate for reaction with another molecule and alteration of the molecular environment of the substrate have all been suggested as activation mechanisms.

Binding to an enzyme can weaken the critical bond in the substrate. As we have seen, substrates and enzymes have to adjust their structures when forming a complex. Substrates are often distorted towards the transition state structure. This is seen in the enzyme

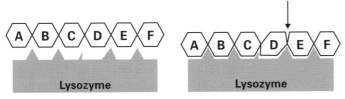

Fig. 25 Binding of substrate to the active centre of lysozyme. Notice how the D ring of the substrate must distort before substrate binding can occur. This ring must assume the half-chair configuration to fit the active centre. The bond cleaved during the reaction is between the D and E rings.

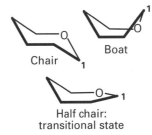

Fig. 26 Transition state in lysozyme catalysis. Ring D in lysozyme substrate adopts the less stable half-chair conformation prior to the cleavage of the glycosidic bond to carbon-1 of the ring.

BOX 4.5
Clinical note: Discovery of lysozyme

Lysozyme was discovered by Alexander Fleming who later discovered penicillin. The antibacterial action of lysozyme has not been used therapeutically. Its presence in tears and other secretions is part of the natural defences of the body.

---

lysozyme, a widely distributed enzyme that kills some bacteria by hydrolysis of their polysaccharide cell wall material. The substrate-binding site on lysozyme lies in a cleft on the surface of the enzyme. This site binds six monosaccharide units in the long polysaccharide chain of the substrate. Five of these six units are not distorted during binding to the enzyme but the other unit is distorted before it can bind (Fig. 25). The mono-saccharide units all contain a six-membered ring containing five carbons and an oxygen atom. This ring is most stable in a puckered configuration, the chair configuration (Fig. 26), with one atom above and one below the plane defined by the other four atoms. This configuration is retained by five of the six bound units. When the other unit binds to lysozyme its ring is forced into the half-chair configuration. Carbon-1 of this ring, the atom that is a partner in the carbon–oxygen bond which is cleaved during reaction, is forced up into the plane of the ring. This weakens the carbon–oxygen bond.

Stabilisation of the products

Once the substrate has bound to the active site with possible activation, the second effect, the promotion of the reaction by nearby chemical groups on the enzyme, comes into play. If the carbon–oxygen bond were to cleave in the lysozyme example, the products would be a carbon atom carrying a positive charge (i.e. an unstable carbanion) and an oxygen carrying a negative charge, also unstable (Fig. 27). There are two carboxyl groups on lysozyme near to where the substrate is bound. One of these, the side chain of an aspartate residue is ionised and has a negative charge. It is close to the carbon atom of the substrate that gains the positive charge on bond cleavage and this favours the

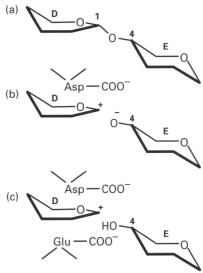

Fig. 27 Stabilisation of the products of bond cleavage during lysozyme catalysis. (a) The D and E rings before bond cleavage. (b) The D and E rings after bond cleavage. There is a carbanion at carbon-1 of the D ring, which is stabilised by the negatively charged carboxyl group on an aspartate side chain at the active centre. (c) The negatively charged oxygen on carbon-4 of the E ring is stabilised by transfer to it of a proton from a protonated glutanate side chain, also at the active centre.

production of this unstable intermediate. The second carboxyl group involved in the catalytic process is on a glutamate side chain. This group must be in the undissociated or protonated state to promote reaction. It gives its proton to the negatively charged oxygen produced by bond cleavage, converting it to the stable hydroxyl group found in the product of the reaction. This is an example of *acid catalysis*. An appropriately positioned amino acid side chain on the enzyme acts as a proton donor to provide the hydrogen ion (proton) needed for facile reaction. The position of such a proton donor may be critical in deciding which of two possible chiral products is formed by the enzyme reaction, that is to determine the stereospecificity of the enzyme.

Proximity and orientation of substrates

Enzymes that have more than one substrate bind these substrates in an orientation suitable for reaction. When the critical bond breaks, new partners are nearby so that the molecular fragments can form new bonds. One of the factors making uncatalysed reactions between two molecules in solution so slow is that collisions between the molecules, although frequent, are almost always in unsuitable orientations for reaction. An enzyme by binding first one substrate and then another can ensure that they are in the optimal orientation for reaction.

Formation of the enzyme–substrate complex explains the stereochemical specificity of enzymes. Substrate-binding sites, being three dimensional, will distinguish between the two optical isomers of a chiral substrate, one will fit the binding site and react, the other will not fit and, therefore, remains unchanged. Enzymes are chiral, so even when a non-chiral substrate is bound, new chemical groupings to be attached to this substrate will always approach from the same direction in space and so produce only one of the two possible stereo-isomers of the product.

Interaction between side chains can enhance their reactivity

Many proteases with different specificities are involved in the digestion of proteins in the gut. One class of digestive protease, the 'serine' proteases, have been studied in great detail and shown to have a common mechanism of action. This class of protease includes trypsin, chymotrypsin and elastase. Thrombin, a protease involved in blood clotting, has a similar mechanism. All these enzymes contain a serine side chain that is uniquely reactive. The hydroxyl group on the side chain displaces the amino group involved in the peptide bond, which is cleaved, and forms a transient ester intermediate with the carboxyl group. The ester intermediate is then hydrolysed leaving the protease free for another round of catalytic action. The enzyme forms an unstable covalent intermediate with part of the substrate. When this intermediate is hydrolysed, the catalytic process is complete.

The serine hydroxyl on its own would not be sufficiently reactive to displace part of the substrate and form a covalent bond with the remainder. In the serine proteases, it has its reactivity enhanced by interaction with an imidazole group on a histidine side chain, which in turn interacts with a negatively charged carboxyl group on an aspartate side chain (Fig. 28). The

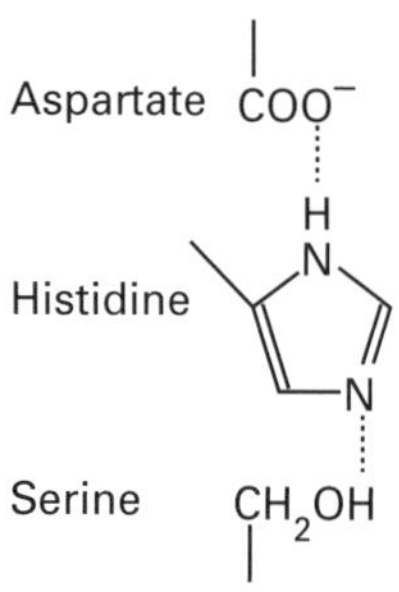

Fig. 28 Activation of the serine side chain of the active site in serine proteases by a charge relay system allowing the negatively charged carboxylate of the aspartate to share its charge with the serine oxygen.

carboxylate 'shares' its negative charge with the serine oxygen, making this atom a stronger nucleophile, more able to attack the carbonyl carbon of peptide and ester substrates. This group of side chains has been called a *charge relay system*. The amino acids contributing to the system are widely separated in the polypeptide sequence but are brought together by the tertiary structure. Nerve gases such as diisopropyl-fluorophosphate inhibit acetylcholine esterase by forming a stable covalent bond between the phosphorus atom of the inhibitor and the oxygen atom on the reactive serine side chain. They do not react with unactivated serines.

4.6 Control of enzyme activity

In every metabolic pathway, the activity of at least one enzyme is subject to regulation so that the flux of material through the pathway can be controlled.

Allosteric control

Some enzymes are reversibly inhibited or activated by the presence of metabolites that are not their substrates or products. These metabolites, if inhibitory, are usually distant products of the pathway, so providing negative feedback for the activity of the pathway. Metabolites that have their concentrations lowered by the pathway may act as activators of the controlling enzyme, giving further control. Enzymes controlled in this way have binding sites additional to those at which they bind their substrates. Binding of inhibitors or activators at these sites changes the conformation of the enzyme molecule, decreasing or increasing its catalytic ability. This form of control is known as allosteric. Allosteric enzymes are always composed of subunits and have multiple interacting active centres. While they can be saturated with their substrates, they often show *sigmoid* graphs of initial rate versus substrate concentration and, therefore, do not obey strict Michaelis kinetics.

Control by reversible covalent modification

This regulation is often in response to a signal coming from outside the cell, for instance response to a hormone. In this case, the enzyme is itself the substrate of other enzymes. One of these modifies the enzyme making it active while another reverses the modification making it inactive again. *Glycogen phosphorylase*, the enzyme that mobilises carbohydrate fuel reserves in animal cells, is activated by addition of a phosphate group to a serine side chain and is inactivated when this phosphate group is removed. The hormones *adrenaline* and *glucagon* trigger the activation of phosphorylase in their respective target cells (pp. 94–95).

Control by irreversible covalent modification

Some digestive enzymes are potentially so damaging to the cells that synthesise them that they are secreted as inactive precursors or *zymogens*. Once secreted, these zymogens are converted into their active forms. This activation process is irreversible. Trypsin, which is a major protease involved in protein digestion in the duodenum, is secreted as the inactive precursor trypsinogen in the pancreatic juice. Once in the duodenum, it is acted on by a specialised peptidase, *enteropeptidase*, secreted by cells in the duodenal wall. Enteropeptidase cleaves a peptide bond in trypsinogen, converting it to trypsin (Fig. 29). Trypsin, once formed, can act on further molecules of trypsinogen so the activation process is autocatalytic. Trypsin also activates other protease precursors from the pancreas, particularly chymotrypsinogen, proelastase and procarboxypeptidase (Fig. 30). Pepsin, the major protease active in the stomach, is secreted as its inactive precursor, pepsinogen. This is activated by an autocatalytic process in the acid conditions of the stomach. Blood clotting also depends on the appropriate activation of protease precursors in the plasma by limited specific proteolysis (Ch. 20).

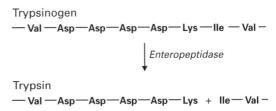

Trypsinogen

— Val — Asp — Asp — Asp — Asp — Lys — Ile — Val —

Enteropeptidase

Trypsin

— Val — Asp — Asp — Asp — Asp — Lys + Ile — Val —

Fig. 29 Activation of trypsin. Enteropeptidase is specific for trypsinogen, which is cleaved at the sequence shown above and thereby activated.

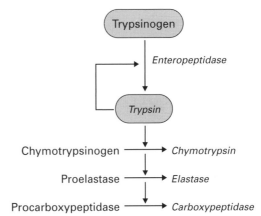

Fig. 30 Activation of digestive proteases.

4.7 **Membrane transport**

Proteins as well as catalysing chemical reactions can also promote transport processes. Ions and hydrophilic molecules cannot, on their own, penetrate the lipid bilayer that is the basis of all biological membranes. Proteins in membranes can form channels that will selectively allow ions to cross the membrane. Transporter proteins can form lipid-soluble complexes with hydrophilic molecules such as glucose. These complexes can pick up their ligands on one side of the membrane and release them on the other side, thus promoting transport. Proteins can also couple transport processes to chemical reactions, so allowing differences in ionic concentration on opposite sides of the membrane to be built up. Proteins involved in transport processes share many of their properties with enzymes. They show specificity, including stereospecificity, they show saturation when the ligand concentration is high and they are susceptible to inhibition, particularly by compounds similar to the ligands they transport.

The involvement of enzymes and other proteins in membrane transport processes will be mentioned again in Chapter 5.

Self-assessment: questions

Multiple choice questions

1. The following statements describe enzyme catalysis:
   a. Enzymes convert all available substrate into product because they do not waste material on side reactions
   b. An enzyme molecule is a true catalyst and remains unchanged after catalysing a reaction
   c. In an equilibrium reaction system, an enzyme that catalyses the forward reaction will also catalyse the back reaction
   d. An enzyme can convert a substrate that is not optically active into a product that is optically active
   e. An enzyme can convert a substrate that is optically active into a product that is not optically active

2. The digestive protease:
   a. Trypsin can cleave peptide bonds involving the carboxyl function of lysine residues
   b. Trypsin can cleave peptide bonds involving the carboxyl function of arginine residues
   c. Chymotrypsin can cleave peptide bonds involving the carboxyl function of phenylalanine and tyrosine
   d. Trypsin and chymotrypsin can cleave ester bonds as well as peptide bonds
   e. Chymotrypsin is active in the duodenum while trypsin is active in the stomach

3. The following statements describe coenzymes and prosthetic groups:
   a. Some enzymes contain metal ions such as zinc or copper that are essential for their activity
   b. Some enzymes contain organic molecules that are derived from vitamins and that are essential for activity. These molecules are called prosthetic groups
   c. Coenzymes are small polypeptides that are involved in transfer reactions catalysed by enzymes
   d. Coenzymes are required in some enzyme-catalysed reactions as carriers of acyl groups or phosphate groups
   e. Coenzymes are required in some enzyme-catalysed oxidation–reduction reactions involving hydrogen transfer

4. In enzyme assays:
   a. Enzymes must be purified before their activity can be measured
   b. Enzymes are usually assayed by measuring the rate of the reaction they catalyse under standardised conditions
   c. The observed rate in an enzyme assay should be proportional to the amount of enzyme present
   d. The catalysed reaction can be followed by measuring the rate of appearance of product or the rate of substrate consumption
   e. The graph of amount of product formed against time is known as a progress curve

5. For the assay of enzymes:
   a. Spectrophotometry is a convenient and sensitive technique for many enzymes
   b. Enzymes that catalyse the formation of polymers such as nucleic acids or glycogen are often assayed using radioactive isotopes
   c. The catalysed reaction must be stopped before the amount of product formed is measured
   d. Since the rate of the catalysed reaction tends to decrease with time during the course of an assay, the rate of reaction is always measured as close to the start of the reaction as possible
   e. pH, temperature and substrate concentration must be controlled during assay

6. In enzyme assays:
   a. NAD and NADP-linked dehydrogenases are readily assayed by spectrophotometry because NAD^+ and $NADP^+$ absorb light at 340 nm
   b. Many enzymes catalysing hydrolysis reactions are readily assayed by spectrophotometry using nitrophenyl derivatives as substrates
   c. Hexokinase cannot be assayed directly by spectrophotometry
   d. In coupled enzyme assay, a purified enzyme that is easy to assay is added to the reaction mixture to act on the product of the enzyme being studied
   e. The purified enzyme that is added for coupled enzyme assay must be present in large enough amount so that the reaction it catalyses is not rate-limiting

7. In enzyme assays:
   a. Enzyme assay is much used in biochemical research but has no practical importance
   b. Enzymes often have an optimum temperature so they should be assayed close to the temperature of the tissue or cell in which they occur
   c. Enzymes often have an optimum pH for activity so they should be assayed at a pH value close to this optimum
   d. Enzymes are denatured if they are not kept close to their optimum pH
   e. Enzymes are inactive outside the pH range 4 to 9

8. The following statements describe the effect of varying substrate concentration, [S], on the rate, v, of an enzyme-catalysed reaction:
   a. K_m, the Michaelis constant, is equal to the substrate concentration at which v is equal to one half of V_{max}
   b. At [S] values below K_m, v is approximately proportional to [S]
   c. At [S] values well above K_m, v is approximately independent of [S]
   d. At high [S] values, v approaches V_{max} as [S] increases
   e. The parameters v, V_{max}, [S] and K_m are related by the Michaelis equation as follows:
   $$v = (V_{max} + [S])/(K_m + [S])$$

9. The Michaelis constant, K_m:
   a. Is measured in the same units as the substrate concentration
   b. For a given substrate is a characteristic of an enzyme
   c. Can be considered to be a measure of the affinity an enzyme has for its substrate
   d. Has a low value to indicate a low affinity for substrate
   e. Often has different values for differing isozymes

10. The following statements describe the inhibition of enzymes:
   a. Many enzymes are non-specifically inhibited by heavy metal ions such as mercury and lead
   b. Many specific inhibitors of enzymes bind reversibly to the active centre and form an unproductive enzyme–inhibitor complex
   c. Some specific inhibitors of enzymes bind covalently to the enzyme that they inhibit
   d. Inhibition by inhibitors that bind reversibly to the active centre is relieved by decreasing the concentration of substrate
   e. Many drugs act by specific enzyme inhibition

11. The following statements describe the mechanism of enzyme action:
   a. Many enzymes have flexible structures that allow them to enfold their substrates
   b. The substrate is often distorted when it enters an enzyme–substrate complex
   c. An enzyme that catalyses the reaction between two substrates often binds them together in an orientation which promotes reaction
   d. Amino acid side chains near the active centre often have a role in the catalytic process
   e. Amino acid side chains involved in the formation of the active centre are usually close together in the amino acid sequence of the enzyme protein

12. In the mechanism of enzyme action:
   a. The two electrons that were shared in the bond which is cleaved in an enzyme-catalysed reaction are usually shared by the atoms that were joined by the bond
   b. Acidic and basic amino acid side chains often play an important role in catalysis
   c. The state of ionisation of acidic and basic groups near the active centre affects the catalytic activity of the enzyme
   d. Amino acid side chains near the active centre can interact to enhance their reactivity
   e. Some enzymes form temporary covalent bonds with part of the substrate

13. Allosteric enzymes have the following features:
   a. An allosteric enzyme has ligand-binding sites other than the active centre; metabolites or other signal molecules can bind at these sites and switch the enzyme on or off
   b. Allosteric enzymes always have subunits and multiple active centres
   c. Allosteric enzymes do not obey Michaelis kinetics
   d. Allosteric control is irreversible
   e. Allosteric enzymes are often involved in negative feedback control mechanisms

14. Zymogens:
   a. Are inactive precursors of enzymes that are activated by specific proteolytic cleavage of critical peptide bonds
   b. Activation is important in the digestion of proteins and in the clotting of blood
   c. Trypsin, chymotrypsin and elastase are proteases produced by activation of their respective zymogens
   d. Those of trypsin, chymotrypsin and elastase are synthesised in the pancreas and reach the duodenum before they are activated
   e. Pepsin, the major protease in the stomach, is secreted as pepsinogen, which is activated by trypsin action

15. In the control of enzyme activity by reversible covalent modification:
   a. Some enzymes are activated by being phosphorylated on a serine side chain and inactivated by the removal of the phosphate group
   b. Some enzymes are inactivated by being phosphorylated on a serine side chain and activated by the removal of the phosphate group
   c. Phosphorylation of serine side chains to control enzyme activity is catalysed by enzymes known as protein kinases, which require ATP
   d. Dephosphorylation of serine side chains to control enzyme activity is catalysed by enzymes known as protein phosphatases
   e. Control of enzyme activity by reversible phosphorylation is an important cellular response to some hormonal signals

True/false questions

Are the following statements true or false?

1. Enzymes are able to work under milder conditions than most chemical catalysts but, because of side reactions, cannot convert as much of the substrate into products.
2. Coenzymes are small, heat-stable molecules containing a nucleotide grouping that are often involved in enzyme-catalysed transfer reactions.
3. Enzymes that contain prosthetic groups can often be separated into a protein part, the holoenzyme, which is inactive, and a non-protein part.
4. Enzymes may have one or more active centres where their substrates bind and undergo chemical change.
5. Purified enzymes are often used to measure the activity of other enzymes.
6. Lactate dehydrogenase can be assayed by following changes in [NADH] by spectrophotometry.
7. Enzyme assays using radioactively labelled substrates are especially useful for measuring the activity of enzymes that synthesise polymers such as glycogen and DNA.
8. Phosphatases are enzymes that synthesise phosphate esters.
9. Liver and heart lactate dehydrogenase are identical.
10. Isoenzymes are distinct molecular forms of enzymes catalysing the same reaction and controlled in the same way.

11. The hydrogen ion concentration (pH) must be controlled during enzyme activity measurements. This is because the catalytic mechanism often involves amino acid side chains that need to be in a particular state of ionisation for reaction to occur.
12. $K_m = V_{max}/2$.
13. The addition of a competitive inhibitor to an enzyme reaction will increase the K_m for substrate.
14. Some enzyme inhibitors are irreversible in their action and others are reversible.
15. The value of V_{max} determined for an enzyme is proportional to the amount of enzyme used when measuring values of the initial rate, v.
16. The value of K_m determined for an enzyme is independent of the amount of enzyme used when measuring values of the initial rate v but will vary from one isoenzyme form to another.
17. Allosteric control of enzyme activity is achieved by the enzyme having an active centre that can bind either the substrate or the end product of the metabolic pathway in which the enzyme is involved.
18. Trypsin, chymotrypsin, elastase and thrombin all act outside cells and are all secreted as inactive proenzymes or zymogens.

Short essay question

What is the evidence that an enzyme forms a complex with its substrate during the course of an enzyme-catalysed reaction? How does this complex formation account for the specificity of enzymes and their potency as catalysts?

Self-assessment: answers

Multiple choice answers

1. a. **False.** Material is not wasted on side reactions but some substrate may not be converted to product because an equilibrium mixture of substrate and product is produced.
   b. **True.** Each enzyme molecule can bring about many rounds of catalysis.
   c. **True.** Otherwise the enzyme would not bring the system to equilibrium.
   d. **True.** For example, pyruvate to L-lactate by lactate dehydrogenase in muscle.
   e. **True.** For example, L-lactate to pyruvate by lactate dehydrogenase in muscle.

2. a. **True.** Trypsin needs a positively charged side chain like that of lysine in its substrate.
   b. **True.** Arginine also has a positively charged side chain.
   c. **True.** These amino acids have bulky hydrophobic side chains needed for substrate binding.
   d. **True.** Esters are cleaved by the same mechanism and are used as substrates in some assays for these enzymes.
   e. **False.** Trypsin is active in the duodenum. It is pepsin which is active in the stomach.

3. a. **True.** For example, carbonic anhydrase contains zinc; cytochrome oxidase contains both copper and haem iron.
   b. **True.** Vitamins provide many enzyme prosthetic groups that cannot be synthesised in the body.
   c. **False.** Coenzymes are involved in transfer reactions but usually have a nucleotide moiety in their structures. They are not polypeptides.
   d. **True.** Transfer reactions of acyl groups often involve coenzyme A. Phosphate transfers often involve ATP.
   e. **True.** Most hydrogen transfer reactions involve NAD or NADP.

4. a. **False.** Enzymes do not need to be purified before being assayed. Assay conditions should be such that only the target enzyme is active.
   b. **True.** This is the principle of enzyme assay.
   c. **True.** Otherwise the assay is not valid.
   d. **True.** It is usually better to follow product formation but for some enzymes substrate consumption is easier to measure.
   e. **True.** By definition.

5. a. **True.** Spectrophotometry is generally used if it is applicable.
   b. **True.** Only isotopic methods can measure the amount of new polymer formed in the presence of polymer present at the start of the assay.
   c. **False.** By using optical methods it is often possible to follow an enzyme-catalysed reaction without stopping it.
   d. **True.** Experimental conditions are only defined at the start of the reaction.
   e. **True.** These factors greatly influence the rate of reaction observed.

6. a. **False.** It is NADH and NADPH which absorb light at 340 nm, not the oxidised forms NAD^+ and $NADP^+$.
   b. **True.** Nitrophenol product is convenient to measure by spectrophotometry.
   c. **True.** There is no useful change in light absorption during the reaction.
   d. **True.** The added enzyme acts as an 'indicator' for the enzyme being assayed.
   e. **True.** Otherwise the added enzyme sets the rate of the observed reaction.

7. a. **False.** For instance, enzyme assay is much used in clinical diagnosis.
   b. **False.** Enzymes have no true optimum temperature for their action, the best temperature for an assay depends on several factors.
   c. **True.** At this pH, the rate is least sensitive to small changes in pH.
   d. **False.** Enzymes vary greatly in their stability to changes in pH.
   e. **False.** Many enzymes are stable outside this range, e.g. pepsin is stable in below pH 4 and alcohol dehydrogenase is active at pH 10.

8. a. **True.** This is a useful working definition.
   b. **True.** At values of [S] well below K_m, v is proportional to [S].
   c. **True.** If [S] $>>$ K_m, the enzyme is saturated with substrate and v is independent of [S].
   d. **True.** At high values of [S], the value of v is a useful working definition of V_{max}.
   e. **False.** The Michaelis equation should be $v = (V_{max}$ and [S])$/ (K_m + $[S]$)$. The numerator is the product of V_{max} and [S] not their sum.

9. a. **True.** Remember K_m and [S] are added together in the denominator of the Michaelis equation.
   b. **True.** Differences in K_m values would indicate the existence of isoenzymes.
   c. **True.** Enzymes with low K_m values are active at low [S] values.
   d. **False.** A low value of K_m indicates a high affinity for substrate.

e. **True.** Measuring of K_m values is one way of distinguishing isoenzymes.

10. a. **True.** This is one reason why such ions are environmental poisons.
    b. **True.** Such an inhibitor has features required for binding to the enzyme but not for reaction.
    c. **True.** For example, nerve gases form covalent derivatives of acetylcholinesterase.
    d. **False.** Inhibition is relieved by increasing [S].
    e. **True.** For example, monoamine oxidase (MAO) inhibitors. This is a basis for rational drug development.

11. a. **True.** This is the concept of 'induced fit'.
    b. **True.** The enzyme often forces the substrate toward the transition state for the reaction.
    c. **True.** This is one factor responsible for efficient catalysis by enzymes.
    d. **True.** The roles of such side chains are often revealed by studies relating the structures and catalytic mechanisms of enzymes.
    e. **False.** The active centre is usually formed by folding, which brings side chains together from widely separate positions in the amino acid sequence.

12. a. **False.** When an enzyme cleaves a bond, both electrons which formed the bond generally remain with one of the atoms in the bond.
    b. **True.** Often they act catalytically as acids or bases; sometimes the charge on the side chain is important for stabilising reaction intermediates.
    c. **True.** Acidic or basic groups cannot play their role in catalysis unless they are in the appropriate state of ionisation.
    d. **True.** For example, the enhanced reactivity of serine side chains at the active centres of serine proteases results from interaction with nearby histidine and aspartic acid side chains.
    e. **True.** For example, covalent bonds with the serine side chains in serine proteases.

13. a. **True.** This describes allosteric control of enzyme activity.
    b. **True.** This applies to all allosteric enzymes so far studied.
    c. **True.** The graph of initial rate v against [S] is often sigmoid.
    d. **False.** Allosteric control is reversible; the activity of an allosteric enzyme depends on the concentrations of allosteric activators and inhibitors that are present at any time.
    e. **True.** Allosteric control with negative feedback is found in many metabolic pathways.

14. a. **True.** By definition.
    b. **True.** These are the major processes in which zymogens are found.

c. **True.** These three proteases have many other similarities.
d. **True.** Most of the proteases active in the gut are synthesised as zymogens in the pancreas.
e. **False.** Pepsinogen is activated by the acidic conditions in the stomach. Trypsin is not active in the stomach.

15. a. **True.** Glycogen phosphorylase is an example.
    b. **True.** Glycogen synthetase is an example.
    c. **True.** Protein kinases transfer phosphate groups from ATP to hydroxyl groups on the side chains of serine, threonine or tyrosine residues.
    d. **True.** Protein phosphatases remove phosphate groups from proteins.
    e. **True.** Control of glycogen synthesis and breakdown by glucagon in liver and by adrenaline in muscle are notable examples.

True/false answers

1. **False.** Side reactions are rarely important in enzyme-catalysed reactions.
2. **True.**
3. **False.** The protein part without the prosthetic group is called the apoenzyme. The holoenzyme is the protein part plus the prosthetic group.
4. **True.**
5. **True.** This is coupled enzyme assay. Usually the added enzyme converts the product of the target enzyme into something that is more readily measured.
6. **True.**
7. **True.** The use of isotopes allows the investigator to distinguish between polymer that was originally present as primer, template or contaminant and polymer which is synthesised during the course of the assay.
8. **False.** They hydrolyse phosphate esters.
9. **False.** Different isoenzymes of lactate dehydrogenase are present in these two tissues.
10. **False.** They catalyse the same reaction but they are usually controlled in different ways.
11. **True.**
12. **False.** K_m is the substrate concentration at which $v = V_{max}/2$.
13. **True.**
14. **True.**
15. **True.** Enzyme assay depends on this proportionality.
16. **True.**
17. **False.** The allosteric activator or inhibitor is bound at a different site from the substrate binding site or active centre.
18. **True.** This prevents unwanted reactions occurring in the cells.

Short essay answer

Several lines of evidence point to complex formation. The phenomenon of saturation with substrate is most easily explained in this way, as is the phenomenon of competitive inhibition. Also the formation of some enzyme–substrate complexes can be detected by optical and other physical methods. Models of enzyme molecules often show plausible binding sites for their substrates.

Complex formation explains enzyme specificity if the substrate binding site on the enzyme makes a large number of specific non-covalent interactions with a large part of the substrate molecule. Complex formation can also explain the potency of enzymes as catalysts. By binding two reactants in a complex, optimal orientation can be achieved for their reaction. Reactants can also be made more reactive within the complex by distortion towards the transition state for the reaction.

Cell membranes

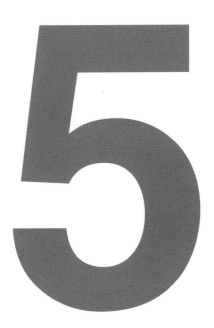

5.1 Membrane structure

Cells need a structure at their boundary to confine what must be kept in the cell. The boundary structure of the cell is the cell membrane, referred to in animals as the *plasma membrane*. Anything inside this membrane is intracellular and anything outside is extracellular. Functions of the membrane include:

- control of intracellular conditions by import and export of materials
- secretion of materials for use outside the cell
- reception of signals from other cells
- identification of the cell to other cells so that cells can interact, e.g. adhere to form structures.

Eukaryotic cells have internal membranes

As well as having plasma membranes, most eukaryotic cells have other membranes within them so that most cells are divided into functional compartments (Fig. 31). For instance, the cell nucleus is surrounded by the nuclear membrane. Every mitochondrion is delimited by two membranes, an outer and an inner membrane, separated by an intermembrane space. Other cellular organelles such as lysosomes and the Golgi apparatus are membranous structures. Table 3 lists some of the more important biochemical processes that occur within the different cellular compartments and organelles.

Cellular membranes are associated with other structural components in a cell: the *cytoskeleton*, a system of protein filaments and microtubules. No attempt has been made to represent the cytoskeleton in Figure 31.

Cell membrane structure

Lipid components

Cell membranes are based on a phospholipid bilayer. In addition, the plasma membrane has oligosaccharide groups attached to its exterior. Lipids are defined as materials that are extracted from living material by non-polar solvents such as chloroform. They are not water soluble, although as we shall see, they can interact with water in important ways. Lipids have diverse chemical structures. Lipids found in membranes include *phospholipids* and *cholesterol* (Fig. 32). Phospholipids such as phosphatidylcholine (PC) are the main constituents of most membranes. The fluidity of the membrane depends on the length and degree of unsaturation of the fatty acid hydrocarbon chains. Short chains and unsaturation increase the fluidity. Fluidity of the membrane is also influenced by temperature: membranes are less fluid at low temperatures. The fatty acid content of membrane lipids varies from one organism to another depending on the temperature at which the organisms live. Cholesterol is found in the plasma membrane of animal cells, where it reduces fluidity. It is not present in the membranes of plant or bacterial cells.

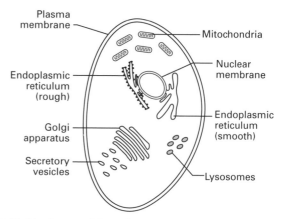

Fig. 31 Membranes of the cell.

Table 3 The main cellular compartments and their functions

Compartment or organelle	Main biochemical functions
Nucleus	Contains DNA DNA replication and packaging RNA synthesis RNA processing
Mitochondria	Most enzymes of the citric acid cycle and fatty acid oxidation
Mitochondrial inner membrane	Oxidative phosphorylation Succinate dehydrogenase Fatty acyl CoA dehydrogenase
Ribosomes	Protein synthesis
Endoplasmic reticulum	Transport of newly synthesised proteins to the Golgi apparatus
Golgi apparatus	Sorting and modifying newly synthesised proteins for transport within the cell and for export
Lysosomes	Hydrolytic enzymes, e.g. proteases, carbohydrases, lipases, nucleases Processing of imported macromolecules
Secretory vesicles	Proteins and other materials for export, en route from Golgi to plasma membrane
Cytosol	Glycolysis Fatty acid synthesis Pentose phosphate pathway

BOX 5.1
Clinical note: Lung surfactant

Dipalmitoyl phosphatidyl choline is a major constituent of lung surfactant which covers the alveolar surfaces in the lung. It exerts a surface pressure which prevents complete collapse of the alveoli when air is expelled from the lung. It is normally first secreted about the time of birth and its absence is responsible for respiratory distress syndrome seen in newborn, especially premature, infants.

Membrane lipid molecules are *amphipathic*, each has a hydrophobic part and hydrophilic part. Such molecules are surface active: they will line up at an air–water or

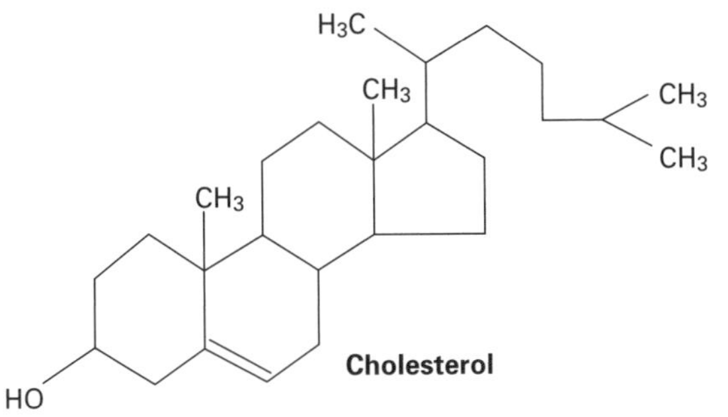

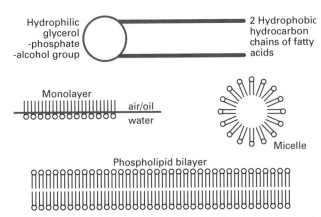

Cholesterol

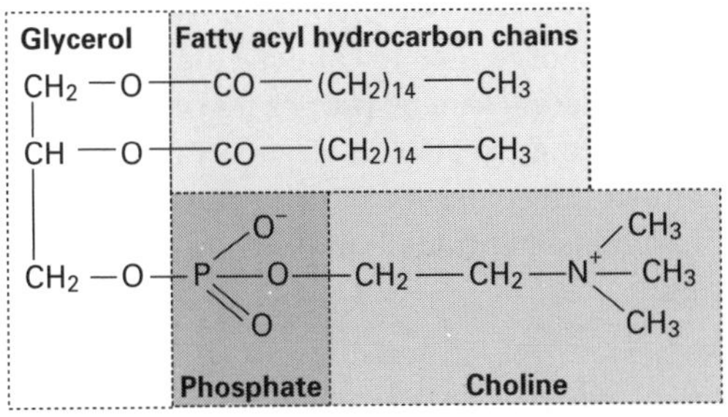

Phosphatidylcholine (lecithin)

Fig. 32 Membrane lipids. Phosphatidylserine and phosphatidylethanolamine are also commonly found.

diffuse laterally within the plane of the bilayer; they can also rotate about an axis perpendicular to the bilayer. However, they cannot move their hydrophilic head groups from one side of the membrane to the other, such a 'flip-flop' motion is energetically impossible. Membrane lipids remain in the orientation in which they are inserted in the membrane and cannot move from one layer of the bilayer to the other. As a result the lipid compositions of the two layers can be, and indeed are, distinct.

The lipid bilayer forms a barrier to the passage of many molecules, particularly hydrophilic and charged molecules such as glucose and amino acids. Any materials that can cross the bilayer itself by diffusion are usually small uncharged molecules such as oxygen, carbon dioxide, short-chain fatty acids in their undissociated forms and water itself.

Phospholipid bilayers are impermeable to polar molecules

A lipid bilayer has at its core a hydrophobic layer which is about 4 nm deep. This core is a barrier that prevents small hydrophilic molecules and ions from entering or leaving the cell. A glucose molecule or an amino acid would have to break its hydrogen bonds with water while it was crossing the bilayer, so the bilayer is impermeable to glucose and amino acids. Similarly potassium, sodium and chloride ions are insoluble in the lipid layer and cannot pass through it. Macromolecules are also unable to cross the membrane on their own. Transport of all these materials across the membrane does occur. It depends on the presence of specific protein *transporters* in the membrane.

Protein components

Proteins are found associated with the membrane. The amount of protein and the nature of membrane proteins vary from one membrane to another. The inner mitochondrial membrane is about 75% protein by weight, most membranes have much less. Membrane proteins have many functions, which include:

- transport of materials across the membrane
- reception and transmission of signals from other cells
- structural, giving shape to the cell or binding the cell to others to form tissues.

Different membrane proteins are associated with the membrane in different ways (Fig. 34). Some proteins

water–oil interface to form a monolayer with the hydrophilic part of the molecule in contact with the water phase and the hydrophobic part projecting into the non-aqueous phase. If no surface is available, the molecules may form *micelles*, spherical aggregates with hydrophobic cores and hydrophilic exteriors. Another stable configuration that these molecules can adopt is a *bimolecular leaflet*: two monolayers back to back with the hydrophobic surfaces in contact (Fig. 33). This structure allows the hydrophilic groups on the molecules to stay in contact with water while minimising contact between the hydrophobic groups and water. Such a planar structure is stable except at its edges. It can become completely stable by forming a closed surface such as a sphere. Cell membranes are based on *lipid bilayers* in the form of closed surfaces. The lipid bilayer is flexible and self-sealing. It is a dynamic structure, rather like a two-dimensional liquid. Individual molecules in the bilayer are able to

Fig. 33 Phospholipid molecules in water can form a monolayer at any unoccupied air–water or oil–water interface. They can also form micelles and bilayers.

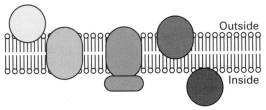

Fig. 34 Proteins in the membrane.

are inserted into the lipid bilayer and have regions that are accessible to both the extracellular and intracellular phases; they are said to 'span' the membrane. Others are anchored in the lipid bilayer so that they remain associated with the membrane but have contact with only one side of the membrane. Still further proteins are attached to the outside or inside of the bilayer. Membrane proteins are sometimes classified as integral or peripheral, the former cannot be removed from the membrane without destroying it while the latter can be removed still leaving the membrane intact.

The orientation of membrane proteins with respect to the membrane is important; regions of a protein must remain in contact with the same phase all the time. While proteins may be mobile within the plane of the membrane and may also be able to rotate around an axis perpendicular to the plane of the membrane, they can never flip-flop or rotate about an axis parallel to the plane of the membrane.

Complex carbohydrate groups

Complex carbohydrate groups are carried on the outer surface of cells. They are involved in cell–cell interactions and allow the *immune* system to distinguish between cells that are 'self' and cells that are 'non-self' and are, therefore, targets. *Blood group* substances, carbohydrates on the surface of the red cell, differ among individuals according to blood group and must be matched between the donor and the recipient of a blood transfusion.

5.2 Transport across membranes

Transport of molecules accross membranes may occur in three ways:

- diffusion: free passage from a high to a low concentration
- facilitated diffusion: transport along a concentration gradient by a carrier system without the expenditure of energy
- active transport: involves carrier proteins and requires energy, often occurs against concentration gradients.

Small molecules

Transport proteins facilitate the transport of molecules that would otherwise be unable to cross the membrane. Every cell that uses glucose as a fuel has *glucose transporter* proteins embedded in its membrane. These proteins bind glucose molecules from the extracellular fluid on the outside of the membrane and release them on the inside of the cell. Amino acids and ions such as chloride, bicarbonate, sodium, potassium and calcium are transferred across the membrane by specific transport proteins.

Transport proteins resemble enzymes:

- they bring about a process which would otherwise be much too slow because it involves a large energy barrier
- they show specificity, including stereospecificity
- they show saturation kinetics
- they are inhibited by specific inhibitors
- their absence owing to a genetic mutation can give rise to an inherited disease
- they occur in distinct forms: just as distinct molecular forms of enzymes, or isozymes, occur within an organism to catalyse the same reaction but have different kinetic properties or control mechanisms, so also do transport proteins occur in distinct molecular forms. The glucose transporters in animals mentioned on p. 76 are an example of this.

Active membrane transport

Transport processes can occur to decrease or increase a concentration difference between one side of the membrane and the other. Transport is energetically favourable when it is downhill, that is from a region where the transported molecule is present in high concentration to a region where its concentration is low. But transport in the opposite direction can occur if the transport protein is able to use metabolic energy to move the transported molecule uphill. Transport of a molecule against a concentration difference or electrical gradient is often referred to as *active transport*. Some transport proteins are also *ATPases* and use the energy from the hydrolysis of ATP; they are often referred to as *pumps* (Fig. 35). ATP hydrolysis and the transport of ions are tightly coupled in ion pumps; one cannot occur without the other. Another way of achieving uphill transport is by cotransport, moving one molecule uphill but at the same time moving another molecule downhill (Fig. 36). This process is referred to as *secondary active transport*. An example is the cotransport of sodium and glucose, which is important during the absorption of glucose in the gut. Glucose, at low concentration in the lumen of the gut, is taken into cells, which may contain a higher concentration. Uphill transport of glucose is achieved by its cotransport with sodium ions, which are moving from a high sodium concentration region to a low sodium

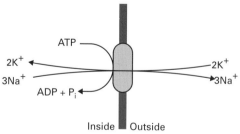

Fig. 35 Active transport: ATPase in the cell membrane acting as an ion pump.

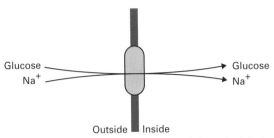

Fig. 36 Cotransport of sodium and glucose is important during the absorption of glucose in the gut. Glucose, at low concentration in the lumen of the gut, is taken into cells, which may contain a higher concentration.

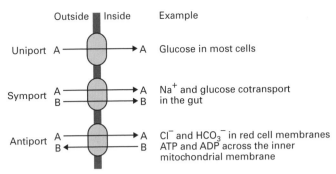

Fig. 37 Transporters classified by the nature of the transport process.

concentration region within the cell. This explains why starvation victims are better treated with glucose solutions that contain salt than with glucose solutions in water alone.

Transport of charged molecules

Materials that are transported are sometimes electrically neutral like glucose but may be charged like sodium or potassium ions; transport of the charged molecules is influenced by membrane potentials. Membranes are barriers to the movement of ions and can act as electrical insulators if ion transport is not allowed. If the distribution of ions is not the same on each side of a membrane, then an electrical potential difference can be established across the membrane. When a charged particle moves across a membrane it will be influenced by the electrical potential that exists across the membrane as well as by any concentration difference. Ions can be transported from regions of low concentration to regions where the concentration is higher if there is a sufficiently large electrical potential gradient that favours the movement. Ionic movement from a region of high concentration to a region where the concentration is low may be energetically unfavourable if the transport is opposed by an adverse electrical potential. Potential differences will be dissipated if ion transporters allow ion transport down the gradient.

Transport and energy conversion

A pump transporting a charged ion can use the chemical energy of ATP hydrolysis to build up a membrane potential. For example, energy from the oxidation of foodstuffs is used to pump hydrogen ions across the mitochondrial inner membrane. This builds up an electrical potential and a pH difference across this membrane. Energy stored in this way is used to drive the synthesis of ATP from ADP and inorganic phosphate (p. 85).

Linked transport

Transport of different molecules is sometimes linked;

for example the cotransport of sodium and glucose in the gut.

Classification of transporters

Membrane transport proteins can be classified according to the nature of the transport process that they promote (Fig. 37).

Uniport. This is the simplest type of transporter. It can transport a single molecule at a time. The glucose transporters found on the plasma membranes of most cells are uniports.

Symport. This is required by its mechanism to transport two different molecular species at the same time, neither species can be transported on its own. The glucose transporter involved in the uptake of glucose from the gut is a symport, it can only transport glucose while it simultaneously transports a sodium ion. Energy from the concentration difference for sodium ions (high sodium concentration outside cells and low inside) is used to move glucose from a region where its concentration may be low, in the lumen of the gut, to a region where its concentration is higher, inside the mucosal cell (Fig. 52).

Antiport. This, like the symport, involves the transport of two molecular species at the same time, but in this case the species move in opposite directions. There is an antiport in the red cell membrane that brings about the exchange of chloride and bicarbonate ions. Another antiport, this time in the mitochondrial inner membrane, allows ATP made inside the mitochondrion to leave by exchanging it for ADP, which enters the inner mitochondrial compartment and can then be phosphorylated to form more ATP.

Macromolecules

Import of macromolecules

Other receptor proteins are involved in the import of macromolecules into the cell by the process known as receptor-mediated endocytosis. Lipoproteins, which distribute cholesterol to cells (see Chapter 10), and transferrin, which carries iron, are examples of macro-

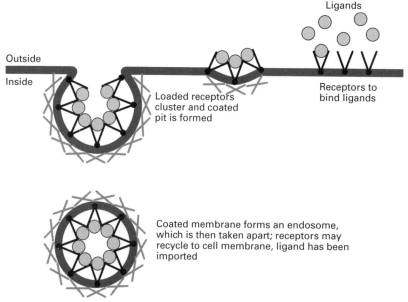

Fig. 38 Receptor-mediated endocytosis, used to import macromolecules into the cell.

molecules that enter cells in this way. These molecules bind to specific receptor molecules that have binding domains on the outside of the plasma membrane. Once loaded, these receptor molecules move in the plane of the membrane to form a cluster. Internal domains of the receptors interact with intracellular proteins, notably *clathrin*, which builds up a structure that makes the membrane invaginate, forming what is known as a coated pit. Eventually a part of the membrane pinches off inside the cell to form an *endosome*, which contains both the receptors and the receptor-bound molecules. The endosome is then taken apart, making the imported molecules available to the cell and releasing the receptors for re-cycling or for breakdown (Fig. 38).

Export of macromolecules

Secretion of macromolecules through the plasma membrane also occurs. Pancreatic cells synthesise the precursors of digestive proteases and secrete them into the pancreatic juice. Other pancreatic cells in the islets synthesise the peptide hormones insulin and glucagon and secrete them as required into the blood. Proteins for secretion are packaged into intracellular membrane-bounded vesicles by the Golgi apparatus. The membranes of these vesicles fuse with the plasma membrane of the cell and the contents of the vesicles are released outside the cell.

Membrane functions like those described above are vital to the functioning of the nervous system. Secretion of neurotransmitters by nerve endings involves the fusion of vesicles that contain the transmitter with the plasma membrane. Detection of these neurotransmitters by another neuron involves receptor proteins. These in turn may activate transport of ions down a potential gradient, resulting in a nerve impulse.

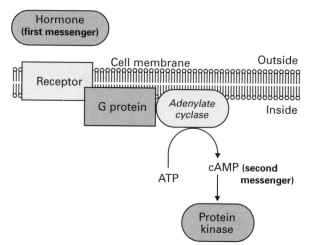

Fig. 39 Role of membrane proteins in the cellular response to hormones.

5.3 **Hormone receptors**

Membrane proteins are involved in the cellular response to some water-soluble hormones, such as adrenaline (epinephrine), and the peptide hormones glucagon and insulin. Target cells that can respond to a particular hormone have receptor proteins for that hormone on the outside of their plasma membranes. These proteins have an extracellular domain that carries binding sites for the hormone. When hormone molecules circulating in the plasma are recognised and bind, a conformational change that occurs in this external domain is transmitted through another domain that spans the lipid bilayer to the inside of the membrane (Fig. 39). This triggers enzymic events inside the cell that amplify and transmit the hormonal message to influence metabolic events (Chapter 18).

Self-assessment: questions

Multiple choice questions

1. The following statements describe membrane function:
   a. Cell membranes carry molecules which are specific for each type of cell
   b. Cell membranes are involved in the response of cells to water-soluble hormones
   c. Cells can export macromolecules but cannot import them
   d. Cells can import small molecules such as building blocks and some metabolites
   e. Cell membranes separate regions with different ionic compositions

2. The following substances are components of plasma membranes in animals:
   a. Phospholipid
   b. Cholesterol
   c. Triacylglycerol
   d. Carbohydrate
   e. Protein

3. Membrane phospholipid molecules:
   a. Are organised in two layers
   b. In each layer are able to rotate freely about axes perpendicular to the plane of the membrane
   c. Diffuse freely within each layer
   d. Move freely between the two layers
   e. Determine the fluidity of a membrane, which depends on its lipid composition and on temperature

4. The following statements describe membrane proteins:
   a. Membranes contain more phospholipid than protein
   b. Protein molecules in membranes can rotate and move laterally; they can also change their direction of insertion in the membrane
   c. Some membrane proteins are in contact with the aqueous phase on both sides of the membrane
   d. Membrane proteins act as receptors and transporters but not catalysts (enzymes)
   e. Some membrane proteins carry complex oligosaccharide groups

5. The following substances are able to cross phospholipid bilayers freely:
   a. Carbon dioxide
   b. Glucose
   c. Glycine
   d. Sodium ions
   e. Chloride ions

6. Protein-mediated transport across membranes:
   a. Shows stereospecificity
   b. Shows saturation
   c. Can be inhibited by specific inhibitors
   d. In different cell membranes involves transporters that sometimes have different kinetics
   e. Never involves chemical change

7. Membrane transport is directly involved in the following processes:
   a. The absorption of nutrients from the gut
   b. The uptake of nutrients by cells
   c. The movement of metabolites between compartments in cells
   d. The generation of ATP by oxidative phosphorylation
   e. The replication of DNA

8. The following statements describe mechanisms of membrane transport:
   a. A uniport is responsible for movement of a single molecule or ion and can only carry out transport down a gradient of concentration or potential between the two sides of the membrane
   b. An antiport is responsible for the linked movement of two molecules or ions, one in one direction and one in the opposite direction
   c. A symport is responsible for the linked movement of two molecules or ions, both in the same direction
   d. Transport of ions across membranes can set up or dissipate membrane potentials
   e. Transport of ions or molecules across membranes can set up or dissipate concentration differences between the two sides of the membrane

Short essay question

Write about the similarities between enzymes and the proteins that are responsible for transport processes in membranes.

Self-assessment: answers

Multiple choice answers

1. a. **True.** Membranes contain transporter proteins and carry hormone receptors and recognition molecules that are specific to each cell type.
    b. **True.** Water-soluble hormones cannot enter through cell membranes. They influence their target cells by binding to specific receptors.
    c. **False.** Cells can both export and import macromolecules. Macromolecules that are imported by cells include transferrin and low-density lipoprotein.
    d. **True.** Cell membranes contain transporters for many small molecules including glucose and amino acids.
    e. **True.** Cell membranes contain ion pumps which maintain higher potassium and lower sodium ion concentrations inside cells than in the surrounding fluid.

2. a. **True.** Phospholipid is the main constituent of the bilayer.
    b. **True.** Cholesterol is found in the membranes of animals but not of plants.
    c. **False.** Triacylglycerol is not found in membranes. It is the energy-storage material of adipose tissue cells and is non-polar, not amphipathic.
    d. **True.** Membrane glycoproteins are present.
    e. **True.** Proteins have many functions in all membranes.

3. a. **True.** The phospholipid bilayer is the basis of membrane structure.
    b. **True.** Phospholipid molecules are free to rotate about their long axis.
    c. **True.** Phospholipid molecules can diffuse in the plane of the membrane.
    d. **False.** Phospholipid molecules remain in whichever layer, inner or outer, they were first inserted.
    e. **True.** Membranes are less fluid at low temperatures. The degree of unsaturation of fatty acyl side chains in the phospholipids controls membrane fluidity.

4. a. **False.** Membranes vary; the mitochondrial inner membrane is 75% protein.
    b. **False.** They cannot change their direction of insertion.
    c. **True.** They are said to span the membrane.
    d. **False.** Some very important enzymes are membrane bound.

e. **True.** Membrane glycoproteins are important in cell–cell interactions.

5. a. **True.** Carbon dioxide is sufficiently lipid soluble to cross without the aid of a carrier.
    b. **False.** Cells that use glucose have a glucose transporter in their membranes.
    c. **False.** Glycine is too polar to cross a bilayer on its own.
    d. **False.** Sodium ions are moved across membranes by specific transporters.
    e. **False.** Most ions including chloride are too insoluble in lipid to cross lipid bilayers.

6. a. **True.** Stereospecificity is found in almost every protein–ligand interaction.
    b. **True.** The kinetics of transport are similar to enzyme kinetics.
    c. **True.** For example, ouabain inhibits the Na^+/K^+ pump (ATPase) in membranes.
    d. **True.** For example, glucose transporters in liver have much higher K_m values than those in brain and most other tissues.
    e. **False.** Transport of ions against a potential or concentration difference is often linked to the hydrolysis of ATP.

7. a. **True.** This is how nutrients enter the body.
    b. **True.** Membrane transporters are needed for almost all nutrients.
    c. **True.** This often controls metabolic processes.
    d. **True.** ATP generation is powered by the transport of hydrogen ions down a potential and concentration gradient into mitochondria. ADP and inorganic phosphate must be transported into mitochondria and ATP transported out.
    e. **False.** The replication of DNA does not involve membrane transport.

8. a. **False.** Uniport transport linked to ATP hydrolysis can set up concentration, or potential differences, for instance, the sodium pump responsible for movement of sodium ions out of many cells.
    b. **True.** By definition.
    c. **True.** By definition.
    d. **True.** For example, setting up the resting membrane potential of nerves and dissipating it during an action potential.
    e. **True.** This is how cells control the composition of their contents and the internal environment of the body.

Short essay answer

Points which should be mentioned include; (i) both promote processes made slow by a large energy barrier; (ii) both can promote uphill as well as downhill processes by coupling their action to ATP hydrolysis; (iii) both show great specificity, including stereospecificity, in the molecules that they can convert or transport; (iv) both show saturation kinetics; (v) both can be inhibited by competitive inhibitors; (vi) both show distinct molecular forms in different cells and tissues. The absence of an enzyme or a transport process caused by a genetic mutation can give rise to an inherited disease.

Gas transport by the blood

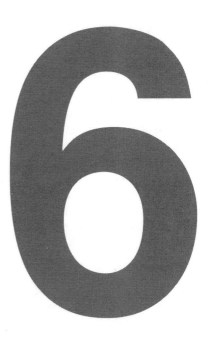

6.1 Red cells

In this chapter, we shall see how red cells circulating in the blood supply oxygen to the tissues and eliminate carbon dioxide. These relatively simple cells contain a few components directly involved in gas transport and not much else. The mature red cell has minimal metabolism, no mitochondria, no nucleus and no ribosomes or protein synthesis. The macromolecules involved in gas transport are:

- haemoglobin, a protein with a haem prosthetic group
- carbonic anhydrase, an enzyme
- chloride/bicarbonate transporter, a membrane protein.

Because the oxygen supply to the tissues limits the rate at which most organisms can use energy, the components of the gas transport system have evolved to become as efficient as possible. The transport processes for oxygen and carbon dioxide are highly integrated.

6.2 Oxygen transport

The supply of oxygen to the tissues is our most immediate physical need. A human adult at rest needs a continuous supply of energy equivalent to about 150 watts, enough to power a large light bulb. This energy is generated by oxidising foodstuffs with molecular oxygen. We take in about 250 ml of oxygen gas per minute and this is our most pressing physical need. If our oxygen supply is interrupted for more than a few minutes, irreversible damage is done to some tissues, notably the brain. Ensuring that the subject is breathing is a top priority in First Aid. Oxygen is abundantly available in the air around us but cannot diffuse into our tissues at a sufficient rate to meet our needs. It must be transported from the *lung*, the specialised organ for gas exchange, by the blood to all the other tissues.

The problem of transporting oxygen

Oxygen is only slightly soluble in water. A litre of water in equilibrium with air at atmospheric pressure dissolves about 5 ml of oxygen. To transport 250 ml of oxygen each minute in solution in water would involved pumping 50 litres of water per minute, a major undertaking that would increase our energy need and hence our oxygen need even further. It is much more efficient to increase the oxygen-carrying capacity of the blood (the pumped liquid) and to pump at a lower rate.

Haemoglobin

Haemoglobin greatly increases the oxygen-carrying capacity of the blood. Blood can carry about 200 ml of oxygen per litre because it contains a large amount of haemoglobin, about 150 g per litre. This amount of protein dissolved directly would make a very viscous solution, which would need much energy to pump it around the body. This is avoided by carrying the haemoglobin in red cells, which are suspended in plasma. The biconcave disc shape of most mammalian red cells is possibly an adaptation to make them more flexible for passing through capillaries. Even though the red cells account for about 45% of the blood volume, the blood is not much more viscous than plasma.

Haemoglobin is a remarkably soluble protein. Red cells contain about 350 g haemoglobin per litre. The disease *sickle cell anaemia* is caused by a mutant form of haemoglobin that has a lowered solubility when deoxygenated. It is precipitated if the partial pressure of oxygen becomes too low. This deforms the red cells and makes them less flexible so that they block capillaries. The red cells are also more fragile than normal and have a decreased lifetime in the circulation.

Haemoglobin has been much studied. This is not only because of its important physiological role, but also because it is so readily available. Red cells are easily isolated from blood by centrifugation and washing with isotonic saline. Haemoglobin accounts for more than 95% of the soluble proteins released from red cells when they are lysed with distilled water. The supernatant from such a lysate has been used for many studies in physical biochemistry. Many studies on haemoglobin are facilitated by its red colour; haemoglobin absorbs blue light very strongly and its absorption of light is influenced by the binding of some ligands. The study of haemoglobin has revealed many features later discovered in other proteins.

Haemoglobin structure and function

The 20 amino acid side chains available in proteins include no group with any capacity for binding oxygen. Haemoglobin has haem groups as binding sites for oxygen: haemoglobin is said to have a *haem* prosthetic group. Haem can be removed from haemoglobin leaving the colourless protein known as *globin* and haemoglobin can be reconstituted by adding haem to globin.

Haemoglobin has a molecular weight of about 65 kilodaltons (kDa) and contains about 600 amino acid residues. These form four polypeptide chains, two identical alpha chains and two identical beta chains. Alpha chains and beta chains are similar in size and have distinct but related sequences. Each chain is folded to form a subunit with a binding site for a haem group. The folded chains or subunits also bind to each other to form the complete molecule (Fig. 40). No covalent bonds are involved in the binding of haem to the globin chains or the assembly of the globin subunits to form the tetrameric haemoglobin molecule. There are two alpha and two beta subunits. Alpha and beta subunits are similar but not identical; they have similar tertiary structures with eight sections of alpha helix. The

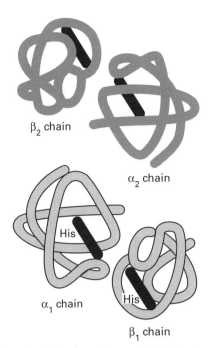

Fig. 40 The subunit structure of haemoglobin. The two pairs of subunits are shown separated for clarity. Normally, the $\alpha_2\beta_2$ pair (shaded above) interlock with the $\alpha_1\beta_1$ pair (outline above). The relative positions of the two alpha–beta pairs changes on oxygenation of the haemoglobin.

haemoglobin molecule can be considered as two equivalent pairs of alpha-beta subunits that lock together. The relative positions of the two pairs of subunits changes on oxygenation of the haemoglobin.

The structure of haem is shown in Figure 83 (p. 114). It is an iron-containing organic group which can combine with oxygen. On its own, it would not be a satisfactory oxygen transporter. It is virtually insoluble in water and it can react with oxygen in more than one way. The oxidation state of the iron atom in haem corresponds to ferrous (Fe^{II}) and in this state it can bind molecular oxygen. The complex which is formed is quickly and irreversibly converted to a compound containing ferric iron (Fe^{III}). Haem on its own can combine with oxygen but it does not give it up again. To be a successful transporter, haem must release its oxygen when oxygen levels are low, i.e. it must be oxygenated not oxidised.

Oxygenation, not oxidation

Haem forms a water-soluble complex when it is bound to globin. It is bound by the protein in such a way that one of the coordination positions on the iron is still available to bind oxygen. It is also held in a chemical environment where the oxidation of its iron atom by molecular oxygen is almost completely inhibited. The iron of each haem group is linked to the side chain of a so-called proximal histidine residue. These histidine residues are shown in two of the subunits depicted in Figure 40. The ligands oxygen and carbon monoxide can bind to the iron of each haem on the other side of the haem from the proximal histidine. There is another histidine side chain, that of the distal histidine,

positioned near the ligands. As a result, haem bound to globin can pick up oxygen in the lungs and release it in the tissue capillaries. The iron atom in haem remains in the ferrous state during oxygen transport. Haemoglobin is said to be capable of *reversible oxygenation*.

Allosteric effects in haemoglobin

The globin parts of the molecule can bind other molecules as well. The binding of oxygen by haemoglobin is influenced by changes of pH and carbon dioxide concentration. This influence is mediated by sites that bind hydrogen ions and carbon dioxide. A further binding site, formed in the crevice between the two beta subunits, binds *2,3-bisphosphoglycerate* (2,3-BPG), which when bound, decreases the affinity of haemoglobin for oxygen.

Haemoglobin is said to show *allosteric* interactions between its ligand-binding sites. Allosteric means 'at another place'. If the other binding site(s) interacts with an identical ligand the effect is said to be *homotropic*, if the other ligand is a different molecule, the effect is *heterotropic*.

Homotropic allosteric effects

The binding of an oxygen molecule at one haem group influences the affinity with which oxygen is bound at another haem group. Since the ligands are identical this is a homotropic effect. Its occurrence can be seen when the oxygen dissociation curve of haemoglobin is examined. This curve is a graph of how the amount of oxygen bound by haemoglobin varies with the concentration or partial pressure of molecular oxygen with which it is in equilibrium. Such a graph (Fig. 41) is useful to demonstrate some of the adaptations that have evolved in haemoglobin to make oxygen transport more efficient. Notice that the dissociation curve is *sigmoid* or S-shaped. Its slope increases as we move away from the origin and reaches a maximum value near the point where the haemoglobin is 50% saturated. Beyond that point, the slope decreases again until at high partial pressures of oxygen, such as the pressure in the atmosphere at sea level or in a ventilated lung, haemoglobin

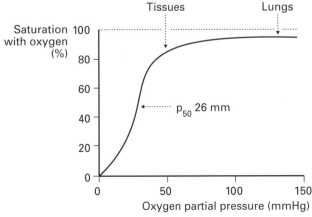

Fig. 41 The oxygen dissociation curve of human blood.

is nearly saturated, with almost every haem group having an oxygen bound to it. Increasing the oxygen pressure beyond this point does not significantly increase the amount carried by the blood.

The sigmoid dissociation curve of haemoglobin shows that the four haem groups on a haemoglobin do not bind oxygen independently. They interact and show a positive cooperativity. The affinity with which oxygen is bound at any haem group is influenced by the binding of other oxygen molecules at the other three haem groups. With all four haem groups unoccupied by oxygen, it is difficult for the first oxygen molecule to bind. However, once it does bind, it changes the shape of the whole haemoglobin molecule making it much easier for the other three haem groups to react. So for each haemoglobin tetramer, the fully deoxygenated and fully oxygenated states are favoured over the partially oxygenated intermediate states. The change in shape of the tetramer is brought about by an amplification of a slight movement of the iron atom when oxygenation occurs. In the deoxygenated state, the iron atom is too large to fit in the space between the four nitrogens of the haem group so it is displaced from the plane of the haem. On oxygenation it shrinks and is held in the haem plane.

The allosteric effect that produces the sigmoid dissociation curve is an important adaptation of haemoglobin to increase the efficiency of oxygen transport. Oxygen is delivered to the tissues without the oxygen concentration in the tissues having to fall too low. Enzymes that use oxygen, particularly *cytochrome oxidase*, have oxygen delivered to them at concentrations sufficient for them to work efficiently. An oxygen transport protein like *myoglobin* with a single haem group needs a high oxygen affinity if it is to be fully oxygenated in the lungs. Not much oxygen dissociates from such a protein unless it is exposed to a very low oxygen concentration (Fig. 42). Were myoglobin to be used instead of haemoglobin, it would deliver oxygen to the tissues at a much lower concentration.

Heterotropic allosteric effects
Haemoglobin also shows heterotropic allosteric interactions, i.e. between the binding sites for different

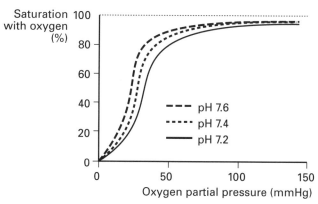

Fig. 43 Effect of pH on the oxygen dissociation curve of haemoglobin (Bohr effect). Notice that acidification, (lowering the pH) decreases the affinity of haemoglobin for oxygen, moving the dissociation curve to the right.

ligands. If oxygen dissociation curves are determined at different pH values or in the presence of different concentrations of carbon dioxide, both of these variables are seen to affect the equilibrium between oxygen and haemoglobin.

Figure 43 shows that at low pH values haemoglobin has a lower affinity for oxygen than it has at high pH values. This is known as the *Bohr effect*. This is a physiological adaptation; it results in an increase in the unloading of oxygen by the blood in tissues where increased energy use has resulted in an increase in the production of carbon dioxide or lactic acid, the respective end-products of aerobic and anaerobic metabolism for the production of ATP.

Regulation by 2,3-BPG
The affinity of haemoglobin for oxygen is affected by the concentration of 2,3-BPG in the red cell (Fig. 44). This substance is produced metabolically from glucose in the red cell (Fig. 176, p. 257). It binds to a site between the beta subunits in deoxyhaemoglobin but not to oxyhaemoglobin. Its presence moves the oxygen dissociation curve to the right. The affinity of haemoglobin for oxygen can, thus, be altered to optimise oxygen transport at high altitude.

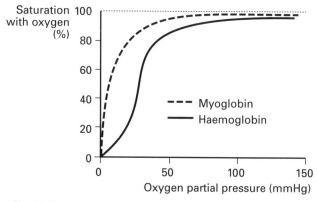

Fig. 42 The oxygen dissociation curves of haemoglobin and myoglobin. Notice how very low partial pressures of oxygen are necessary for appreciable dissociation of oxymyoglobin.

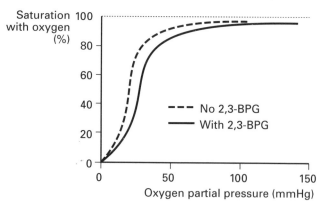

Fig. 44 Effect of addition of 2,3-BPG to the oxygen dissociation curve of haemoglobin. 2,3-BPG binds only to the deoxy form of haemoglobin, stabilising it. In the absence of 2,3-BPG, the dissociation curve is moved to the left.

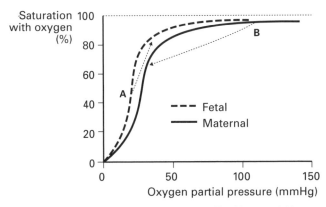

Fig. 45 Oxygen exchange in the placenta. Fetal haemoglobin, HbF, has no binding site for 2,3-BPG so it has a higher affinity for oxygen than the HbA of the mother. This is essential for efficient transfer of oxygen from mother to fetus. Maternal arterial blood (point B above) loses oxygen while fetal blood (point A) gains oxygen until they both have the same partial pressure of oxygen.

2,3-BPG is also important in promoting oxygen transport across the *placenta*. Fetal haemoglobin has the two beta subunits of normal adult haemoglobin replaced by two *gamma subunits*, which do not form any binding site for 2,3-BPG. It, therefore, has a higher oxygen affinity than maternal haemoglobin and oxygen transfers readily from mother to fetus (Fig. 45).

Haemoglobin was the first protein studied that showed allosteric effects. These effects are also important in many other proteins as we will discover when we consider how the catalytic activity of enzymes is controlled in metabolism.

Carbon monoxide binding to haemoglobin

A few other small molecules, notably carbon monoxide, can bind to the haem groups in competition with oxygen. Haemoglobin has a 250-fold higher affinity for carbon monoxide than it has for oxygen, so exposure to low concentrations of carbon monoxide, from car exhaust fumes or from badly ventilated gas heaters, can have fatal results. Therapy for carbon monoxide poisoning includes treatment with pure oxygen to increase the partial pressure of oxygen in the lungs, allowing it to compete with and displace the carbon monoxide.

BOX 6.1
Clinical note: Carbon monoxide poisoning

A patient with 30% of their haemoglobin gas-binding capacity occupied by carbon monoxide is much more seriously incapacitated than a patient who has lost 50% of their haemoglobin through anaemia. Bound carbon monoxide triggers the allosteric effect and the remaining haem groups have such a high affinity for oxygen that its transport to the tissues is seriously compromised.

6.3 Carbon dioxide transport

While oxygen has to be transported from lungs to tissues, carbon dioxide must be transported from the tissues for excretion by the lungs. Carbon dioxide has physicochemical properties that make its transport less difficult than the transport of oxygen. Nevertheless, haemoglobin has adaptations that facilitate this process also. Carbon dioxide can be transported in the blood in three ways:

- in simple solution (~10%)
- by reversible conversion to bicarbonate and hydrogen ions (> 50%)
- by reversible combination with amino groups on haemoglobin to form carbamino haemoglobin (~ 30%).

Simple solution

Carbon dioxide is much more soluble than oxygen and about 10% of its transport can be accounted for as transport of the dissolved gas.

Bicarbonate and hydrogen ions

Carbon dioxide can also react with water to form bicarbonate and hydrogen ions.

$$CO_2 + H_2O \rightleftharpoons HCO_3^- + H^+$$

The reaction is reversible and slow, taking minutes to approach equilibrium even at body temperature. In pure water, the equilibrium is very much in favour of carbon dioxide, only about one part in a thousand being converted to carbonic acid. Carbonic acid is a stronger acid than acetic acid and ionises to form *bicarbonate* ions and hydrogen ions. At pH 7.4, the pH of blood, if a buffer species is present that can take up the hydrogen ions then more than 90% of carbon dioxide can be converted to bicarbonate before equilibrium is achieved. One of the adaptations of haemoglobin is that it is a powerful buffer at pH 7.4, so carbon dioxide can be converted to bicarbonate in the red cell. More than one half of the carbon dioxide transported from the tissues to the lungs is transported as bicarbonate ions.

Carbonic anhydrase
The uncatalysed reaction between carbon dioxide and water is slow and would be unable to produce enough carbon dioxide from bicarbonate during the second or less that the red cell spends in the lung capillary. Red cells contain an enzyme, carbonic anhydrase, which catalyses the reversible hydration of carbon dioxide to form bicarbonate ions and hydrogen ions. Carbonic anhydrase is a zinc protein with a molecular weight of about 30 kDa. The single zinc atom is essential for activity. The enzyme is very active in red cells but absent from the plasma. Production of bicarbonate and

hydrogen ions is, therefore, confined to the red cells so that negligible change in pH of the plasma occurs as a consequence of carbon dioxide transport. Haemoglobin, as well as its other adaptations for gas transport, has a high content of the amino acid histidine. This amino acid has an imidazole group on its side chain that acts as a powerful buffering group so that the pH change within the red cell owing to carbonic anhydrase action is minimised. Some other buffering groups on haemoglobin are oxygen-linked, their buffering action is influenced by the state of oxygenation of the haem groups. This accounts for the Bohr effect, the effect of pH on the oxygen dissociation curves of haemoglobin (Fig. 43). Increased carbon dioxide concentrations lower the pH and promote the dissociation of oxygen from combination with haemoglobin. Tissues that are metabolically most active and which produce the most carbon dioxide, therefore, receive the greatest supply of oxygen.

Chloride/bicarbonate transporter

The amount of carbon dioxide that can be converted into bicarbonate in the red cell is also increased by the ability of the red cell to 'share' its bicarbonate ions with the plasma. The red cell membrane contains an ion transporter that promotes the exchange of chloride and bicarbonate ions between the red cell and plasma. In tissue capillaries, when carbon dioxide is converted to bicarbonate in the red cell, some of the bicarbonate ions can leave the red cell and enter the plasma (Fig. 46). Chloride ions must move in the opposite direction to avoid any net transport of charge. In the lung capillaries, some of the bicarbonate in the red cell is converted to carbon dioxide, which is expired, and more bicarbonate enters the red cell from the plasma. There is a corresponding movement of chloride ions from red cell to plasma. The carbon dioxide–bicarbonate system, as well as accounting for removal of about 60% of carbon dioxide produced by the body, is also important in regulation of acid–base balance.

Combination with haemoglobin

Carbon dioxide can react with some N-terminal amino groups on haemoglobin directly (no enzyme is required) to form labile carbamino compounds or *carbamates*, which release carbon dioxide in the lungs.

$$Hb\text{-}NH_2 + CO_2 \rightleftharpoons Hb\text{-}NH\text{-}COO^- + H^+$$

The reaction only involves N-terminal groups, which must be unprotonated. Lysine side chain amino groups, which are much more basic, are fully protonated at physiological pH values.

This process is allosterically linked to oxygenation so that combination of haemoglobin with carbon dioxide favours deoxygenation and combination with

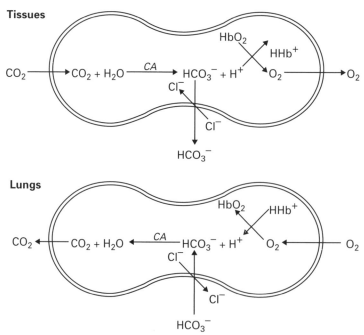

Fig. 46 Movement of bicarbonate and chloride ions during gas transport. Chloride ions enter the red cell to keep electrical balance. When hydrogen ions are produced by hydration of carbon dioxide (in the tissues) they promote the dissociation of oxyhaemoglobin (HbO_2), CA, carbonic anhydrase.

oxygen favours release of carbon dioxide. Carbamate formation accounts for about 30% of carbon dioxide transport.

6.4 Abnormal haemoglobins and haemoglobinopathies

The important inherited disease sickle cell anaemia is caused by a change in the structure of the haemoglobin molecule. This change makes sickle cell haemoglobin, HbS, electrophoretically distinguishable from the normal adult form of haemoglobin, HbA. Haemoglobin is readily obtained from human subjects so many samples have been screened by electrophoresis and hundreds of mutant haemoglobins discovered. Some of these haemoglobins are associated with disease states, particularly anaemia; others show normal function. In many cases, the amino acid sequence of the mutant haemoglobin differs from the normal at only two positions in the 600 or so of total sequence. For example, HbS has the same amino acid sequence as HbA except at position 6 in each of its two beta chains, where it has valine residues instead of the glutamates found in HbA. This seemingly slight change creates a 'sticky' patch on the molecule that promotes aggregation of the deoxy form and decreases its solubility. The resulting aggregates distort the red cell, shortening its lifetime and make the cell less flexible and thus unable to negotiate tissue capillaries. Replacing a glutamate residue, which has a negatively charged side chain, with a valine residue, which has no charge on its side chain, incidentally alters the charge and the electrophoretic mobility of the protein.

The presence of HbS in red cells, even with HbA also present as in heterozygotes, makes them less likely to be invaded by the malaria parasite. This gives the individual a significant resistance to malaria and accounts for the high incidence of the gene for this form of haemoglobin in areas of the world where malaria is rife.

Much has been learnt about the relationship between haemoglobin structure and function by identifying the differences between HbA and a large number of mutants. The role of two histidine residues in each subunit is particularly important. The side chains of these residues are close to the haem iron and their replacement by tyrosine side chains gives forms of haemoglobin (HbM) in which the haem group is instantly oxidised to the ferric state when it reacts with oxygen. This destroys the ability of the haem groups to act as an oxygen carrier.

Self-assessment: questions

Multiple choice questions

1. In gas transport by the blood:
   a. Oxygen is the substance most urgently needed for human survival
   b. An adult at rest uses about 250 ml of oxygen per hour
   c. A litre of water in equilibrium with air at atmospheric pressure dissolves about 50 ml of oxygen
   d. The oxygen-carrying capacity of normal blood is about 20 ml of oxygen per litre
   e. Normal blood contains about 375 g haemoglobin per litre

2. The haemoglobin molecule:
   a. Contains four atoms of iron which must be in the Fe^{II} oxidation state for it to bind oxygen
   b. Has each iron atom combined in a haem group
   c. Contains four identical polypeptide chains per molecule
   d. Has each polypeptide chain associated with a haem group
   e. Is approximately spherical in shape

3. Haemoglobin:
   a. Is the only protein contained in red blood cells
   b. Is contained in red cells because it is not very soluble in water
   c. Appears red because the haem groups strongly absorb blue light
   d. Changes colour when it reacts with oxygen or carbon monoxide
   e. Changes colour when its iron atoms are oxidised from the Fe^{II} to the Fe^{III} state

4. Haem:
   a. Contains one atom of iron which is in the Fe^{II} state
   b. Does not react with oxygen unless the haem is combined with globin
   c. Is very insoluble in water
   d. Has an iron atom that can be readily converted into the Fe^{III} state
   e. In haemoglobin occurs as four identical molecules

5. In haemoglobin:
   a. There are two kinds of globin chain in each haemoglobin molecule
   b. Each haem is attached to a globin chain by a covalent bond
   c. The globin chains are joined by disulphide bonds
   d. The four globin chains have similar tertiary structures
   e. The tertiary structure of each globin chain contains eight sections of alpha helix

6. The following substances are ligands of haemoglobin:
   a. Oxygen
   b. Carbon monoxide
   c. Carbon dioxide
   d. 2,3-Bisphosphoglycerate
   e. Lactate

7. The ligand binding-capacity of haemoglobin is:
   a. Up to four molecules of oxygen
   b. Up to four molecules of carbon monoxide
   c. Four molecules of oxygen and four of carbon monoxide
   d. A total of four molecules of oxygen or carbon monoxide
   e. Only one molecule of 2,3-bisphosphoglycerate

8. When oxygen combines with haemoglobin:
   a. Oxygen binding at one haem group in a haemoglobin molecule influences oxygen binding at the other haem groups
   b. Oxygen binding at one haem group in a haemoglobin molecule makes it more difficult for oxygen to bind at the other haem groups
   c. Increases in carbon dioxide concentrations in the red cell decrease the affinity of the haemoglobin for oxygen
   d. Binding of 2,3-bisphosphoglycerate to haemoglobin makes it bind oxygen with lower affinity
   e. Increase in pH in the red cell makes haemoglobin bind oxygen with higher affinity

9. When carbon dioxide is transported in the blood:
   a. A significant quantity of carbon dioxide is carried in solution in the blood
   b. A significant quantity of carbon dioxide is carried as bicarbonate in the blood
   c. The interconversion of carbon dioxide and bicarbonate is catalysed by carbonic anhydrase
   d. Carbonic anhydrase is present in the plasma and not in the red cell
   e. Carbon dioxide can react directly with haemoglobin

10. The following statements describe sickle cell haemoglobin:
    a. It differs from normal adult haemoglobin in every subunit

b. It is less soluble than normal adult haemoglobin when oxygenated
c. It is only found in subjects suffering from sickle cell anaemia
d. Individuals possessing sickle cell haemoglobin are less likely to contract malaria
e. It does not have a sigmoid oxygen dissociation curve

Short essay question

Haemoglobin has been called an 'honorary' enzyme. Write about the properties which haemoglobin shares with enzymes.

Self-assessment: answers

Multiple choice answers

1. a. **True.** Oxygen deprivation can kill in minutes.
   b. **False.** We need about 250 ml per minute.
   c. **False.** It only dissolves about 5 ml of oxygen.
   d. **False.** Blood carries about 200 ml of oxygen per litre.
   e. **False.** Blood contains about 150 g haemoglobin per litre.

2. a. **True.** Haemoglobin cannot function as an oxygen carrier unless the four iron atoms are in the Fe^{II} oxidation state.
   b. **True.** Four haem groups each containing an iron atom.
   c. **False.** Each molecule contains two alpha and two beta chains.
   d. **True.** Each of the four subunits consists of a polypeptide chain and a haem group.
   e. **True.** The overall shape is close to spherical.

3. a. **False.** It is the predominant but not the only protein in the red cell.
   b. **False.** Haemoglobin is very soluble in water. Haem is almost insoluble.
   c. **True.** Haemoglobin has a very strong absorption band in the blue.
   d. **True.** The colour changes are useful to show the state of the haemoglobin.
   e. **True.** Methaemoglobin, the oxidised form of haemoglobin, is found in some clinical conditions. The extent of its formation can be measured by spectrophotometry.

4. a. **True.** Haematin, which contains Fe^{III} is the oxidised form of haem.
   b. **False.** Haem is oxidised irreversibly by oxygen.
   c. **True.** It is almost completely insoluble.
   d. **True.** Many oxidising agents will convert the iron to Fe^{III}.
   e. **True.** They are chemically identical.

5. a. **True.** Two alpha chains and two beta chains.
   b. **False.** The binding of haem to globin involves only non-covalent forces.
   c. **False.** There are no disulphide bonds in haemoglobin. Only non-covalent forces are involved in the aggregation of the four subunits.
   d. **True.** Their tertiary structures resemble each other and that of myoglobin.
   e. **True.** About 75% of the amino acid residues are contained in the eight alpha helical segments, the A, B, C, D, E, F, G and H helices.

6. a. **True.** The main function of haemoglobin is reversible binding of oxygen.

b. **True.** Carbon monoxide binds with higher affinity than oxygen, which is why it is such a poisonous gas.
   c. **True.** Carbon dioxide binds to the N-terminal amino groups, not the haems.
   d. **True.** 2,3-Bisphosphoglycerate binds to deoxyhaemoglobin.
   e. **False.** Haemoglobin does not bind lactate.

7. a. **True.** Haemoglobin is saturated when it binds four molecules of oxygen.
   b. **True.** A molecule of carbon monoxide can bind at each haem group.
   c. **False.** Each haem group can bind a molecule of oxygen *or* carbon monoxide, not both together.
   d. **True.** One molecule of oxygen or carbon monoxide at each haem group.
   e. **True.** There is one binding site for 2,3-bisphosphoglycerate between the beta subunits in each haemoglobin tetramer.

8. a. **True.** This is known as haem–haem interaction or cooperativity.
   b. **False.** Binding of oxygen at one haem group makes it easier for the other groups to react.
   c. **True.** This makes oxygen transport by haemoglobin more efficient.
   d. **True.** 2,3-Bisphosphoglycerate stabilises deoxyhaemoglobin.
   e. **True.** Removal of H^+ ions by reaction with bicarbonate to produce CO_2 in the lung increases affinity of Hb for oxygen.

9. a. **True.** About 10% of the total.
   b. **True.** About 60% of the total.
   c. **True.** Unless it is catalysed, this reaction is too slow to allow carbon dioxide to be unloaded by the blood in the lungs.
   d. **False.** Carbonic anhydrase in the blood is confined to the red cells.
   e. **True.** It can react reversibly with the N-terminal alpha amino groups.

10. a. **False.** Only the beta subunits are affected.
    b. **False.** It is the deoxygenated form of sickle cell haemoglobin that has the low solubility.
    c. **False.** Subjects with one sickle gene have approximately 50% mutant and 50% normal haemoglobin in each red cell. They have no clinical symptoms.
    d. **True.** This makes possession of one sickle gene an advantage in malarial areas and accounts for the high incidence of the gene.
    e. **False.** Its oxygen affinity is very similar to that of normal haemoglobin.

Short essay answer

The following points should be mentioned. Haemoglobin and enzymes have binding sites where small molecules are bound reversibly. Both show specificity of binding and exhibit saturation. Both can occur as different molecular forms in different tissues and at different stages of development. These forms often show different affinities for their ligand. Both can have their binding sites blocked by competitive inhibitors. Some enzymes have binding sites like those on haemoglobin that interact or show cooperativity. Some enzymes have allosteric sites like those on haemoglobin. When these sites are occupied they can alter the affinity with which the protein binds its main ligand. Both occur as mutant forms where function is altered or lost.

Carbohydrate and fat catabolism

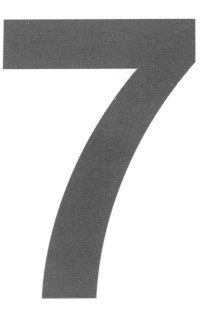

7.1 Basic concepts of metabolism

Metabolism is an enormous topic within biochemistry and it is easy to become lost in a mountain of detail. The aim of this 'core' text is to present essential material on metabolism that will explain the design of the major metabolic pathways and their control in the fed and fasted states. The first question to answer is: 'what is metabolism?'.

Metabolism is the sum of all of the enzyme-catalysed reactions that take place in cells and can be viewed as having two contrasting processes, *catabolism* and *anabolism*.

- catabolism: energy-yielding reactions in which complex molecules are broken down to small molecules
- anabolism: energy-requiring reactions in which simple precursor molecules are converted into complex molecules.

Catabolism produces chemical energy (usually ATP) and reducing power (NADPH) which is needed for maintenance of the body and for anabolic processes.

Catabolism

The catabolism of complex nutrient molecules (lipids, carbohydrates and amino acids) to simpler end-products such as carbon dioxide, water and ammonia is accompanied by the synthesis of ATP (Fig. 47). ATP is frequently described as the 'energy currency' of cells as it can be transported to those sites in the cell where it is utilised for various cellular functions:

- synthesis of proteins, RNA, DNA for growth, adaptation and repair
- synthesis of fats and glycogen
- performance of mechanical work
- transport of ions against a gradient
- absorption of nutrients against a gradient.

The reaction ATP $\rightleftharpoons$ ADP + inorganic phosphate (P_i) is displaced far from equilibrium in cells; this enables otherwise unfavourable reactions in metabolic pathways to proceed. It does not depend on special properties of the pyrophosphate bonds (so-called 'high-energy' bonds) in ATP! The very high ratios of ATP to ADP are possible because of the very efficient synthesis of ATP in cells.

The oxidation of fuels such as glucose and fatty acids (Fig. 48) results in the production of the reduced coenzymes NADH and $FADH_2$. Electrons and hydrogens are lost by the substrates being oxidised and are gained by the coenzymes produced. Electrons provide a means for transfer of chemical energy from the energy-yielding reactions of catabolism to the energy-requiring reactions of ATP synthesis and the biosynthesis of hydrogen-rich molecules such as fatty acids. Within mitochondria, the oxidation of NADH and $FADH_2$ by the electron transport chain (p. 85) establishes a proton gradient that drives the reverse reaction ADP + P_i → ATP.

Anabolism

Anabolism refers to biosynthetic processes in which simple precursor molecules are enzymatically converted into the molecular components of cells, such as nucleic acids, proteins, lipids, and polysaccharides. Biosynthesis requires the input of chemical energy (usually ATP), which is provided by catabolism. There is also often a requirement for 'reducing power' in the form of NADPH (Fig. 48).

The source of our dietary fuels

We are *heterotrophs*, which means that we 'feed on others' and can synthesise our organic molecules only from *other* organic compounds that we obtain from *autotrophs* (plants), which are 'self-feeding'. Autotrophs and heterotrophs live together in a symbiotic relationship where autotrophs use solar energy and atmospheric carbon dioxide to build complex organic molecules. Heterotrophs use these complex molecules as fuel and, in the case of aerobic organisms, return carbon dioxide to the atmosphere. Hence, carbon and oxygen are continuously cycled between the plant and animal world.

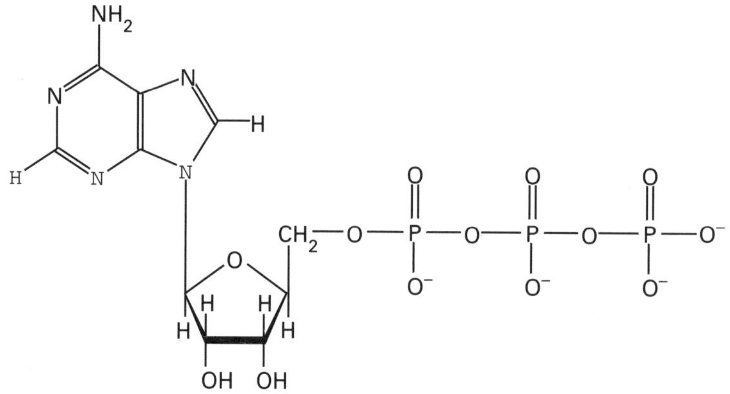

Fig. 47 The structure of ATP.

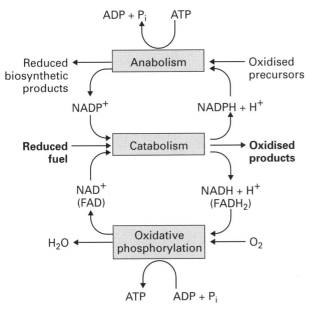

Fig. 48 Transfer of reducing power in the overall strategy of metabolism.

Stages of metabolism

Although metabolism involves hundreds of different compounds (metabolites) and enzymes, the central pathways are few in number and common to most forms of life. Krebs and Kornberg showed the simplicity of this arrangement when they placed all of the major metabolic pathways within a scheme called 'The three stages of metabolism'.

- Stage 1: digestion giving monomeric units that are absorbed from the gut

- Stage 2: conversion of the monomeric units into simple molecules within cells
- Stage 3: simple molecules oxidised to carbon dioxide and water; most of the ATP is generated at this stage.

The monomeric units within Stage 2 are *amino acids*, *glucose* and *fatty acids*. The key metabolic intermediate *acetyl co-enzyme A* is produced at the end of Stage 2. Figure 49 outlines these stages and shows how biosynthetic pathways can be superimposed upon the catabolic pathways. These pathways will share some enzymes and have others that can only catalyse an anabolic or a catabolic reaction. Stage 3 constitutes an *amphibolic* pathway in that it can be used catabolically to degrade small molecules from Stage 2 or can be used anabolically to provide precursor molecules for biosynthesis.

Enzymatic and thermodynamic aspects of metabolism

Much of the information gleaned from studying enzymes (Chapter 4) needs to be reviewed if one is to understand the operation and control of the key metabolic pathways in the body. You should also review thermodynamic aspects of chemical reactions and be aware that every reaction in a metabolic pathway must have a free energy change, ΔG, that is negative (or very close to zero in the case of those reactions which are effectively at equilibrium). The free energy change for the entire pathway must therefore be negative! On purely thermodynamic grounds, it should be clear that catabolic and anabolic pathways cannot be simply the

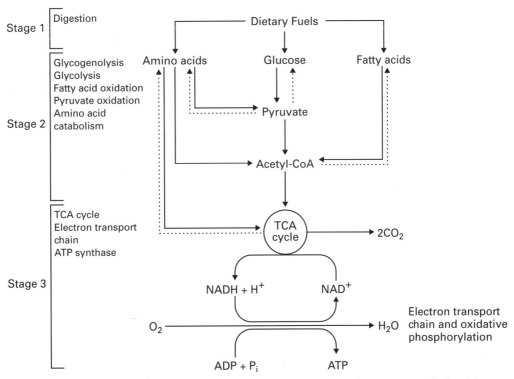

Fig. 49 Integration of carbohydrate; amino acid and fatty acid metabolism. Pyruvate, acetyl-CoA and the TCA cycle have central roles for all three fuels. The dashed lines indicate biosynthetic pathways.

reverse of each other. For example, the conversion of glucose to pyruvic acid (glycolysis) must be different from the reverse process where glucose is synthesised from pyruvic acid (gluconeogenesis). Although glycolysis and gluconeogenesis are *parallel* pathways, three of the steps are unique to each pathway. An important advantage of *parallel* pathways is that they can be independently regulated. For example, the flux of metabolites between glucose and pyruvic acid can be regulated in both directions. If the catabolic pathway is 'turned on', the anabolic pathway is 'turned off' and vice versa. *Dual regulation* is common to all parallel anabolic and catabolic pathways and is the key to gaining an understanding of the control of metabolism in the fed and fasting state (Chapter 11).

Compartmentalisation is critical for regulation

Metabolic regulation is enhanced by compartmentalisation, in which opposing reactions/pathways are physically separated. For example, fatty acid synthesis occurs within the cytosol of the cell whereas fatty acid oxidation occurs in the mitochondria. There are many other examples.

Energy charge

Parallel routes for ATP-yielding and ATP-requiring pathways are necessary since the pathway followed in catabolism is energetically impossible for anabolism. These parallel pathways can be independently controlled by the *energy charge* of the cell. The compounds involved in calculating energy charge – ATP, ADP and AMP – are allosteric effectors for many enzymes.

$$\text{Energy charge} = \frac{[\text{ATP}] + 0.5[\text{ADP}]}{[\text{ATP}] + [\text{ADP}] + [\text{AMP}]}$$

Most cells maintain a steady-state charge in the range 0.8 to 0.95. When ATP is utilised in a muscle cell ADP + P_i are formed. *Adenylate kinase* action can result in regeneration of one ATP plus AMP from two ADP. The ATP is used to perform work but the (relatively) large increase in [AMP] activates both glycogen breakdown (p. 95) and the first controlled step in glycolysis (p. 79), thus providing even more ATP.

Coenzymes and prosthetic groups contain water-soluble vitamins

Coenzymes and prosthetic groups are special molecules (Table 4) in that they act along with enzymes in many reactions in metabolism (pp. 28–29). They increase the types of reaction that can occur in the body and provide links by which energy and reducing power can be transferred from reaction to reaction. An important point to recognise is that most of the coenzymes and prosthetic groups are derivatives of water-soluble (B) vitamins. Patients with deficient intake of certain B vitamins will have defects in metabolic pathways, leading to altered metabolism that can have serious consequences (Chapter 19).

Table 4 Coenzymes in intermediary metabolism

Enzymatic reaction	Coenzymes/cofactors
Oxidation–reduction	Nicotinamide adenine dinucleotide (NAD$^+$)
	Nicotinamide adenine dinucleotide phosphate (NADP$^+$)
	Flavin adenine dinucleotide (FAD)
	Flavin mononucleotide (FMN)
	Lipoic acid
Amino acid catabolism	Pyridoxal phosphate
Oxidative decarboxylation	Thiamine pyrophosphate
Carboxylation	Biotin
Reductive biosynthesis	NADPH
	Tetrahydrobiopterin
	NADH
Acyl transfer	Coenzyme A
	Acyl carrier protein (ACP)
1-Carbon metabolism	Tetrahydrofolate (FH$_4$)
Methylation reactions	S-Adenosyl-methionine
	Tetrahydrofolate (FH$_4$)
	Methylcobalamin (B$_{12}$)

Coenzymes and prosthetic groups should be categorised according to the type of reaction that they are involved with, the metabolic pathways where they participate, the specific B (or other) vitamin source and any associated defects caused by vitamin deficiency (Chapter 19).

7.2 Digestion and absorption of dietary carbohydrates and fats

Digestion and absorption of carbohydrates, fats and proteins give rise to the monomeric units glucose, fatty acids and amino acids that are used for subsequent reactions within the cells.

Dietary carbohydrate

About 50–60% of the calories consumed by the average Western adult is in the form of carbohydrate. Only a small fraction of the total carbohydrate of the plant world can be utilised for nutrition by humans since we lack the digestive enzymes for the degradation of cellulose and some other plant polysaccharides that are present in our diets. This indigestible carbohydrate forms a large part of the so-called *dietary fibre* thought to be beneficial in reducing the incidence of diseases of the colon and some metabolic diseases.

Polysaccharides

The polysaccharides that mammals can digest include *starch*, which consists of glucose units (Fig. 50). It has amylose and amylopectin components, the former being a long chain of glucoses joined by α-1:4-linkages. Amylopectin has α-1:4- and also α-1:6-linkages, which result in branching. *Glycogen* (animal starch) is similar in structure to amylopectin but with a greater frequency of branching. A specific digestive enzyme is required to

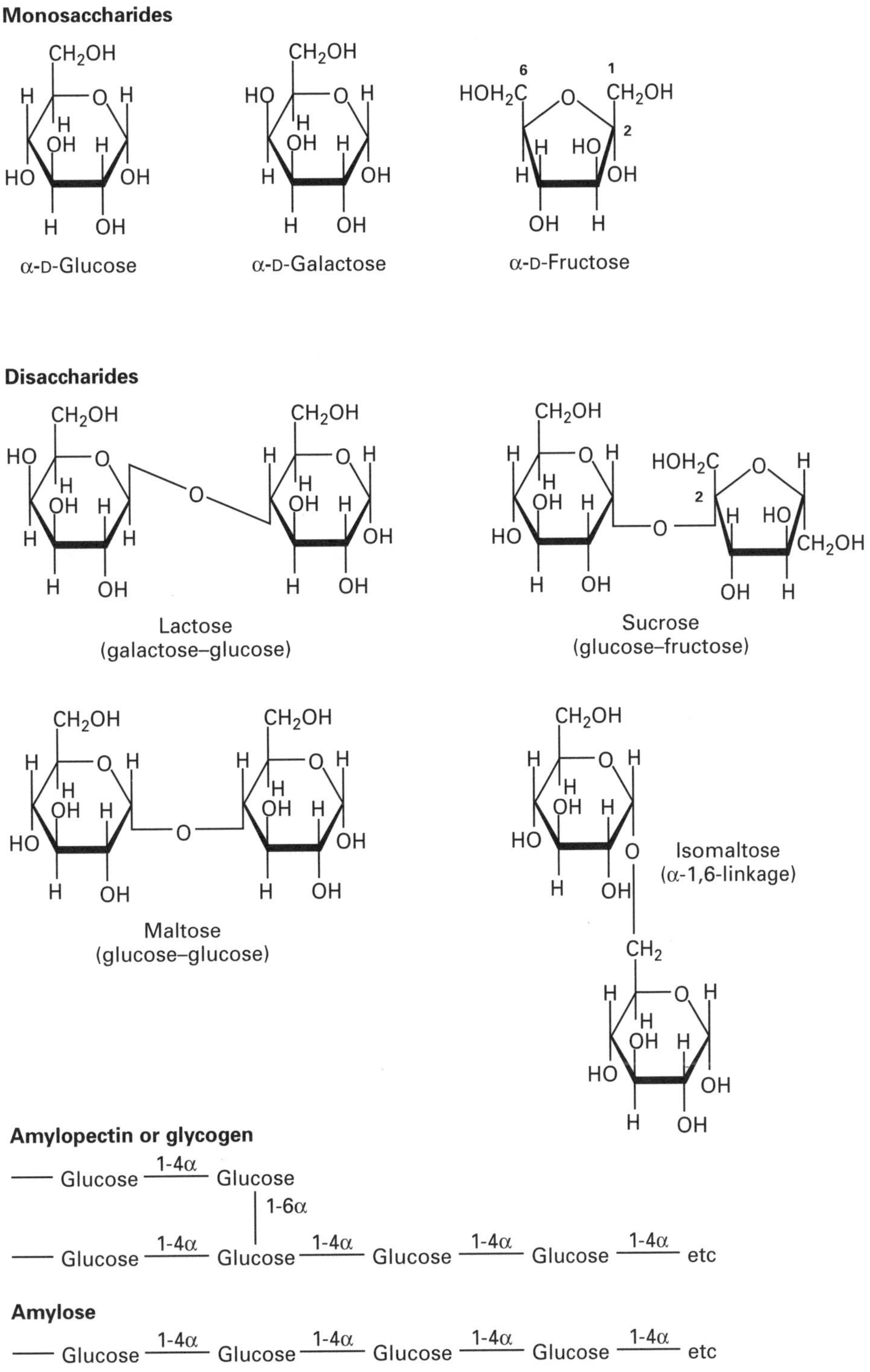

Monosaccharides

α-D-Glucose α-D-Galactose α-D-Fructose

Disaccharides

Lactose
(galactose–glucose)

Sucrose
(glucose–fructose)

Maltose
(glucose–glucose)

Isomaltose
(α-1,6-linkage)

Amylopectin or glycogen

—— Glucose $\xrightarrow{1\text{-}4\alpha}$ Glucose
|
| $1\text{-}6\alpha$
|
—— Glucose $\xrightarrow{1\text{-}4\alpha}$ Glucose $\xrightarrow{1\text{-}4\alpha}$ Glucose $\xrightarrow{1\text{-}4\alpha}$ Glucose $\xrightarrow{1\text{-}4\alpha}$ etc

Amylose

—— Glucose $\xrightarrow{1\text{-}4\alpha}$ Glucose $\xrightarrow{1\text{-}4\alpha}$ Glucose $\xrightarrow{1\text{-}4\alpha}$ Glucose $\xrightarrow{1\text{-}4\alpha}$ etc

Fig. 50 The structure of carbohydrates in the diet.

deal with the α-1:6-linkages in amylopectin and glycogen. Only a single glucose residue in amylopectin and glycogen will have a free reducing group on carbon-1. The glucose moieties at the ends of branches are referred to as *non-reducing* ends.

Dissacharides

Disaccharides include *sucrose*, consisting of one fructose and one glucose; *lactose* made up of one galactose and one glucose; and *maltose* made of two glucoses.

Monosaccharides

Monosaccharides found in our dietary carbohydrates include *glucose*, *fructose* and *galactose*. All of the monosaccharides are reducing sugars, since they possess a reducing group at carbon-1 or carbon-2.

Carbohydrate digestion

Carbohydrates are digested by a process of glycoside hydrolysis, with the resultant monosaccharides being

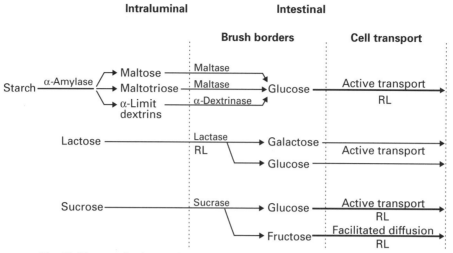

Fig. 51 The overall scheme of carbohydrate digestion and absorption. RL indicates a rate-controlling step in the process.

absorbed by the intestinal mucosal cells (Fig. 51). Dietary polysaccharides are hydrolysed to disaccharides and oligosaccharides within the lumen of the gastro-intestinal tract by *salivary α-amylase* and by *pancreatic α-amylase*. Both of these enzymes have a pH optimum around 7.0; consequently, the action of salivary amylase is quickly stopped by the acidity in the stomach. However, in the small intestine, where the pH has been increased through the buffering action of pancreatic juice and bile, pancreatic amylase continues the digestion of starch and glycogen in the food. Products of amylase action on starch include the disaccharide maltose and various oligosaccharides, which includes limit dextrins (which are small branched oligosaccharides that contain α-1:6- and α-1:4-linkages) and maltotriose (Fig. 51).

Oligosaccharides and disaccharides are then hydrolysed to monosaccharides by enzymes confined to the brush border of intestinal epithelial cells. The *carbohydrases* of the brush border are *sucrase-α-dextrinase*, *glucoamylase* and *lactase*. The products of their action upon α-limit dextrins, maltotriose, maltose, sucrose and lactose are the three monosaccharides glucose, fructose and galactose (Fig. 51).

Carbohydrate absorption

The monosaccharides produced by the action of oligo- and disaccharidases of the brush border of the intestinal cells are absorbed into the cells by several types of transport mechanism (Chapter 5). Fructose moves into

> **BOX 7.1**
> **Clinical note: Lactose intolerance**
>
> Lactase is quite different from the other carbo-hydrases in that it catalyses the hydrolysis of a β-1:4-linkage, as found in lactose. Many people have delayed-onset lactose intolerance caused by a significant fall in the levels of intestinal lactase by the early teens. If such individuals consume a large lactose load (e.g. milk) it leads to abdominal full-ness, bloating, cramping, pain and profuse watery diarrhoea since the unhydrolysed disaccharide is an osmotic load. Metabolites of lactose produced by colonic bacteria increase the osmotic load further and include acids and gases. Eliminating lactose from the diet prevents these problems.

the cell on a membrane carrier but is not actively trans-ported against a concentration gradient, i.e. facilitated diffusion. Glucose and galactose are actively trans-ported and this is accomplished by a sodium symport system (Fig. 52). This transport process ensures that the intracellular glucose concentration is maintained at a higher level than that in the intercellular space on the vascular side of the cell, thus ensuring that glucose will be transported passively into the bloodstream. The carrier-bound sodium ions and glucose are internalised along an electrochemical gradient that results from the low intracellular sodium concentration. On the luminal side, one molecule of glucose and two molecules of

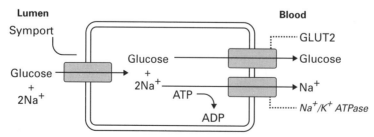

Fig. 52 The glucose–sodium symport (see text for details).

sodium bind to the membrane carrier. Presumably the binding of the sodium ions produces a conformational change such that glucose now binds with greater affinity to the carrier. Inside the cell, the sodium ions are released from the carrier, and diminished affinity allows the glucose to dissociate. A Na^+/K^+ ATPase allows the sodium ions to be transported into the lateral intercellular spaces against a concentration gradient using the free energy of ATP hydrolysis. Since glucose transport does not involve ATP directly, it can be considered as secondary active transport. Glucose is transported from the mucosal cell into the intercellular space by a high-capacity glucose transporter (GLUT2) (pp. 76–77).

Dietary fats

The major dietary lipids are *triacylglycerols (triglycerides)*, which are esters of an alcohol (glycerol) and fatty acids (Fig. 53). Naturally occurring fats usually have different long-chain fatty acids in all three ester positions. The fatty acids can be saturated, e.g. palmitate or stearate, or unsaturated, e.g. oleate. Other fatty acids are polyunsaturated. Fats are hydrophobic molecules.

BOX 7.2
Clinical note: Cholera and dysentery

A practical use of co-transport is the administration of a mixture of NaCl and glucose by mouth to subjects with cholera or dysentery who are sodium depleted as a result of diarrhoea. The provision of glucose along with the NaCl enables them to reestablish their sodium levels.

Fat digestion and absorption

Dietary triacylglycerols are absorbed after undergoing partial hydrolysis, with bile salts playing a key role. The key steps are listed.

1. Salivary and lingual lipases preferentially hydrolyse triacylglycerols composed of short- and medium-chain fatty acids (as found in cow's milk).
2. In the small intestine, bile salts emulsify fats.
3. *Pancreatic lipase* and *co-lipase* are secreted from the pancreas. Co-lipase provides an anchor for pancreatic lipase at the triacylglycerol–bile

---

Saturated fatty acids: $CH_3 - (CH_2)_n \underset{\beta}{\overset{3}{-}CH_2} - \underset{\alpha}{\overset{2}{CH_2}} - \overset{1}{COO^-}$ (ω under CH_3)

Examples:	Butyrate	C_4
	Palmitate	C_{16}
	Stearate	C_{18}

Monounsaturated fatty acids: $CH_3 - (CH_2)_n - CH = CH - (CH_2)_n - COO^-$

| Examples: | Palmitoleate | $C_{16:1;9}$ (or Δ^9) |
| | Oleate | $C_{18:1;9}$ (or Δ^9) |

Polyunsaturated fatty acids:

Examples:	Linoleate	$C_{18:2;9,12}$
	a-Linolenate	$C_{18:3;9,12,15}$
	Arachidonate	$C_{20:4;5,8,11,14}$

Triacylglycerols (triglycerides):

Glycerol

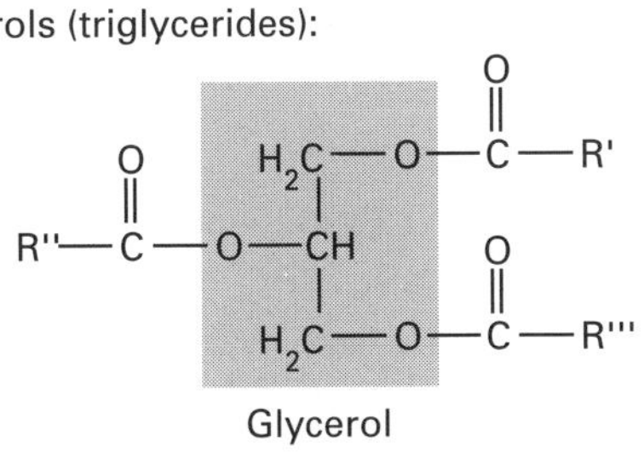

Fig. 53 Fatty acid and triacylglycerol structures. Two different nomenclatures are shown for fatty acids. In one, the carboxyl carbon is carbon-1 and the rest of the carbons follow from that, with the terminal methyl group carbon having the number corresponding to the number of carbons in the fatty acid. The other scheme uses Greek letters starting from the carbon following the carboxyl carbon. In that scheme, the terminal methyl group is referred to as the omega (ω) carbon. In unsaturated fatty acids the number that follows the colon (:) refers to the number of double bonds and is followed by a number that refers to the location of the double bonds. In most unsaturated fatty acids found in the body, the double bonds are *cis*.

salt–water interface. In the small intestine, pancreatic lipase catalyses the hydrolysis of triacylglycerols to 2-monoacylglycerols by removing fatty acids from the 1 and 3 positions.

4. Bile salt micelles are formed that contain triacylglycerols, monoglycerides, fatty acids and fat-soluble vitamins, and these allow for the lipids to be absorbed into the mucosal cells.

5. Fatty acids of less than 10–12 carbons go directly to the liver via the portal vein.

6. Triacylglycerols are reformed in intestinal mucosal cells from long-chain fatty acids and monoglycerides and are then incorporated into *chylomicrons*, which are lipoproteins involved in the delivery of fatty acids (p. 124).

7. *Cholesteryl esters* in the diet are hydrolysed by the action of *cholesteryl ester hydrolase*. Unesterified cholesterol and cholesteryl esters are included in the fat micelles.

8. *Phospholipids* in the diet are hydrolysed by the action of *pancreatic phospholipase A$_2$*, which removes the fatty acid at the carbon-2 position leaving a lysophospholipid, a powerful detergent. The fatty acids released and the lysophospholipids are incorporated into micelles and transported into mucosal cells and appear in chylomicrons.

Gastrointestinal hormones have an important role in digestion

These hormones ensure that digestive enzymes are present in sufficient quantity in the stomach or small intestine and that the conditions are correct for the action of these enzymes. Key points include:

- *gastrin*, made in the G cells found in the pyloric glands of the antrum and the proximal duodenum, stimulates acid and pepsinogen secretion in the stomach (p. 106). Protein meals, large peptides and distension of the stomach increase gastrin secretion.

- *secretin*, made in S cells which are found between crypts and villi of the upper intestine, stimulates water and bicarbonate secretion by pancreatic ductal cells and therefore ensures that the acidity produced in the stomach is neutralised. Acidification, achieved when the acid chyme enters the small intestine during the digestion of a meal, is the only known stimulus for its secretion.

- *cholecystokinin*, made chiefly in the duodenum and proximal jejunum, stimulates acinar cells to secrete digestive enzymes such as amylase and lipase as well as the zymogen forms of proteolytic enzymes. It also brings about dilation of the sphincter of Oddi, allowing bile to flow from the gallbladder into the duodenum. Thus, it has a very important role to play in dietary fat digestion and absorption. CCK secretion is increased by fats, peptides and amino acids present in the lumen of the small intestine.

7.3 Carbohydrate catabolism

Carbohydrates, mainly in the form of the monosaccharide glucose, are important fuels for tissues in the body. An important concept is that glucose can be used as a fuel by all tissues but there is considerable variation in the ability of different tissues to use other fuels (Chapter 11).

Glucose transport into cells

Following a meal that contains carbohydrate, there is efficient digestion and absorption leading to a significant increase in blood glucose concentration. Glucose is taken up by all tissues in the body, with a high percentage entering liver and muscle where it can be stored as glycogen. The transport of glucose across animal cell membranes involves transport proteins that span the plasma membrane.

Glucose transporters (GLUTs)

There are two distinct gene families of glucose transporters (Fig. 37). One group are the Na$^+$/glucose cotransporters involved in glucose and galactose absorption in the intestine (p. 74). The other comprises facilitated-diffusion glucose transporters that are ubiquitously expressed in mammalian cells. These proteins are passive systems that equilibrate glucose across membranes. They are responsible for the movement of glucose from the blood into cells, supplying cellular glucose for energy metabolism and the biosynthesis of carbohydrate-containing macromolecules (glycogen, glycoproteins, glycolipids, nucleic acids, etc.). Glucose uptake into cells is of great physiological significance and glucose transporters facilitate the achievement of glucose homeostasis in the fed and fasting states (Chapter 11). The key points (summarised in Table 5) are:

- GLUT1 is the 'housekeeping' glucose transporter functioning in all tissues including those which are

Table 5 Glucose transport into cells

Transporter	Location	Characteristics
Na$^+$/glucose transporters	Gut	Glucose–sodium symport
Facilitated-diffusion transporters		
GLUT1	Brain All cells	Low *Km*
GLUT2	Liver, beta cells of pancreas, kidney, intestine	High *Km*
GLUT3	Most cells	Low *Km*
GLUT4	Muscle Adipose tissue	Insulin-dependent translocation to plasma membrane
GLUT5	Intestine, liver	Fructose absorption

solely dependent upon glucose for their fuel (such as the brain). It operates at low blood glucose concentrations, i.e. it has a low K_m.

- GLUT2 has a high K_m for glucose. Its presence in the liver means that the liver will take up glucose effectively only when the blood glucose concentration is raised, such as after a meal. It also operates to allow for the export of glucose from the liver (to maintain blood glucose levels).
- GLUT3 is another low K_m glucose transporter also present in the brain.
- GLUT4 occurs in adipose tissue and muscle cells, tissues that have little need for GLUT4 to be present in the plasma membranes of these tissues during the fasting state since these tissues are not glucose manufacturers/exporters. Their GLUT4 transporters are sequestered in intracellular membranes until an increase in blood insulin concentration leads to recruitment of GLUT4 molecules to the plasma membrane; this is complete within 5 minutes.
- GLUT5 is a fructose transporter present in the small intestine and the liver.
- Other glucose transporters occur in the endoplasmic reticulum in liver and are important in glucose production.

Glycolysis

The glycolytic pathway is the series of reactions that occurs in the cytosol of cells and allows glucose to be converted to pyruvate (Stage 2 reactions). Glycolysis results in limited ATP synthesis but, in addition, some of the intermediates have critical roles in other pathways and systems.

Relative importance in tissues and organs. This should be obvious since glucose is a fuel for all tissues in the body and under normal conditions is the only fuel for the brain. Glycolysis is an essential precursor to the oxidative phase of glucose metabolism that occurs in the mitochondria of cells. Also the pyruvate formed can provide the oxaloacetate required for operation of the vitally important TCA cycle. Clearly, in cells which lack mitochondria (such as erythrocytes), glycolysis is the only pathway that has the potential to generate ATP for these cells.

Overall design of the pathway

Figure 54 shows the overall design of the pathway and Figure 55 the series of reactions.

In the first phase of glycolysis, glucose is converted to fructose 1,6-bisphosphate (F-1,6-BP). The two kinases involved are *hexokinase or glucokinase* and then *phosphofructokinase-1* (PFK-1). Hexokinase and glucokinase have differing kinetic properties (Fig. 21, p. 33). Hexokinase has a low K_m for glucose and catalyses the conversion of glucose to glucose 6-phosphate (Reaction 1) in all tissues of the body. Glucokinase is present in the liver and in the beta cells of the islets of Langerhans

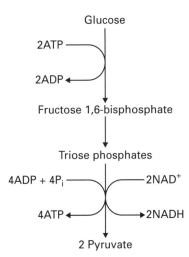

Fig. 54 Overall design of glycolysis.

in the pancreas. The product of the reaction, glucose 6-phosphate, inhibits hexokinase but not glucokinase. Glucokinase has a K_m much higher than the normal blood glucose concentration. This ensures that during the fasting state the liver is not metabolising blood glucose. Additionally, the high K_m is consistent with the role of the liver in the fed state where the liver takes up glucose and stores it as glycogen. PFK-1 catalyses a second phosphorylation (Reaction 3) which is often described as the first committed step of glycolysis, and is subjected to allosteric control.

In the second phase of glycolysis, F-1,6-BP is converted to two interconvertible triose phosphates (Reaction 4) and one of these, 3-phosphoglyceraldehyde, is oxidised in the single oxidative step of glycolysis (Reaction 6). The enzyme involved, *3-phosphoglyceraldehyde dehydrogenase*, is NAD$^+$-dependent. It is important to recognise that there are limited amounts of NAD$^+$ in cells and, therefore, it has to be regenerated if glycolysis is to proceed. Because NADH cannot cross the inner mitochondrial membrane, 'shuttles' serve to carry this out during oxidative metabolism (p. 85). During vigorous exercise in muscle, *lactate dehydrogenase* serves to regenerate NAD$^+$ in a reaction in which pyruvate is reduced to lactate (Reaction 11).

In the third phase of glycolysis, reactions occur in which ATP is synthesised by a process known as substrate-level phosphorylation, contrasting with ATP formation in oxidative phosphorylation in mitochondria.

PFK-1 and pyruvate kinase are important in the control of glycolysis

Flux control through the glycolytic pathway is 'distributed' (it is invalid to consider that one of the steps is the rate-limiting step!) and involves the reactions catalysed by hexokinase, PFK-1 and PK, each of which have large negative $\Delta G^{0\prime}$ values. Understandably, it is these reactions that are subjected to some degree of regulation. In addition, control of glucose transport into

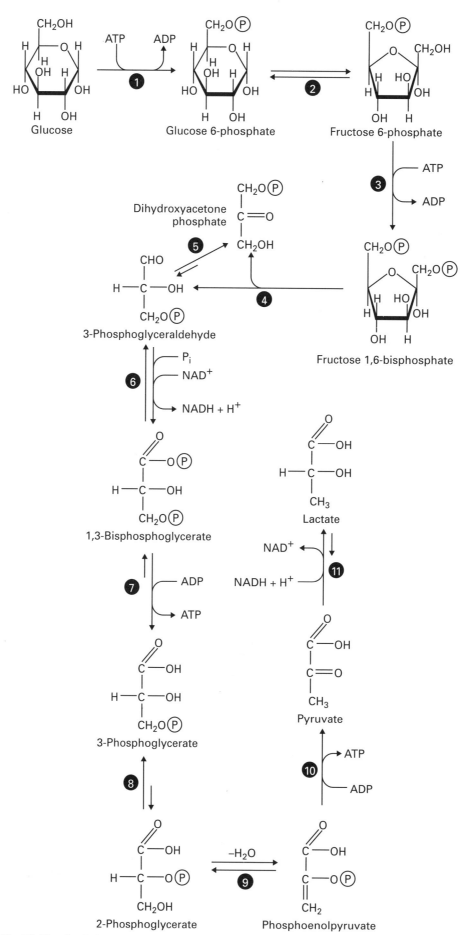

Fig. 55 The glycolytic pathway. Phosphate groups are indicated by a circled P. The enzymes catalysing the numbered reactions are discussed in the text.

the cell will affect the potential maximum flux through the pathway. Most attention has been given to PFK-1 since it catalyses the first committed step in glycolysis.

Regulation of PFK-1

PFK-1 is inhibited by ATP and citrate and activated by AMP and F-2, 6-BP. Under resting conditions, the level of ATP in a cell is sufficient to inhibit PFK-1. An increase in AMP is a signal that ATP is being used at a high rate and that catabolism is necessary to replenish ATP used for whatever reason. The AMP effect is insufficient to activate PFK-1 unless F-2, 6-BP levels also increase. Increased citrate in a cell is a signal that fatty acids are being utilised as fuel and, logically, this should lead to decreased need for glucose catabolism. PFK-1 is also inhibited by an increase in hydrogen ion concentration and this safeguards cells against over-accumulation of pyruvate or lactate. The rationale for the effects of F-2, 6-BP on glycolysis and the opposing reactions of gluconeogenesis in the liver are discussed in Chapter 8.

Net reactions of glycolysis

Summation of all of the reactions gives the following equations for aerobic and anaerobic glycolysis. Note that under anaerobic conditions, the equation shows that lactate formation leads to oxidation of NADH.

Aerobic glycolysis

$$Glucose + 2\,ADP + 2\,P_i + 2\,NAD^+ \rightarrow 2\,Pyruvate + 2\,ATP + 2\,NADH + 2H^+ + H_2O$$

Anaerobic glycolysis

$$Glucose + 2\,ADP + 2\,P_i \rightarrow 2\,Lactate + 2\,ATP + 2\,H_2O$$

Aerobic metabolism of pyruvate

Pyruvate enters the mitochondria along with H^+ using a symporter. Within mitochondria, it can be completely oxidised to carbon dioxide and water with the associated production of ATP but first it has to be oxidised to acetyl-CoA. The PDC is huge: it comprises three enzymes involved in the actual reaction plus enzymes involved in its control (Fig. 56). There is a core of 60 E_2 monomers plus 30 E_1 dimers and 6 E_3 dimers. PDC is frequently referred to as pyruvate dehydrogenase (PDH) but it is clear that the first reaction is a decarboxylation catalysed by E_1 that has thiamine pyrophosphate (TPP) as cofactor. E_2, which has lipoate covalently linked, has two functions; one is the dehydrogenation of the 2-carbon unit to give an acetyl group and the second is the transfer of the acetyl group to a third coenzyme, coenzyme A. If the acetyl group (which serves as a precursor of, amongst others, fatty acids and cholesterol) remained attached to the lipoate that is covalently linked to E_2, it would be less available

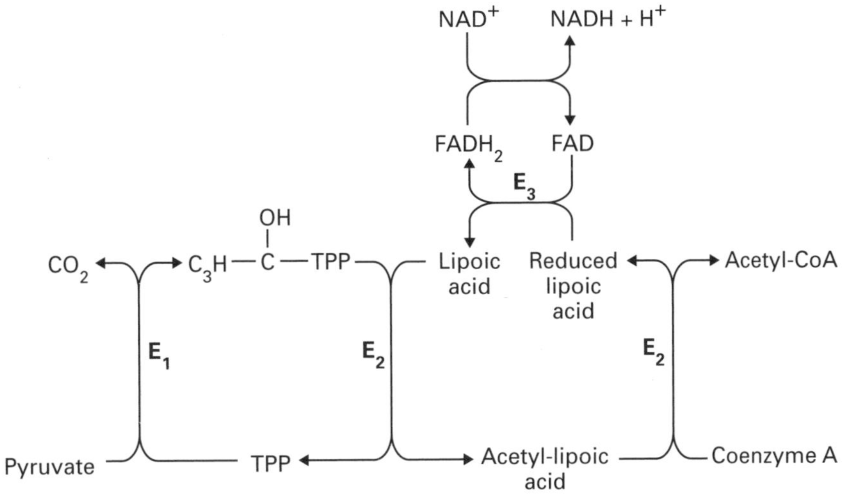

Overall reaction

$$Pyruvate \ + \ NAD^+ \ + \ CoA \longrightarrow Acetyl\text{-}CoA \ + \ CO_2 \ + \ NADH$$

Participating enzymes		Participating Cofactors/coenzymes
E_1	Pyruvate dehydrogenase (PDH)	TPP, thiamine pyrophosphate (B_1)
E_2	Dihydrolipoyl transacetylase	Lipoic acid
E_3	Dihydrolipoyl dehydrogenase	CoA, Pantothenate-containing factor
		FAD, flavin adenine dinucleotide (B_2)
		NAD, nicotinamide adenine dinucleotide (niacin)

Fig. 56 Reactions of the pyruvate dehydrogenase complex.

for other metabolic pathways. In the last group of reactions lipoate is regenerated to its oxidised form by E_3, a flavoprotein that utilises FAD as cofactor. Finally, the $FADH_2$ is reoxidised to FAD using NAD^+ giving the final products of the reaction: acetyl-CoA, carbon dioxide and NADH. The PDC reactions have three important features.

1. The PDC-catalysed reaction is **irreversible**. This has very important consequences for intermediary metabolism in that acetyl-CoA cannot be converted to pyruvate and, therefore, fatty acids are not glucogenic (cannot be used to make glucose).
2. The activity of PDC is the major determinant of glucose oxidation in well-oxygenated tissues in vivo. The conversion of the glycolytic metabolites of glucose to acetyl-CoA enables them to enter Stage 3 of metabolism, leading to the generation of several molecules of ATP.
3. The control of PDC is multi-faceted in that the reaction is critical to energy metabolism thus it responds to nutritional state and hormones and also to levels of intrinsic metabolites (Fig. 57). A mixture of covalent and allosteric mechanisms are involved. E_1 of the complex is inhibited by phosphorylation and activated when dephosphorylated. A kinase and a phosphatase are involved and their activities are affected by the ratios of acetyl-CoA/CoA, $NADH/NAD^+$, and ATP/ADP. In every case, a high ratio activates the kinase leading to decreased PDC activity and vice versa. In addition, Ca^{2+} enhances phosphatase activity both by facilitating the association of the phosphatase with the complex and by decreasing the K_m for the protein substrate, the phosphorylated E_1 component. Insulin (in adipocytes) and catecholamines (in cardiac tissue) increase pyruvate conversion to acetyl-CoA by activation of the E_1 phosphatase. The physiologic

wisdom of the control of PDC will become apparent in Chapter 11.

7.4 Fat catabolism

Fatty acids have a higher energy content per gram than glucose since they are more reduced. The body has limited carbohydrate storage capacity but enormous capacity to store fats (Chapter 11). This means that fatty acids are usually available as fuel and if a tissue can utilise them (e.g. the heart), then less glucose is required. Also, when undergoing long-term exercise, a worker or athlete will use fatty acids as a preferred fuel. This occurs particularly in muscles that have a high content of mitochondria (red muscle).

Fatty acid are mobilised from stored triacylglycerols

Fatty acids are stored as triacylglycerols mainly in adipose tissue. Their mobilisation as fuels for use by other tissues involves the action of several lipases with the end products of their action being glycerol plus three fatty acids (Fig. 58). One of the lipases, *triacylglycerol lipase*, is active when phosphorylated; it is called hormone-sensitive lipase because phosphorylation occurs when hormones such as glucagon, growth hormone and adrenaline are produced in increased amounts in the fasting state or during exercise (Chapter 11). Glycerol, the other product of triacylglycerol hydrolysis, can be phosphorylated in the liver and then metabolised as a glycolytic intermediate.

Oxidation of fatty acids

The overall design of the beta-oxidation pathway is shown in Figure 58. The key points are:

- fatty acids are taken up by tissues in which they can be oxidised and the action of *fatty acyl-CoA synthase* generates fatty acyl-CoA derivatives.
- this introduces a problem of the impermeability of the inner mitochondrial membrane to long-chain fatty acyl-CoA derivatives. This is solved by converting them to acyl-carnitines catalysed by *carnitine palmitoyltransferases I (CPTI)*, transferring the acyl-carnitines using a translocase membrane, and then *carnitine palmitoyltransferases II* catalyses the regeneration of the fatty acyl-CoA derivatives, now located in the proximity of the enzymes of the beta-oxidation pathway.
- beta-oxidation involves reactions (Fig. 58) that are similar to the sequence succinate $\rightarrow$ fumarate $\rightarrow$ malate $\rightarrow$ oxaloacetate of the TCA cycle.
- $FADH_2$ and NADH are formed in the two oxidation steps (Reactions 1 and 3) and in the final step the cleavage of the β-ketoacyl CoA with a second molecule of CoA (Reaction 4), which yields acetyl-

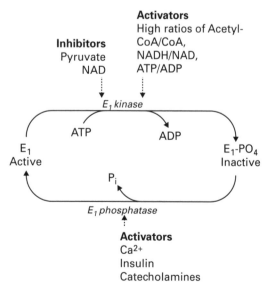

Fig. 57 Control of the PDC by both covalent modification and allosteric mechanisms.

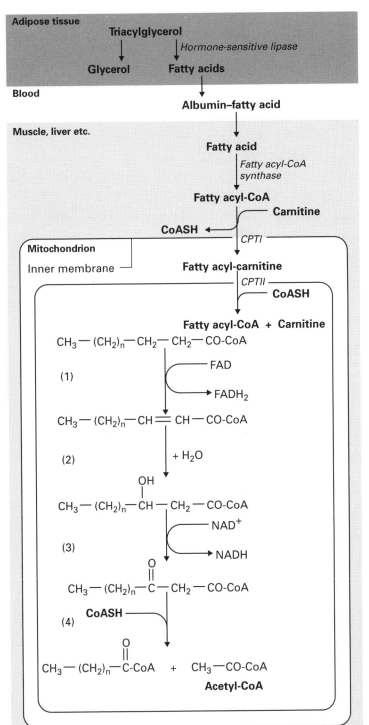

Fig. 58 Fat mobilisation and fatty acid beta-oxidation. The rate of fatty acid release from adipose tissue affects the total amount of fatty acid available as a fuel for tissues such as liver and muscle.

CoA and a fatty acyl-CoA shortened by two carbons. Hence, activation is only required once.

The oxidation of palmitate, a 16-carbon fatty acid, would result in the following:

$$Palmitoyl\text{-}CoA + 7FAD + 7NAD^+ + 7CoASH + 7H_2O \rightarrow$$
$$8\ Acetyl\text{-}CoA + 7FADH_2 + 7NADH + 7H^+$$

Seven (not eight!) oxidation cycles will be required in the degradation of palmitoyl-CoA to 8 molecules of acetyl-CoA. Remember, you only need to cut a string once to get two pieces!

The oxidation of $FADH_2$ and NADH involves the electron transport chain and is coupled to ATP synthesis.

Beta-oxidation is controlled by malonyl-CoA

All the evidence points to CPTI being an important control point. Malonyl-CoA, an intermediate in fatty acid biosynthesis, inhibits CPTI and this suggests an understandable link between these opposing pathways. However, another determinant of the amount of fatty acid that can be utilised by, for example, liver, cardiac or skeletal muscle must be the supply of fuel to these

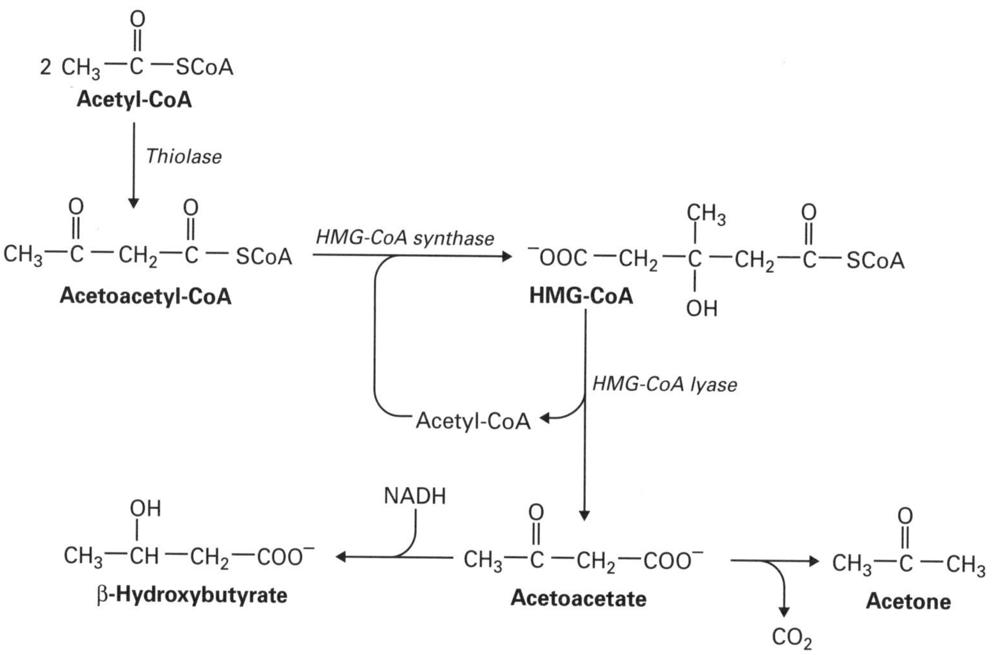

Fig. 59 Ketone body biosynthesis pathway in liver mitochondria.

tissues. That is determined by the rate of fatty acid mobilisation from the fat stores in adipose tissue. Here is another example of control of flux through a pathway being distributed rather than focussed on a single rate-limiting step.

Oxidation of odd-numbered fatty acids

Beta-oxidation of a fatty acid with an odd number of carbon atoms yields successive molecules of acetyl-CoA and one equivalent of propionyl-CoA; the propionyl group has three carbons. The major pathway of propionyl-CoA metabolism occurs in mammalian mito-chondria and involves its conversion to a TCA cycle intermediate, succinyl-CoA, by three steps, one of which requires a vitamin B_{12} coenzyme. One difference between propionyl-CoA and acetyl-CoA is that the former is capable of being converted to glucose whereas acetyl-CoA is not.

Oxidation of unsaturated fatty acids

Most unsaturated fatty acids in biology have *cis* double bonds. This means that one has to have special reactions (not dealt with in this text) to deal with such compounds. The potential for an unsaturated fatty acid to generate ATP is less than for a saturated fatty acid with the same number of carbons. Modified beta-oxidation again yields acetyl-CoA.

Ketone body biosynthesis and metabolism

Ketone bodies were originally thought to be inter-mediates of fatty acid oxidation that could accumulate under abnormal conditions, e.g. in diabetes mellitus. It is now clear that ketone bodies are important fuels

made from fatty acids in the liver and then transported via the blood to many tissues to be used as fuels. In effect, this enables the energy of fats to be utilised by many tissues. The ketone bodies are acetoacetic acid, β-hydroxybutyric acid and acetone (Fig. 59). In contrast to the fatty acids from which they are derived, they provide an alternative fuel for the brain. Key points on ketone body synthesis and metabolism are:

- they are formed in the mitochondria of the liver with β-hydroxy-β-methylglutaryl-CoA (HMG-CoA) being a key intermediate (Fig. 59).
- acetoacetate is the primary ketone body, but in the liver some is reduced to β-hydroxybutyrate by the action of *β-hydroxybutyrate dehydrogenase*; the proportion of these two ketone bodies secreted is dependent upon several factors, including the glycogen status of the liver and the ratio of NADH to NAD+.
- acetoacetate can also be decarboxylated (spontaneously) to yield acetone. Acetone is not a fuel; as it is volatile its production will be indicated by the presence of its characteristic odour in expired air.
- the key enzyme of ketone body utilisation is *3-ketoacyl-CoA transferase* which catalyses the raction where CoA is transferred from succinyl-CoA to acetoacetate (Fig. 60).
- ketone body production is directly related to the rate of fatty acid mobilisation from adipose tissue and their oxidation in liver. Also, low levels of OAA, associated with low rates of glucose metabolism, increase the potential for acetyl-CoA to be converted to ketone bodies rather than enter the TCA cycle.

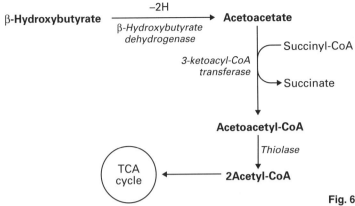

Fig. 60 Ketone body utilisation in extra-hepatic tissues.

BOX 7.3
Clinical note: Type 1 diabetes mellitus

Impaired utilisation resulting from deficiency of insulin (or reduced effectiveness) is associated with excessive formation of ketone bodies. Patients with type 1 diabetes mellitus have the potential to develop ketoacidosis. Acetone production gives the breath a characteristic odour. If untreated, keto-acidosis can result in coma and death.

7.5 The tricarboxylic acid cycle

The tricarboxylic acid (TCA) cycle (Krebs cycle; citric acid cycle) is a part of Stage 3 of metabolism. It allows for intermediates derived from carbohydrate, fat or amino acids to be completely oxidised to carbon dioxide and water. The pathway occurs in mito-chondria where the electron transport chain and ATP synthase are also located.

Overall design of the pathway

The overall design of the pathway is shown in Figure 61. In the TCA cycle the acetyl group in acetyl-CoA can be oxidised to carbon dioxide and water. Citrate formed by the interaction of acetyl-CoA and oxaloacetate is subjected to a series of reactions, four of which are oxidations catalysed by dehydrogenases. In addition to acetyl-CoA, other metabolites, including those derived from amino acids, can feed into the TCA cycle at various

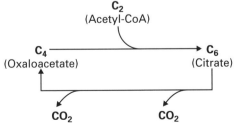

Fig. 61 Four oxidation steps give rise to 3NADH and 1 $FADH_2$. At another step GTP is generated.

points. Also, the TCA cycle provides intermediates for the synthesis of biomolecules; it is amphibolic. Key points about the TCA cycle are:

- oxaloacetate, which reacts with acetyl-CoA entering the cycle, is regenerated in the last step so it functions like a catalyst
- all of the reactions of the TCA cycle (Fig. 62) are catalysed by enzymes dissolved in the fluid of the mitochondrial matrix with the exception of *succinate dehydrogenase*, which is an integral protein of the mitochondrial inner membrane.
- *isocitric dehydrogenase* (3) catalyses the oxidative decarboxylation of isocitrate to α-ketoglutarate (2-oxoglutarate). This is the first of four dehydrogenase reactions that occur in the cycle.
- the 3 NADH and 1 $FADH_2$ produced per acetyl-CoA molecule are, in turn, oxidised via the electron transport chain coupled to *ATP synthase* that results in the production of 9 ATPs; the single GTP is produced by substrate-level phosphorylation
- *α-ketoglutarate dehydrogenase* (4) catalyses an oxidative decarboxylation by a mechanism similar to that of PDC. Thiamine pyrophosphate, lipoic acid, CoASH, FAD and NAD^+ are involved in the catalytic mechanism (Fig. 56). α-Ketoglutarate represents a significant point of convergence in metabolism. Several amino acids can be converted to glutamate, which if transaminated or oxidatively deaminated yields α-ketoglutarate. Conversely, these amino acids can be synthesized from α-ketoglutarate (p. 110).

Net reaction

The net reaction of acetyl-CoA metabolism in the TCA cycle is:

$$\text{Acetyl-CoA} + 3\,\text{NAD}^+ + \text{FAD} + \text{GDP} + \text{P}_i + 2\text{H}_2\text{O} \rightarrow$$
$$2\text{CO}_2 + 3\text{NADH} + 2\text{H}^+ + \text{FADH}_2 + \text{GTP} + \text{CoASH}$$

Citrate synthase, isocitrate dehydrogenase and α-ketoglutarate dehydrogenase are control points of the TCA cycle

Flux through the TCA cycle will be determined by several parameters. Within the actual pathway, isocitrate dehydrogenase and α-ketoglutarate dehydrogenase are

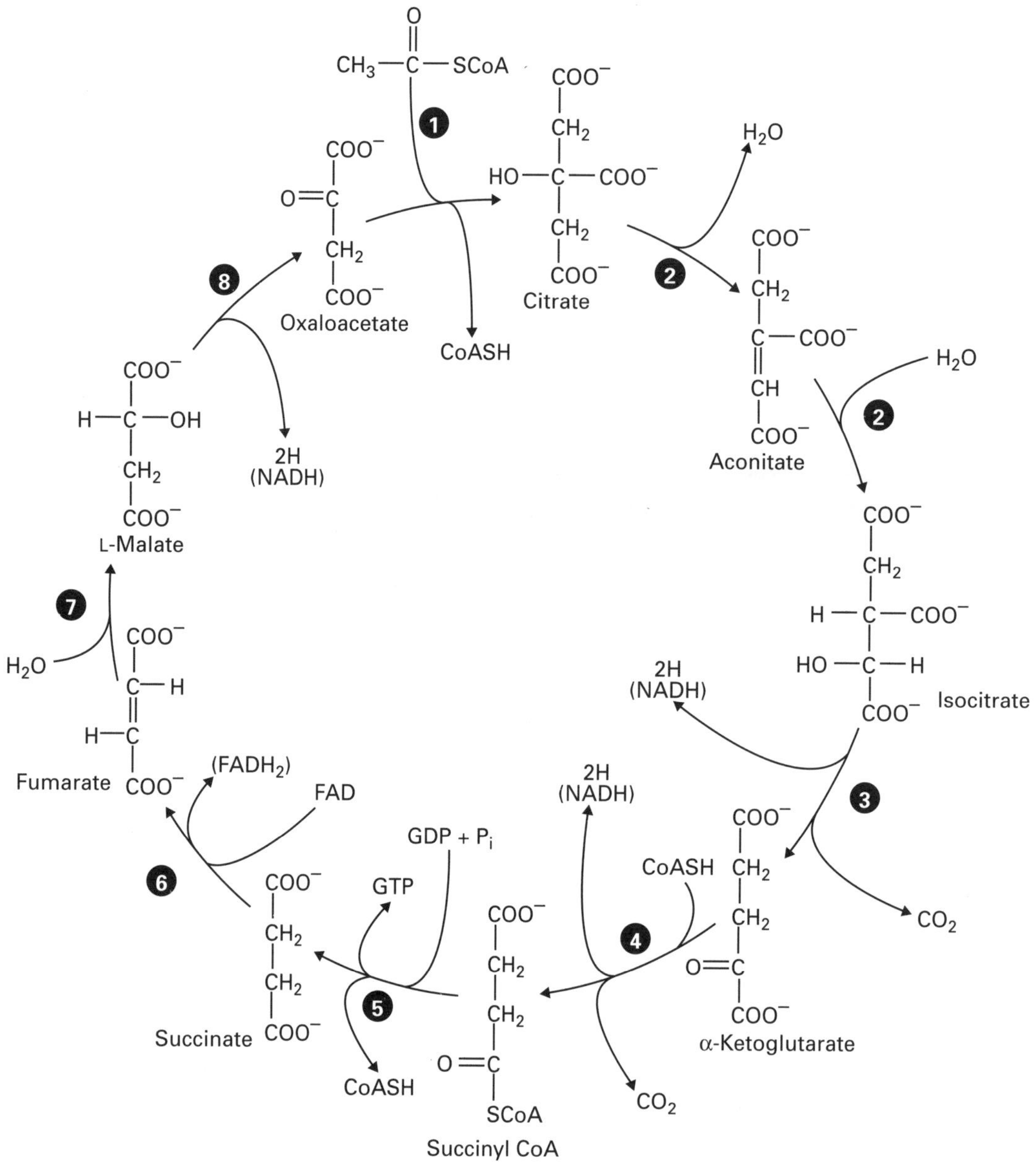

Fig. 62 The reactions of the TCA cycle. The enzymes 1–8 are described in the text.

sensitive to energy charge and to the ratio of $NAD^+/NADH$. However, the flux through the pathway is more complicated and is related to the activity of pathways that supply acetyl-CoA, including the PDC and fatty acid beta-oxidation.

Supramolecular organisation of TCA cycle enzymes as a *metabolon* has been proposed by Srere since they are at very high concentration in the mitochondrial matrix. This arrangement would allow for channelling of intermediates.

7.6 Electron transport and oxidative phosphorylation

Transfer of energy-rich molecules

Products of the TCA cycle include $NADH + H^+$ and

$FADH_2$, which are 'energy-rich' molecules because they contain a pair of electrons of high transfer potential. Transfer of these electrons to oxygen through a series of carriers has the potential to generate ATP. Oxidative phosphorylation is the process in which ATP is formed as electrons are transferred by this series of carriers from $NADH + H^+$ and $FADH_2$ to oxygen. The formation of a proton gradient is critical to this process.

Shuttles are used for NADH generated in the cytosol

NADH is also generated in the glycolytic pathway in a reaction catalysed by glyceraldehyde 3-phosphate dehydrogenase. If aerobic metabolism of glucose is to occur – for example to support the performance of muscular work – then cytosolic NADH must be reoxidised to NAD^+. One possibility would be to reoxidise the NADH in mitochondria using the respiratory assemblies that are located in the inner membrane of the mitochondria. However, neither NAD$^+$ nor NADH can pass across the inner mitochondrial membrane. Reoxidation of NADH formed in the cytoplasmic oxidation of glyceraldehyde 3-phosphate by NAD$^+$ occurs by the operation of two shuttles. The principle of both shuttles is that NADH reduces a metabolite and therefore NAD$^+$ is regenerated. Then, the reduced metabolite is oxidised by mitochondrial enzyme but in this case the FADH$_2$ or NADH produced can be oxidised via the electron transport chain. The shuttles in question are the *glycerol 3-phosphate shuttle* with the net reaction being:

$$\text{NADH(cytosol)} + \text{FAD(mitochondria)} \rightarrow$$
$$\text{NAD}^+\text{(cytosol)} + \text{FADH}_2\text{(mitochondria)}$$

and the *malate-aspartate shuttle* with the net reaction being:

$$\text{NADH(cytosol)} + \text{NAD}^+\text{(mitochondria)} \rightarrow$$
$$\text{NAD}^+\text{(cytosol)} + \text{NADH(mitochondria)}$$

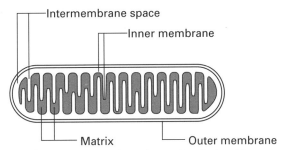

Fig. 63 Compartments and membranes in mitochondria.

Mitochondrial electron transport

The mitochondria of the cell consist of two membranes: the outer and inner membranes (Fig. 63). The outer membrane is 6–7 nm thick and is freely permeable to molecules with molecular weights under 10 000. The intermembrane space contains the enzymes that catalyse the interconversion of adenine nucleotides. The inner membrane is 6–8 nm thick and has many folds directed towards the mitochondrial matrix. These invaginations (called cristae) increase the surface area of the inner membrane and are increased in cells with high rates of respiratory activity. Much of the lipid in the inner membrane consists of phospholipid with phosphatidylcholine (PC) predominating on the cytoplasmic side and phosphatidylethanolamine (PE) on the matrix side. Most of the cardiolipin is on the matrix side.

The electron transport system is composed of five protein–lipid–enzyme complexes, which contain flavins, ubiquinone (coenzyme Q$_{10}$), iron–sulphur clusters, cytochromes (haem proteins) and protein-bound copper (Fig. 64). Complexes I and II are the 'electron gatherers' transferring electrons to ubiquinone. Then the electrons are transferred through the complexes containing cytochromes and eventually react with molecular oxygen in

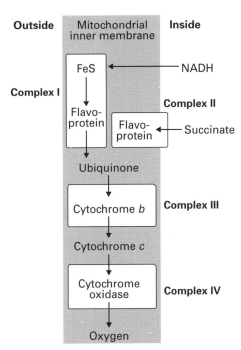

Fig. 64 Respiratory chain complexes of mitochondria.

the reaction catalysed by cytochrome *c* oxidase. Characteristics of these complexes include:

- complex I accepting reducing equivalents in the form of NADH, derived from the action of NAD$^+$-linked dehydrogenases in the major pathways of intermediary metabolism. The transfer of electrons to ubiquinone involves FMN and multiple iron-sulphur clusters (FeS).
- complex II deriving reducing equivalents in the form of FADH$_2$ from succinate dehydrogenase and, among others, fatty acyl-CoA dehydrogenase of fatty acid beta-oxidation. Electrons are transferred to ubiquinone.
- complex III being the cytochrome *b-c*$_1$ complex which receives electrons from ubiquinone and passes them on to complex IV.
- complex IV comprising cytochrome *c* oxidase which donates the electrons that have traversed the electron transport chain to oxygen, producing water. It consists of 13 polypeptide subunits. Subunits I, II and III are encoded by the mitochondrial genome and the others by nuclear DNA. Subunits I and II contain the two copper atoms of cytochrome oxidase as well as haems a and a$_3$. Cytochrome oxidase is inhibited by carbon monoxide, which binds to the Fe^{II} form and also by cyanide, which binds to the Fe^{III} form.

ATP synthesis makes use of a proton gradient

The chemiosmotic hypothesis of Mitchell states that oxidation and phosphorylation are coupled by a *proton gradient* (a proton motive force). In this model, it is proposed that an electrochemical gradient (proton

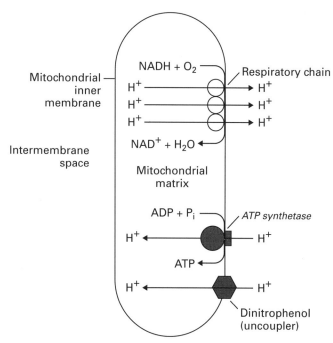

Fig. 65 The proton circuit in oxidative phosphorylation. Note that the electron transport chain and ATP synthase are separate entities in the inner mitochondrial membrane!

gradient) is generated by a proton pump in the inner membrane of the mitochondria. The proton pump is operated by electron flow and causes protons to be expelled through the membrane from the matrix space. Protons flow back into the matrix down their electrochemical gradient and the energy released is used to drive the synthesis of ATP (Fig. 65). Protons are pumped across the inner mitochondrial membrane into the intermembrane space at complexes I, III and IV. This generates a proton gradient and the potential energy of this gradient is used in complex V (ATP synthase) to drive the formation of ATP from ADP + P_i.

- In complex V, ATP synthesis is carried out by a molecular assembly in the inner membrane shown schematically in Figure 66. The spheres, which project on the matrix side of the inner membrane of the mitochondria, are referred to as F_1. Solubilised F_1, in the absence of a proton gradient, hydrolyses ATP. F_0 is the hydrophobic component of ATP synthase and it spans the inner membrane; this is the proton channel of the complex. The stalk

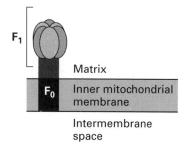

Fig. 66 ATP synthase of mitochondria.

between F_1 and F_0 contains several proteins, one of which is sensitive to oligomycin. This antibiotic inhibits ATP synthesis by interfering with the utilisation of the proton gradient.

Phosphorylation can be uncoupled from oxidation

- Oxidation can be uncoupled from ATP synthesis by uncoupling agents, such as 2,4-dinitrophenol. These compounds are weak acids with lipid-soluble acidic and basic forms, which collapse the proton gradient by becoming protonated, traversing the inner mitochondrial membrane and, thus, dissipate the proton gradient. Under these conditions, electron transport and oxygen utilisation run unchecked at their maximal rates but ATP synthesis through ATP synthase ceases.
- A unique mitochondrial protein – the uncoupling protein (UCP) – gives *brown adipose tissue* (BAT) the ability of facultative heat production. BAT differs from energy-storing white adipose tissue in having an abundance of mitochondria. UCP is a proton translocator that also uncouples oxidation from ATP synthesis in BAT cells. BAT is found in mammals mainly in the interscapular, subscapular, axillary and suprasternal regions of the body. Babies have more BAT than adults.

ATP yield

In intact, coupled mitochondria, the yield of ATP processed through oxidative phosphorylation has been calculated to be 2.5 ATP per NADH and 1.5 ATP per $FADH_2$ (older editions of the standard textbooks will use slightly higher values, 3 for NADH and 2 for $FADH_2$). These are also expressed as P/O ratios, where P refers to the number of ATPs synthesised and O to an oxygen atom (one half O_2).

ATP from glucose oxidation
Using these data and a knowledge of glucose metabolism, one can calculate that the complete oxidation of glucose can yield 32ATP, assuming handling of cytosolic NADH by the malate shuttle. The 32ATP are generated since glucose oxidation to carbon dioxide and water produces 2NADH and 2ATP from glycolysis, 2NADH from PDC, and 6NADH, 2FADH$_2$ and 2GTP from TCA cycle activity. If the glycerol 3-phosphate shuttle is used, the yield from glucose will be 30ATP.

ATP from fatty acid oxidation
The complete oxidation of an 18-carbon fatty acid to carbon dioxide and water will generate 120ATP. Please note that 120ATP is significantly more than the 96 (3 × 32) ATP produced from the complete oxidation of three glucoses. This is a good indication of the higher energy content of the more reduced fuel!

Self-assessment: questions

Multiple choice questions

1. Stage 3 of metabolism:
   a. Is common to the oxidation of all fuel molecules
   b. Involves the breakdown of dietary fuels into smaller units, such as monosaccharides, amino acids and fatty acids
   c. Produces most of the ATP and carbon dioxide in cells
   d. Is localised to the mitochondria of cells
   e. Is very active in mature erythrocytes

2. The following are reasons why the biochemical pathway for the catabolism of a molecule is almost never the same as the pathway for the biosynthesis of that molecule:
   a. It would be extremely difficult to regulate the pathway if it served both functions
   b. Enzyme-catalysed reactions are always irreversible
   c. The free-energy change would be unfavourable in one direction
   d. Biochemical systems are usually at equilibrium

3. The following processes require ATP:
   a. Synthesis of glycogen in liver and muscle
   b. Stage 3 of metabolism
   c. Transport of ions against a gradient
   d. Synthesis of proteins
   e. Performance of mechanical work

4. The following enzyme(s) is required for the digestion of amylopectin but is *not* required for the digestion of amylose:
   a. Lactase
   b. Maltase
   c. Sucrase-α-dextrinase
   d. Alpha amylase
   e. All of the above

5. Pancreatic and salivary amylase:
   a. Both catalyse reactions where water is one of the reactants
   b. Both have pH optima less than 3.0
   c. Both catalyse the hydrolysis of α-1,4-linkages within amylose with maltose being the major product
   d. Both are located on the brush border of the small intestine
   e. Their actions on amylopectin and/or glycogen lead to the production of limit dextrins

6. Glucokinase in the liver:
   a. Is a hexokinase isozyme
   b. Because of its high K_m, ensures that significant liver glycogen synthesis does not occur until blood glucose levels are elevated
   c. Is not inhibited by glucose 6-phosphate
   d. Is induced in the fasted state

7. Phosphofructokinase-1 activity is enhanced by increased levels of:
   a. Citrate
   b. 5'-AMP
   c. Hydrogen ions
   d. Fructose 2,6-bisphosphate (F-2,6-BP)
   e. ATP

8. Lactate:
   a. Is formed from pyruvate in a reaction catalysed by a dehydrogenase
   b. Formation is favoured by a high $[NADH]/[NAD^+]$ ratio in the cytosol of muscle cells
   c. Is a major product of glucose metabolism in red blood cells
   d. Formation occurs when the TCA cycle is operating at capacity

9. The following statements describe pyruvate dehydrogenase and α-ketoglutarate dehydrogenase:
   a. Both enzymes are multi-enzyme complexes with multiple coenzymes and cofactors
   b. The action of either enzyme on its substrate results in the formation of a product which contains coenzyme A
   c. Neither enzyme is present in red blood cells
   d. NADH is a product of the action of either enzyme on its substrate
   e. Pyruvate dehydrogenase is a cytosolic enzyme whereas α-ketoglutarate dehydrogenase is found in the mitochondria

10. Identify the single correct statement concerning general aspects of energy metabolism in the body:
    a. Glucose is the only fuel that can be oxidised to produce ATP in the body
    b. The TCA cycle, the electron transport chain and ATP synthase are all located in mitochondria of cells
    c. The overall free energy change in a catabolic pathway need not be negative
    d. ATP has only one pyrophosphate bond
    e. The Na^+/K^+ pump does not use ATP

11. The following statements describe the mobilisation and utilisation of fatty acids in the body:
    a. Fatty acids are transported in plasma bound to albumin

b. On a molar basis, fatty acid oxidation to carbon dioxide and water yields more ATP than do carbohydrates

c. Fatty acid oxidation to carbon dioxide and water requires a functional TCA cycle

d. Fatty acids are excellent fuels for skeletal muscle

e. It is coenzyme A derivatives of fatty acids that are beta-oxidised

12. Acetoacetate:
   a. Is the immediate precursor of both β-hydroxybutyrate and acetone in the body
   b. Cannot be used by the brain as a fuel
   c. Levels in blood increase in the fasted state
   d. Is produced by a metabolic pathway in which HMG-CoA is a key intermediate
   e. Formation is critical in long-term starvation

13. The oxidation of long-chain fatty acids (such as palmitate):
   a. Provides much of the ATP required by cardiac muscle
   b. In a tissue requires the presence of carnitine
   c. Provides much of the ATP used by red blood cells
   d. Occurs in the smooth endoplasmic reticulum of liver and muscle cells
   e. Can lead to increased production of ketone bodies

True/false questions

Are the following statements true or false?

1. Glycogen, cellulose and starch are all polymers of glucose.
2. Maltose is a disaccharide, with the monosaccharide units being glucose and fructose.
3. Hexokinase is inhibited by glucose 6-phosphate, the product of the reaction that it catalyses.
4. In most adults, the gut has a greater ability to hydrolyse lactose than it does starch.
5. Insulin action on adipocytes increases the amount of GLUT4 in the plasma membrane of these cells.
6. GLUT2 has a higher K_m for glucose than does GLUT1.
7. Pyruvate dehydrogenase is a key enzyme in the anaerobic pathway of glucose metabolism in the body.
8. The metabolism of one glucose to pyruvate through the glycolytic pathway produces 2NADH.
9. ATP synthase is localised to the matrix of mitochondria.
10. Carbon monoxide binds to both haemoglobin and cytochrome oxidase.

11. The pyruvate dehydrogenase complex is subject to control by allosteric and phosphorylation/dephosphorylation mechanisms.
12. The reaction in glycolysis catalysed by pyruvate kinase is an example of substrate-level phosphorylation.
13. Most of the oxygen used in animal tissues is used by cytochrome oxidase.
14. The respiratory chain in mitochondria contains several proteins that contain metal atoms, including copper and iron.
15. Proton transport associated with the respiratory chain in mitochondria moves protons (hydrogen ions) outwards across the inner mitochondrial membrane when the chain is functioning.
16. Cyanide reacts with cytochrome oxidase in a similar fashion to carbon monoxide.
17. 5'-AMP levels increase when ATP is being utilised at a high rate in cells.
18. Glucose utilisation per gram of tissue is higher in brain than in muscle in a subject at rest.
19. Each complete beta-oxidation cycle for fatty acid oxidation leads to the production of one molecule of NADH and one of $FADH_2$.
20. All of the enzymes of the TCA cycle are located in the mitochondrial matrix.
21. Isocitrate dehydrogenase and α-ketoglutarate dehydrogenase are important control points in the TCA cycle.

Short essay questions

1. Discuss the role of glucose oxidation as it relates to our ability to oxidise fatty acids completely.
2. In 1861, Pasteur observed that when yeast that had been under anaerobic conditions was switched to aerobic conditions, its glucose consumption (and ethanol production) decreased dramatically. Explain this observation using your knowledge of the control of glycolysis.
3. Explain one way in which cells that are carrying out aerobic metabolism of glucose deal with the impermeability of the inner mitochondrial membrane to NADH.
4. Discuss how the process of oxidative phosphorylation in mitochondria is affected by the presence of 2, 4-dinitrophenol.
5. Prepare 'balance sheets' that explain the number of ATPs generated when (a) three molecules of glucose and (b) a molecule of an 18-carbon, saturated fatty acid are completely oxidised in cells capable of oxidative phosphorylation and utilising the malate shuttle.

Self-assessment: answers

Multiple choice answers

1. a. **True.** Stage 3 consists of the TCA cycle plus electron transport and ATP synthase. All of the fuels used in the body can feed into the TCA cycle of cells that contain mitochondria. Usually, the fuels are converted by Stage 2 to intermediates such as acetyl-CoA, which is then oxidised in the TCA cycle to carbon dioxide and water, with the attendant production of NADH and $FADH_2$.
   b. **False.** Carbohydrates, fats and protein in our food are digested to monosaccharides, amino acids and fatty acids by the process of digestion in Stage 1 of metabolism.
   c. **True.** Stage 3 occurs in mitochondria where the TCA cycle coupled to electron transport and ATP synthase results in the greatest production of ATP in cells.
   d. **True.** Mitochondria are 'the power houses' of cells.
   e. **False.** Mature erythrocytes do not contain mitochondria.

2. a. **True.** Usually when a catabolic pathway is active, the corresponding anabolic pathway is inhibited and vice versa. This is evidence of the sensible control of opposing pathways.
   b. **False.** This would imply that every step in a pathway has a large negative ΔG, which would make it necessary to have completely unique enzymes for every step in opposing pathways.
   c. **True.** The overall free energy change for a pathway must be negative and, clearly, that would not be possible if catabolic and anabolic pathway were the same, i.e. one of them would have an overall positive ΔG.
   d. **False.** Although many reactions in a pathway may be close to equilibrium, none of the reactions in a pathway are at equilibrium since this would mean no net flux through the pathway.

3. a. **True.** Two of the reactions in glycogenesis from glucose require ATP or UTP.
   b. **False.** This is the stage in metabolism resulting in the generation of most ATP.
   c. **True.** Ions would have to be pumped against the concentration gradient and this is usually associated with the hydrolysis (use) of ATP.
   d. **True.** The formation of amino-acyl-tRNA molecules involves the use of ATP.
   e. **True.** The breakdown of ATP by an ATPase allows for actin and myosin to interact in muscular contraction.

4. a. **False.** Lactase is not involved in the digestion of either amylopectin or amylose. It is involved in the digestion of lactose!
   b. **False.** Maltase activity, present in sucrase, α-dextrinase and glucoamylase, is not involved in the digestion of either. This activity is involved in the digestion of maltose produced from amylopectin and amylose by amylase action.
   c. **True.** The α-dextrinase activity of this complex carbohydrase is required for the hydrolysis of the α-1,6-linkages found in amylopectin but not in amylose.
   d. **False.** Alpha amylase is involved in the digestion of *both* amylopectin and amylose.
   e. **False.** Clearly, this is not the case.

5. a. **True.** Almost all of the reactions involved in the digestion of our dietary fuels are hydrolytic, i.e. the second substrate is water!
   b. **False.** Their optimum pH is close to 7.0 and they have little or no activity in the stomach at pH 3.0.
   c. **True.** It is internal α-1,4-linkages that are hydrolysed (not α-1,6) and there is virtually no production of free glucose.
   d. **False.** Both of these enzymes act in the lumen of the gut.
   e. **True.** Limit dextrins that contain α-1,6-linkages are products (in addition to maltose).

6. a. **True.** Glucokinase is a hexokinase isozyme restricted to liver, gut and beta cells of the islets of Langerhans.
   b. **True.** Only at high concentrations of glucose, as seen following a carbohydrate meal, will large quantities of glucose be metabolised in the liver. When glucose levels are low, the liver is a glucose producer!
   c. **True.** It is hexokinase that is inhibited by glucose 6-phosphate.
   d. **False.** Glucose entry into glycolysis is low except when blood glucose levels are high.

7. a. **False.** Citrate is a negative modulator.
   b. **True.** AMP is a positive modulator.
   c. **False.** Increased hydrogen ion concentration, i.e. low pH, is a negative modulator of PFK-1. This effect relates the acid end-products of glycolysis (pyruvic and lactic acids) to the activity of a rate-controlling step.
   d. **True.** F-2,6-BP and AMP are the most important physiologic positive modulators.
   e. **False.** ATP is both a substrate for PFK-1 and a negative modulator of the enzyme. In fact, the

[ATP] in cells is sufficient to inhibit PFK-1 unless positive modulators such as 5'-AMP and F-2,6-BP are present.

8. a. **True.** The enzyme involved is lactate dehydrogenase.
   b. **True.** The conversion of pyruvate to lactate requires NADH.
   c. **True.** Because red blood cells lack mitochondria, they are dependent upon anaerobic glycolysis for the supply of ATP. In order to maintain an adequate rate of glycolysis, NAD$^+$ must be regenerated by the conversion of pyruvate to lactate.
   d. **True.** Under these circumstances, some pyruvate will be converted to lactate and this allows for ATP production to be supplemented by anaerobic glycolysis.

9. a. **True.** They both have three enzymes catalysing oxidative decarboxylations with five coenzymes or cofactors involved. Pyruvate dehydrogenase is often used when the whole pyruvate dehydrogenase complex (PDC) is intended (of which PDH is one enzyme, E_1).
   b. **True.** The products are acetyl-CoA and succinyl-CoA, respectively.
   c. **True.** Red blood cells do not contain mitochondria.
   d. **True.** NAD$^+$ is the final hydrogen acceptor, with the product being NADH in both cases.
   e. **False.** Both enzymes are sited in the mitochondria of cells.

10. a. **False.** Fatty acids and amino acids are also fuels. The confusion is that glucose is usually the only fuel for cells such as erythrocytes, and the brain.
    b. **True.** These together comprise Stage 3 of metabolism.
    c. **False.** The overall free energy change in all pathways must always be negative!
    d. **False.** ATP has two pyrophosphate bonds and ADP has one.
    e. **False.** The Na$^+$/K$^+$ pump, present in all cells of the body, is the major user of ATP when we are at rest.

11. a. **True.** They are hydrophobic molecules.
    b. **True.** Fatty acids are more reduced fuels than carbohydrates and generate more ATP per carbon when completely oxidised in the body.
    c. **True.** The acetyl-CoA produced by fatty acid beta-oxidation is oxidised in the TCA cycle.
    d. **True.** They are important as fuels in the fasted state and during long-term exercise.
    e. **True.** CoA derivatives of fatty acids are formed and these are beta-oxidised.

12. a. **True.** Reduction of acetoacetate yields β-hydroxybutyrate and spontaneous decarboxylation of acetoacetate produces acetone.
    b. **False.** The brain can use both acetoacetate and β-hydroxybutyrate.
    c. **True.** The level of free fatty acids increase and they are the precursors of ketone bodies in the liver.
    d. **True.** HMG-CoA produced in liver mitochondria is the immediate precursor of acetoacetate. (N.B. Cytosolic HMG-CoA is the precursor of cholesterol.)
    e. **True.** In long-term starvation, the use of acetoacetate by the brain helps survival.

13. a. **True.** Since cardiac muscle never rests, it is sensible that it uses the major fuel of the body for most of its ATP requirements
    b. **True.** Carnitine is required since carnitine palmitoyl transferase I (CPTI) catalyses the formation of acyl-carnitines, which can cross the mitochondrial inner membrane whereas long-chain acyl-CoAs cannot.
    c. **False.** Please remember that red blood cells do not have mitochondria.
    d. **False.** Beta-oxidation occurs in the mitochondria of tissues that can utilise fatty acids as fuels.
    e. **True.** Fatty acid oxidation in the liver can lead to ketone body production there.

True/false answers

1. **True.** Although cellulose is not digested by humans, like starch and glycogen it is a polymer of glucose.
2. **False.** Maltose is a disaccharide formed during the digestion of starch. It has an α-1,4-linkage between two glucoses.
3. **True.** This property distinguishes hexokinase from glucokinase.
4. **False.** Many adults from several ethnic groups show a large decrease in brush border lactase activity as they enter their teens. As a result, they have problems handling the lactose in milk.
5. **True.** Insulin action recruits GLUT4 molecules to the plasma membrane of adipocytes (and muscle), leading to greatly increased glucose uptake.
6. **True.** GLUT2 occurs in tissues that take up glucose from blood when glucose levels are high.
7. **False.** The pyruvate dehydrogenase complex catalyses a reaction that is the main determinant of aerobic metabolism of glucose in well-oxygenated tissues.
8. **True.** The glycolytic pathway has a single NAD$^+$-dependent dehydrogenase.

9. **False.** It spans the inner mitochondrial membrane, allowing it to utilise the proton gradient to drive its reversible ATPase and thus produce ATP from ADP + P_i.

10. **True.** Both are haem proteins and carbon monoxide binds to the ferrous (Fe^{II}) form, thus competing with oxygen!

11. **True.** It is E_1 of the multi-enzyme complex that is controlled by phosphorylation–dephosphorylation. The E_1-kinase and E_1 phosphatase involved are subject to allosteric control by metabolic intermediates.

12. **True.** The reaction phosphoenolpyruvate to pyruvate can be coupled to the formation of ATP from ADP. This is termed 'substrate level' phosphorylation, contrasting it with oxidative phosphorylation.

13. **True.** Cytochrome oxidase catalyses the terminal reaction of the electron transport chain, where molecular oxygen is involved.

14. **True.** In addition to iron-containing cytochromes *b* and *c*, there is cytochrome oxidase, which contains both iron and copper. There are also iron–sulphur proteins.

15. **True.** The proton gradient generated then drives ATP synthesis using ATP synthase.

16. **False.** Cyanide reacts with the ferric (Fe^{III}) form of cytochrome oxidase (and haemoglobin), whereas carbon monoxide reacts with the ferrous (Fe^{II}) form of these haem proteins.

17. **True.** 5'-AMP is formed from ADP in the reaction catalysed by adenylate kinase.

18. **True.** Muscle at rest utilises significant amounts of fatty acids, whereas brain can only use glucose.

19. **True.** NAD$^+$- and FAD-linked dehydrogenases are involved in each beta-oxidation cycle.

20. **False.** Succinate dehydrogenase is located in the inner mitochondrial membrane.

21. **True.** Both are affected by the levels of NADH and ATP.

Short essay answers

1. Fatty acids are oxidised to carbon dioxide and water in the mitochondria of tissues such as liver, skeletal muscle and cardiac muscle. The process of beta-oxidation produces many molecules of acetyl-CoA, which are then oxidised in the TCA cycle leading to the production of NADH and FADH$_2$. However, this process is very dependent upon an adequate supply of oxaloacetate to operate the first step in the TCA cycle. Without the concomitant metabolism of glucose, oxaloacetate is not maintained at adequate

levels. This is one of the reasons for excess ketone body production in type I diabetes mellitus. This question is covered by the old phrase 'fat burns in the flame of carbohydrate'.

2. The introduction of oxygen opens up the great potential for ATP synthesis in mitochondria. As a consequence, the amount of glucose that has to be metabolised to support the same level of work must drop by about 94% (32 ATP aerobic versus 2 ATP anaerobic per glucose). The point of control is the conversion of fructose 6-phosphate to fructose 1,6-bisphosphate, catalysed by phosphofructokinase-1 (PFK-1). ATP is a negative modulator of this enzyme. Therefore, when ATP production from oxidative metabolism increases, PFK-1 will be inhibited and the glycolytic rate will fall. Similar observations have been made using in vitro skeletal muscle preparations that are 'twitching' and glucose metabolism is measured under anaerobic and then aerobic conditions.

3. The glycerol 3-phosphate and malate shuttles are used to overcome this problem. In the former, dihydroxyacetone phosphate is reduced to glycerol 3-phosphate by a cytosolic glycerol 3-phosphate dehydrogenase. A similar dehydrogenase located on the inner mitochondrial membrane reforms dihydroxyacetone phosphate; FADH$_2$ is produced, which has the potential to generate ATP. Thus, NAD$^+$ is regenerated to maintain glycolysis and ATP is also produced. The malate shuttle is more complicated but the principle is similar. Oxaloacetate is reduced to malate in the cytosol and the opposing reaction in mitochondria regenerates oxaloacetate, producing mitochondrial NADH. The complication of this shuttle is that oxaloacetate does not cross the inner mitochondrial membrane and its equivalent amino acid, Aspartate has to be an intermediate to allow this to occur.

4. 2,4-Dinitrophenol (DNP) is a lipid-soluble compound that has acidic and basic forms. When it is added to mitochondria that are actively respiring, it becomes protonated and can pass through the inner mitochondrial membrane. The result is that the proton gradient is collapsed and this will be reflected in a sharp drop in ATP synthesis by ATP synthase (which depends upon that proton gradient!). If one is measuring both ATP synthesis and oxygen utilisation in the mitochondrial preparation, one can see the drop in ATP production accompanied by an increase in oxygen utilisation (respiration). For this reason, DNP is described as an uncoupler: it uncouples oxidation (electron transport chain activity) from phosphorylation (ATP synthesis).

5. (a) **Glucose**

Glycolysis → 2 pyruvate + 2NADH 2ATP

2NADH   malate shuttle   5ATP

2Pyruvate → 2 acetyl-CoA + 2NADH
2 NADH   5ATP

2 Acetyl-CoA   TCA cycle,   20ATP
               ETC,
               ATP synthase

Total ATP for 1 glucose   **32**

Total ATP for 3 glucose   **96**

(b) **Stearate**

Activation of stearate   Uses equivalent
                                of 2ATP

8 Beta-oxidations 9 acetyl-CoA
                   $8FADH_2$
                   8NADH

$8FADH_2$ 12ATP
8NADH   20ATP
9Acetyl-CoA   TCA cycle,   90ATP
                   ETC
                   ATP
                   synthase

Total ATP for 1 stearate   **122 − 2 = 120**

In conclusion: **The complete oxidation of stearate yields more ATP per carbon than glucose.**

Other pathways of carbohydrate metabolism

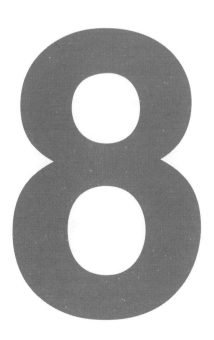

8.1 Glycogen metabolism

Glycogen is found in many cell types in the body but only in high concentration in liver and muscle. A fed man weighing 70 kg will have about 1.6 kg liver containing about 100 g glycogen and 35 kg of muscle containing approximately 400 g glycogen. At a caloric value of 17 kJ/g, the stores of glycogen represent about 8500 kJ of fuel. Relative to the fat stores, this is a small reserve yet it has great functional significance. Glycogen is stored in the fed state and utilised during fasting and exercise. Synthesis (*glycogenesis*) and breakdown (*glycogenolysis*) occur by separate but related pathways (Fig. 67) and are controlled in an integrated fashion via allosteric and covalent mechanisms; hormonal control is very critical. The enzymes of glycogen metabolism are associated with the glycogen granules in cells.

Glycogenesis

The key points about the storage of glycogen are:

- a step unique to glycogenesis is the formation of UDP-glucose from G-1-P and the pyrimidine nucleotide, UTP
- the glucose moieties added to form glycogen come directly from UDP-glucose
- each glycogen molecule contains a protein, *glycogenin*. The identification of this protein explained how the synthesis of the large glycogen molecule is initiated. Glycogenin has enzymatic activity catalyzing the addition of the first 4–8 glucose moieties to a tyrosine in glycogenin, using UDPG as the source of the glucoses

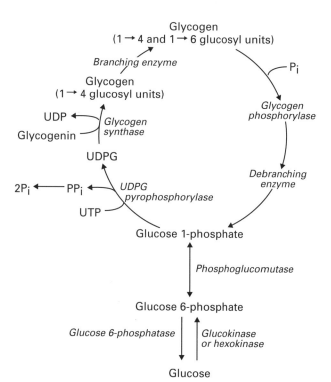

Fig. 67 Pathways of glycogenesis and glycogenolysis.

- glycogen synthase transfers the glucose moiety of UDPG to the non-reducing end of the primer, giving a polymer with α-1,4-linkages
- glycogen is branched and the *branching enzyme* involved is a 4:6-transferase.

Glycogenolysis

Key points about the breakdown of stored glycogen are:

- *glycogen phosphorylase* catalyses the interaction of inorganic phosphate (P_1) with terminal α-1:4-glycosidic bonds at the multiple non-reducing ends of glycogen to yield G-1-P
- phosphorylase contains the coenzyme pyridoxal phosphate
- the branching of glycogen means that there are many sites (ends) for phosphorolysis and this allows for rapid production of G-1-P, which is beneficial in both liver and muscle
- *debranching enzyme* has two distinct catalytic sites and is important for complete utilisation of glycogen. Glucoses are removed from a branch by phosphorylase action until there are only four glucoses attached. Then, a *4:4 glucan transferase* transfers the trisaccharide attached to the glucose in a 1,6- linkage to a different chain. This leaves a single glucose attached at the branch point and the α-1,6-linkage is hydrolysed by *α-1:6-glucosidase* to yield free glucose
- there are different end-products in liver compared with muscle. Muscle lacks *glucose 6-phosphatase (G-6-Pase)* so the end-products of increased muscle glycogenolysis will be pyruvate and lactate (following glycolysis); liver contains G-6-Pase which means that the end product is glucose
- clearly this is consistent with the role of glycogen in muscle, which is to supply that tissue with ATP and the role of glycogen in liver to maintain blood glucose levels.

Glycogenesis and glycogenolysis are controlled in an integrated fashion

It is essential to consider the control of the synthetic and breakdown pathways together (Fig. 68). The control steps in glycogenesis and glycogenolysis are catalysed by *glycogen synthase* and *glycogen phosphorylase*, respectively. They are both subject to control by allosteric and covalent modification.

Allosteric control

ATP and G-6-P levels high	glycogen synthase active; phosphorylase inactive
AMP levels high	glycogen synthase inactive; phosphorylase active

High [ATP] in muscle is indicative of high energy charge and is a signal that there is less need for

(a) The fasting state: low insulin levels, elevated glucagon and/or adrenaline

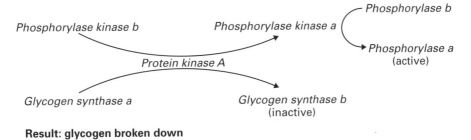

Result: glycogen broken down

(b) The fed state: high insulin levels, low glucagon levels

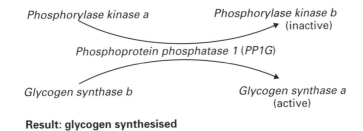

Result: glycogen synthesised

Fig. 68 Control of glycogenesis and glycogenolysis in the fasted (a) and fed (b) states.

glycogen breakdown. In contrast, increased [AMP] is a signal that ATP utilisation is high. Elevated [G-6-P] in both liver and muscle is associated with the fed state and increased availability of glucose (for storage).

Covalent control

cyclic AMP-dependent	glycogen synthase inactive;
protein kinase A active	phosphorylase active
phosphoprotein phosphatase	glycogen synthase active;
active	phosphorylase inactive

Both enzymes exist in active and inactive states. In each case, the active form is designated 'a', and the inactive form is 'b'. Phosphorylation occurs when there is an increase in cyclic AMP. Dephosphorylation involves a phosphoprotein phosphatase.

Hormonal control

Glucagon (liver) and adrenaline (muscle) action results in increased concentration of cyclic AMP within these cells and activation of PKA. This results in activation of phosphorylase and inactivation of glycogen synthase. Further description of these control mechanisms can be found in Chapters 11 and 18.

Insulin release in the fed state leads to the dephosphorylation of both phosphorylase and glycogen synthase. This results in inactivation of phosphorylase and activation of glycogen synthase (Chapter 11).

Effects of calcium

Phosphorylase kinase is also activated by increased concentrations of calcium. This is explained by the fact that phosphorylase kinase has four subunits – αβγδ – and the δ-subunit is the calcium-binding polypeptide *calmodulin*. Binding of calcium activates the enzyme

> **BOX 8.1**
> **Clinical note: Glycogen storage disease**
>
> Defects in enzymes of glycogenolysis usually result in a glycogen storage disease. Subjects with defective branching enzyme in liver have a tendency to develop hypoglycaemia, but the most severe form is seen in those with defective liver G-6-Pase. Subjects with defective muscle phosphorylase cannot support high levels of physical activity.

leading, finally, to increased phosphorylation of the α- and β-subunits of phosphorylase kinase (and, thus, to activation). Calcium is an important signal for muscle contraction; activation of glycogen breakdown will lead to the increased ATP formation required to support this. Adrenaline action on the liver is mediated via α_1-adrenoceptors, leading to increased levels of inositol trisphosphate (p. 230) and calcium.

8.2 Gluconeogenesis

This pathway is defined as 'the formation of glucose from non-carbohydrate sources'. Gluconeogenesis is vital to normal brain function in the fasting state in that the brain receives its principal fuel, glucose, directly from the blood. Despite the high concentration of glycogen in the liver, its total content would be used up by about 16–24 hours of fasting. As a result, glucose synthesis is vital. The liver is the principal site for gluconeogenesis although the kidney also has the pathway (and it is stimulated in response to acidosis!).

Glucogenic precursors include amino acids, lactate and glycerol

Amino acids. Many amino acids are glucogenic (Chapter 9). The metabolism of their carbons results in a net increase in oxaloacetate. This means that any amino acid whose carbons enter the TCA cycle at any point other than acetyl-CoA or whose carbons are converted to pyruvate will be glucogenic.

Lactate and glycerol. Lactate and glycerol are released during anaerobic glycolysis in muscle and fat mobilisation from adipose tissue, respectively, as are other significant gluconeogenic substrates. Lactate dehydrogenase in liver converts lactate to pyruvate. The liver contains a kinase that converts glycerol to glycerol 3-phosphate, the oxidation of which yields dihydroxyacetone phosphate, a gluconeogenesis intermediate. Glycerol is the substrate most easily converted to glucose.

The gluconeogenesis pathway

Most of the reactions of gluconeogenesis are catalysed by the enzymes of the glycolytic sequence (Fig. 69). Because glycolysis and gluconeogenesis are opposing pathways, there has to be control so that glucose

formation or breakdown will occur in a physiologically sound fashion. The flux through the respective pathways is governed by:

a. allosteric effectors
b. covalent modification of enzymes
c. enzyme concentrations.

Covalent modification of key enzymes is brought about (in the main) by fluctuations in the ratio of insulin to glucagon in blood. Insulin is the principal modulator in the fed state when glycolysis should be active; glucagon in the fasting state when gluconeogenesis should be active. Three steps in glycolysis are virtually irreversible and have to be bypassed in gluconeogenesis; three substrate cycles are involved where control can be imposed (Fig. 70).

PEP/pyruvate substrate cycle

- requires two enzymes, acting in sequence
- the first step from pyruvate is catalysed by *pyruvate carboxylase* (PC), a biotin-requiring enzyme of mitochondria, and yields oxaloacetate. PC utilises ATP and has an absolute requirement for acetyl-CoA as an allosteric activator
- the next reaction in this substrate cycle is catalysed

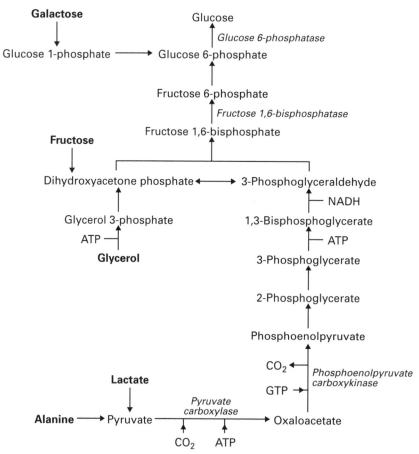

Fig. 69 The gluconeogenesis pathway. Enzymes catalysing reactions unique to gluconeogenesis are shown. The reactions are shown that are involved in the conversion of lactate, alanine, glycerol, fructose and galactose to glucose. This pathway mainly occurs in the liver.

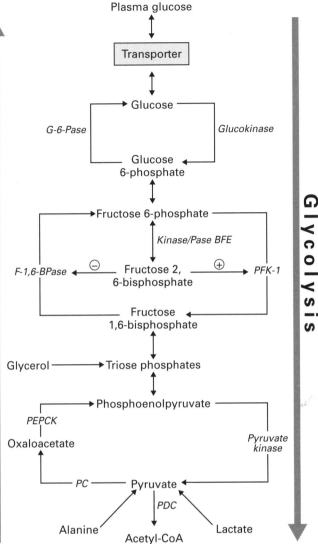

Gluconeogenesis / **Glycolysis**

Fig. 70 Integrated control of hepatic gluconeogenesis and glycolysis. (This schematic is based upon Granner & O'Brien (1992) *Diabetes Care* 15: 369–395.)

by *phosphoenolpyruvate carboxykinase* (PEPCK), which uses GTP

- control is through activation of PC by an increase in the level of acetyl-CoA; the acetyl-CoA is derived from increased utilisation of fatty acids in the liver during fasting. Also involved is induction of PEPCK by glucagon action
- liver-type pyruvate kinase is allosterically activated by F-1,6-BP and inhibited by alanine and ATP; it is also inactivated by phosphorylation. Therefore, the increase in alanine and glucagon in the fasted state results in complete inhibition of pyruvate kinase, avoiding a futile cycle and promoting gluconeogenesis.

F-6-P/F-1,6-BP substrate cycle

- *fructose-1,6-bisphosphatase* (F-1,6-BPase) converts F-1,6-BP to F-6-P and inorganic phosphate
- the level of fructose 2,6-bisphosphate (F-2,6-BP) determines the flux through this substrate cycle.

- F-2,6-BP is controlled by a bifunctional enzyme (BFE) which has kinase and phosphatase activities and is itself subjected to control by phosphorylation/dephosphorylation
- phosphorylation of BFE occurs when glucagon has increased PKA activity; the F-2,6-BPase of the BFE is activated, F-2,6-BP levels fall and gluconeogenesis is turned on
- dephosphorylation of BFE occurs when insulin levels are high, F-2,6-BP rises, leading to inhibition of gluconeogenesis and activation of glycolysis; the resulting increase in F-1,6-BP will activate glycolysis at the pyruvate kinase step.

G-6-P/glucose substrate cycle

- *glucose-6-phosphatase* (G-6-Pase), located on the cisternal surface of the endoplasmic reticulum, catalyses the hydrolysis of G-6-P to give free glucose and inorganic phosphate
- clearly, G-6-Pase is essential for glucose production to occur from both glycogenolysis and gluconeogenesis. It is not present in muscle!
- there is no evidence as yet for short-term regulation of this cycle but the complete details of the G-6-Pase system are only now being determined in the late 1990s.

In summary. It is the PEP/pyruvate cycle which limits the rate of gluconeogenesis, since the rate of glucose synthesis is much greater for substrates that enter the pathway at the triose phosphate level (e.g. glycerol) than for substrates such as alanine and lactate that enter the pathway through pyruvate. Pyruvate kinase is inhibited when glucose production should be favoured (i.e. in the fasted state) and is active when glucose is being processed in the fed state towards pyruvate, acetyl-CoA and fatty acid synthesis. The importance of modulating the level of F-2,6-BP is that it provides a mechanism for controlling F-1,6-BP, which is itself a major modulator of pyruvate kinase.

Sources of glucose

The glucose–alanine cycle connects muscle and liver metabolism

The glucose–alanine cycle (Fig. 71) describes the movement of alanine from muscle in the fasting state, where it is produced by increased protein turnover. Gluconeogenesis from the alanine in the liver allows for increased glucose secretion into the blood where it can be used by the CNS as fuel. This process also occurs during exercise and the glucose produced from alanine can return to muscle to be used as a fuel.

The Cori cycle also connects muscle and liver metabolism

The Cori cycle (Fig. 72) involves lactate leaving skeletal muscle during vigorous exercise, being converted to

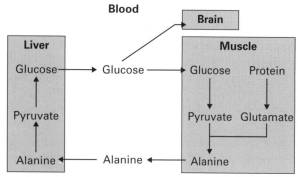

Fig. 71 The glucose–alanine cycle.

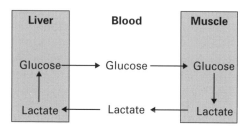

Fig. 72 The Cori cycle. In the Cori cycle, lactate released from muscle is reconverted to glucose in the liver.

glucose in the liver and returning to muscle to be used as a fuel.

Galactose and fructose are glucogenic

Glucose can also be synthesised from galactose and fructose in the liver (Figs 73 and 74).

8.3 Pentose phosphate pathway

The pentose phosphate pathway (also called the hexose monophosphate shunt) is an important alternative pathway for the oxidative metabolism of G-6-P leading to the production of pentose phosphate and NADPH. It is important to distinguish this pathway from glycolysis in that it is a significant pathway of glucose metabolism but does not result in ATP synthesis. The pentose phosphate pathway is important because:

- it produces ribose 5-phosphate, which is required for the biosynthesis of purine and pyrimidine nucleotides and, therefore, for RNA and DNA and the numerous nucleotides that play key roles in intermediary metabolism including ATP, UTP, CTP, GTP, S-adenosyl-methioninine, FAD, NAD and NADP
- it produces 'reducing power' in the form of NADPH, which is required for the synthesis of fatty acids, cholesterol and steroid hormones
- it interconverts 3-,4-,5-,6-, and 7-carbon sugars
- in plants, the pathway is modified to participate in the formation of glucose from carbon dioxide in photosynthesis.

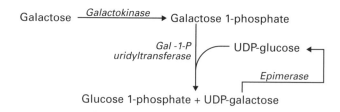

Fig. 73 Glucose production from galactose.

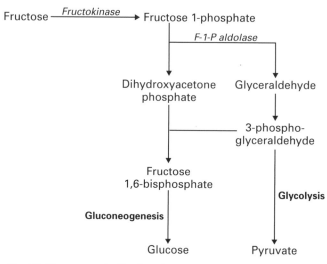

Fig. 74 Glucose production from fructose.

BOX 8.2
Clinical note: Galactosaemia

Newborn babies are tested to ensure that they do not have excessive levels of galactose in their blood since galactosaemia can be dangerous. It is readily treated by avoiding lactose in the diet.

The overall design of the pathway

It is convenient to divide the pathway (Fig. 75) into two phases:

The oxidative phase

- yields pentose phosphate and NADPH
- consists of three reactions, two catalysed by NADP+-linked dehydrogenases, including the rate-controlling step involving *G-6-P dehydrogenase* (G-6-PDH)
- net reaction is 6 G-6-P → 6 (ribulose 5-phosphate) + 12NADPH + 6CO$_2$.

The cycling phase

- allows for the conversion of pentose phosphate to F-6-P and, therefore, G-6-P

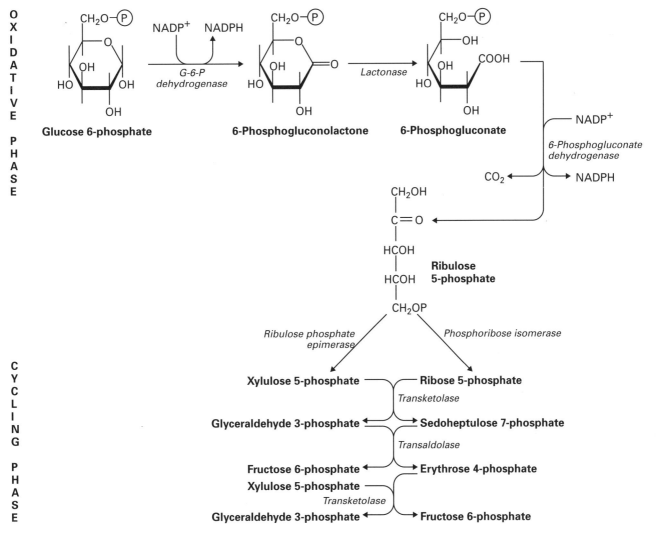

Fig. 75 The pentose phosphate pathway. The main function of this pathway is production of NADPH used in reductive biosynthesis and ribose 5-phosphate needed for nucleotide synthesis.

- pentose phosphates are converted to the glycolytic intermediates F-6-P and glyceraldehyde 3-phosphate through a series of reactions catalysed in sequence by transketolase, transaldolase and, again, transketolase
- transketolase has thiamine pyrophosphate (TPP) as coenzyme
- net reaction is 6 (ribulose 5-phosphate) → 5 G-6-P (via F-6-P).

Cells that have a high requirement for both ribose 5-phosphate and NADPH will have low activity of the 'cycling phase'. In cells that mainly require NADPH, both phases occur, which, in effect, means that six complete cycles occur for each molecule of G-6-P and 6 molecules of carbon dioxide and 12 molecules of NADPH are produced.

Self-assessment: questions

Multiple choice questions

1. When cyclic AMP levels in liver increase:
   a. Glycogen synthase is activated
   b. Phosphoprotein phosphatase 1 (PP1G) is phosphorylated and, therefore, activated
   c. Phosphorylase kinase b is rapidly converted to phosphorylase kinase a
   d. Phosphorylase a is converted to phosphorylase b
   e. The rate of glycogenolysis is increased

2. Glycogen synthase activity:
   a. Is increased by dephosphorylation
   b. Is low when protein kinase A activity is high
   c. In cooperation with branching enzyme yields a polysaccharide that is highly branched
   d. Is present both in muscle and liver
   e. In liver is increased in the fasted state

3. Which of the following statements correctly describe what happens when acetyl-CoA is abundant in a liver cell:
   a. Pyruvate carboxylase is activated
   b. If ATP levels are low, oxaloacetate is diverted to gluconeogenesis
   c. If ATP levels are high, oxaloacetate is diverted to gluconeogenesis
   d. Pyruvate dehydrogenase is activated

4. During the operation of the Cori cycle, which of the following enzymes are directly involved:
   a. Hexokinase (muscle)
   b. Pyruvate kinase (liver)
   c. Pyruvate carboxylase (liver)
   d. Glucose- 6-phosphatase (liver)
   e. Lactate dehydrogenase (muscle)

5. A decrease in the level of fructose-2,6-bisphosphate (F-2,6-BP) in hepatocytes:
   a. Activates fructose-1,6-bisphosphatase
   b. Is brought about by phosphorylation of the bifunctional enzyme (BFE)
   c. Accompanies an increase in blood insulin levels
   d. Is brought about by the action of a phosphatase on F-2,6-BP
   e. Accompanies the fasting state

6. Which of the following would be a consequence of a lack of glycogen phosphorylase in skeletal muscle:
   a. Fasting hypoglycaemia and increased muscle glycogen
   b. Pain from muscle cramps upon exercise and increased muscle glycogen
   c. Fasting hyperglycaemia and increased muscle glycogen
   d. Fasting hyperglycaemia and decreased muscle glycogen
   e. Increased ability to run sprints

7. The following statements describe the control of glycogen metabolism in the body:
   a. In both liver and skeletal muscle, insulin action leads to phosphorylation of glycogen synthase
   b. In both liver and skeletal muscle, insulin action leads to phosphorylation of glycogen phosphorylase
   c. Glycogen phosphorylase and glycogen synthetase are chiefly controlled by hormones such as insulin and glucagon affecting the transcription of the genes coding for the enzymes
   d. An increase in calcium ions in muscle leads to stimulation of glycogen phosphorylase
   e. Cyclic 3',5'-AMP is the second messenger for glucagon action on liver glycogen metabolism

8. The following enzymes should have high activity in the liver during the fasting state in order for gluconeogenesis to proceed at a high rate:
   a. Phosphoenolpyruvate carboxykinase (PEPCK)
   b. Pyruvate carboxylase
   c. Pyruvate dehydrogenase
   d. Pyruvate kinase
   e. Fructose 1,6-bisphosphatase

9. If a cell requires NADPH but does not require ribose 5-phosphate:
   a. Only the oxidative phase of the pentose phosphate pathway would be operational
   b. The ribose 5-phosphate produced is destroyed
   c. Glycolytic intermediates would flow into the reversible (cycling) phase of the pentose phosphate pathway
   d. In effect, all of the carbons of G-6-P would be converted to carbon dioxide
   e. Both the oxidative and cycling phases of the pathway would operate

10. Glucose 6-phosphate dehydrogenase:
    a. Is a mitochondrial enzyme
    b. Is a key enzyme in an ATP-yielding pathway
    c. Catalyses a reaction that produces ribose 5-phosphate
    d. Is an NADP-linked dehydrogenase
    e. Is present in hepatocytes and erythrocytes

True/false questions

Are the following statements true or false?

1. The gluconeogenic pathway from pyruvate requires input of both NADH and ATP.
2. Thiamine pyrophosphate is a coenzyme for transketolase of the pentose phosphate pathway.
3. Even-numbered fatty acids are glucogenic in the liver.
4. The pyruvate kinase activity in liver is inhibited by alanine and by phosphorylation.
5. In glycogenolysis, debranching produces one free glucose per branch point.
6. Glucagon activates glycogenolysis in both liver and skeletal muscle.
7. 5'-AMP is a positive modulator of glycogen phosphorylase and phosphofructokinase-1.
8. Glycogenesis and glycogenolysis occur in different intracellular compartments of the liver and muscle.
9. Acetyl-CoA activates pyruvate carboxylase and thus increases gluconeogenesis.
10. The pentose phosphate pathway produces ribose 5-phosphate required for nucleotide synthesis.

Short essay questions

1. Describe the active form of the enzyme catalysing the rate-limiting step of glycogenesis and then derive from that the nature of the inactive form. Repeat for the enzyme catalysing the rate-limiting step in glycogenolysis. Describe how these changes fit logically into a system to control glycogen metabolism.
2. Describe how gluconeogenesis in the liver is controlled in order to maintain glucose homeostasis during the fasting state.

Case history

The following data were obtained from a patient.

A liver biopsy sample when incubated in the presence of 10^{-9} M adrenaline or glucagon showed increased production of pyruvate and lactate. Incubation with uniformly-labelled [^{14}C]-alanine showed that radioactivity could be incorporated into glycogen but not into glucose. A muscle biopsy sample when incubated in the presence of 10^{-9} M adrenaline showed a large increase in lactate production. The glycogen isolated from muscle and liver had normal structure. Liver glycogen concentrations were significantly above normal.

What diagnosis are these observations consistent with?

Self-assessment: answers

Multiple choice answers

1. a. **False.** The increase in cyclic AMP leads to activation of protein kinase A. This in turn phosphorylates glycogen synthase, giving the inactive form.
    b. **False.** PP1G becomes phosphorylated when insulin acts on liver.
    c. **True.** The activation of protein kinase A brings about the conversion of phosphorylase kinase b to the a form (which is active).
    d. **False.** Since phosphorylase kinase has been activated, phosphorylase b will be converted to the active a form.
    e. **True.** Since phosphorylase has been converted to its active form, then the rate of glycogenolysis will increase.

2. a. **True.** The activation involves enhanced activity of PP1G, a phosphatase that removes a phosphate from glycogen synthase, and glycogen synthesis is 'turned on'.
    b. **True.** Protein kinase A action would lead to phosphorylation and, therefore, inactivation of glycogen synthase.
    c. **True.** The branching serves several functions, most important being that it gives multiple points of attack on any one glycogen molecule – something that is a plus when one needs to turn on glycogenolysis quickly.
    d. **True.** Its function in muscle is to store fuel for that tissue. Its function in liver is connected with glucose homeostasis.
    e. **False.** In the fasted state, one needs to break down liver glycogen to glucose not synthesise more glycogen.

3. a. **True.** Activation of this enzyme starts gluconeogenesis from pyruvate.
    b. **False.** Low ATP would be a signal for catabolism and synthesis of ATP.
    c. **True.** Gluconeogenesis requires ATP.
    d. **False.** PDC is inhibited by high acetyl-CoA levels. The consequence of such an activation would be for even more acetyl-CoA to be formed and gluconeogenesis would be inhibited.

4. a. **True.** Hexokinase catalyses the first step in glycolysis leading to the production of lactate in muscle.
    b. **False.** The pyruvate kinase-catalysed reaction is part of glycolysis not gluconeogenesis.
    c. **True.** Pyruvate carboxylase catalyses the formation of oxaloacetate from the pyruvate derived from lactate.

d. **True.** This enzyme is required to enable glucose to be produced and secreted from the liver.
e. **True.** This enzyme allows lactate to be made in muscle, from which it is secreted.

5. a. **True.** It is critical that F-2,6-BP levels fall in order for gluconeogenesis to proceed at a high rate.
    b. **True.** Phosphorylation of PFK-2/F-2,6-BPase (BFE) activates the phosphatase, leading to a fall in F-2,6-BP.
    c. **False.** Insulin action leads to an increase in F-2,6-BP, activation of glycolysis and inhibition of gluconeogenesis.
    d. **True.** The phosphatase is in BFE.
    e. **True.** Glucagon increase leads to cyclic-AMP-dependent protein kinase A activation, which phosphorylates BFE.

6. a. **False.** Muscle glycogen does not contribute in a significant way to blood glucose homeostasis.
    b. **True.** During exercise the breakdown of muscle glycogen contributes in an important way to the support of exercise and the lack of glycogen phosphorylase will compromise this, resulting in pain (cramps) during exercise. The low rate of glycogen breakdown results in increase levels of glycogen in muscle (this is McArdle's syndrome).
    c. **False.** Again, blood glucose is not affected (and is certainly not increased) if muscle glycogen breakdown is impaired.
    d. **False.** For the reasons cited above. Also, glycogen levels will be increased.
    e. **False.** Since muscle glycogen metabolism is used to support sprinting, the defect in glycogen breakdown will reduce the ability to sprint.

7. a. **False.** Insulin action leads to dephosphorylation (and activation) of glycogen synthase.
    b. **False.** Insulin action leads to dephosphorylation of both glycogen synthase and glycogen phosphorylase.
    c. **False.** Although there are effects of the hormones on gene transcription, the major control is by changes in phosphorylation/dephosphorylation of the enzymes themselves.
    d. **True.** One subunit of phosphorylase is calmodulin, a calcium-binding protein. Calcium binding promotes phosphorylation of other subunits and activation of phosphorylase.
    e. **True.** Increased cyclic AMP (caused by glucagon) activates protein kinase A, which in

turn brings about phosphorylation of phosphorylase kinase and then phosphorylase.

8. a. **True.** This is a key enzyme in the pyruvate/PEP substrate cycle, which allow PEP to be formed from pyruvate.
   b. **True.** Another enzyme in the pyruvate/PEP substrate cycle, it catalyses the formation of oxaloacetate from pyruvate.
   c. **False.** If this enzyme were active, then pyruvate formed from alanine or lactate would be converted to acetyl-CoA and, therefore, be unable to generate glucose.
   d. **False.** If this enzyme were active then a 'futile' cycle would be set up, with any PEP formed being reconverted to pyruvate.
   e. **True.** This enzyme activity allows for F-1,6-BP formed from gluconeogenic substrates to be converted to F-6-P en route to glucose.

9. a. **False.** The oxidative phase gives 2NADPH plus pentose 5-phosphate.
   b. **False.** This is not the solution.
   c. **False.** That would result in ribose 5-phosphate synthesis and no NADPH.
   d. **True.** The end result would be oxidation of G-6-P to $6CO_2$ with 12NADPH being formed per glucose.
   e. **True.** This would give NADPH plus carbon dioxide as products.

10. a. **False.** This enzyme is localised to the cytosol of cells.
    b. **False.** The pentose phosphate pathway does not generate ATP.
    c. **False.** The product is NADPH plus 6-phosphogluconolactone.
    d. **True.** Remember a key function of this pathway is to produce NADPH.
    e. **True.** NADPH is required in both types of cell.

True/false answers

1. **True.** NADH is required to convert 1,3-bisphosphoglycerate to 3-phosphoglyceraldehyde and ATP (or GTP) is required at three of the steps.
2. **True.** Thiamine deficiency results in decreased activity of the pentose phosphate pathway.
3. **False.** Since they are converted entirely to acetyl-CoA, they are ketogenic rather than glucogenic.
4. **True.** These are important signals leading to inhibition of pyruvate kinase, meaning that gluconeogenesis will then proceed more effectively.
5. **True.** The debranching system includes a 1,6-glucosidase that catalyses the hydrolysis of 1,6-bonds, yielding one free glucose per bond.
6. **False.** Glucagon has no effect on muscle glycogen metabolism. Adrenaline is the hormone that activates muscle glycogenolysis.

7. **True.** An increase in intracellular AMP is a signal that cells require to turn on ATP synthesis; it activates both phosphorylase b, the rate-controlling step in glycogen breakdown, and phosphofructokinase-1, an important rate-controlling step in glycolysis.
8. **False.** The enzymes involved are found in the cytosol associated with glycogen granules.
9. **True.** This enzyme is almost inactive without bound acetyl-CoA.
10. **True.** Its major function is to make NADPH and ribose 5-phosphate.

Short essay answers

1. (a) Glycogen synthase catalyses the rate-determining step in glycogenesis and it is active when it is dephosphorylated. Logically, since it would be inefficient for glycogenolysis to be active when glycogenesis is active, the enzyme catalysing the rate-determining step in glycogenolysis, glycogen phosphorylase, must be inactive when dephosphorylated. (b) Similarly in glycogenolysis, phosphorylase is active when it is phosphorylated and glycogen synthase, in contrast, must be inactive when phosphorylated.

   Under conditions when glycogen should be synthesised -- the fed state and when insulin and glucose levels are high – glycogen synthase and phosphorylase are both dephosphorylated, with the former then being active and the latter inactive. Under conditions when glycogenolysis should be promoted – the fasted state as far as liver glycogen is concerned and exercise as far as muscle glycogen is concerned – both control enzymes are phosphorylated, leading to activation of phosphorylase and inactivation of glycogen synthase.

2. Gluconeogenesis is controlled at the level of two of the substrate cycles that involve the opposing pathways of glycolysis and gluconeogenesis (Fig. 70).

   The pyruvate/PEP substrate cycle. Fasting conditions should lead to increased conversion of pyruvate to PEP via oxaloacetate. This is mediated largely by the action of glucagon, alanine and acetyl-CoA. Glucagon stimulates an increase in cyclic AMP, leading to activation of protein kinase A (PKA). This activity results in the phosphorylation of pyruvate kinase and to its inactivation. Alanine, which enters liver at an enhanced rate during fasting (the source is muscle protein turnover), also inhibits pyruvate kinase. Inhibition of pyruvate kinase means that any PEP formed from alanine or lactate via pyruvate and oxaloacetate will not be dissipated and futile cycling is avoided. Also, during fasting, more fatty acids are mobilised to the liver and their oxidation yields acetyl-CoA, an activator of pyruvate carboxylase, resulting in increased production of oxaloacetate from which PEP, and eventually glucose, is formed. The increase in acetyl-CoA production also inhibits the PDC and this will also increase the overall efficiency of gluconeogenesis. Glucagon increases the transcription of the PEPCK gene. This induction increases the conversion of oxaloacetate to PEP.

The F-6-P/F-1,6-BP substrate cycle. The major control of this substrate cycle is via the control of the level of F-2,6-BP, an inhibitor of fructose 1,6-bisphosphatase (F-1,6-BPase) (and activator of phosphofructokinase (PFK) 1). Under fasting conditions, increased activity of PKA leads to phosphorylation of a bifunctional enzyme (BFE) – PFK-2/F-2,6-BPase – and this results in inactivation of PFK-2 and activation of the F-2,6-BPase, with the latter decreasing the levels of F-2,6-BP. The end result is relaxation of the inhibition of F-1,6-BPase and production of F-6-P, which then is converted to G-6-P and, finally, to glucose. The last reaction is catalysed by the essential G-6-Pase. This is a classic example of combined allosteric and covalent control. The BFE (and, therefore, the level of F-2,6-BP) is subjected to control by phosphorylation/dephosphorylation. The F-6-P/F-1,6-BP substrate pair is subjected to allosteric control of PFK-1 and F-1,6-BPase by the level of F-2,6-BP.

Case history answer

It is clear that both liver and muscle are able to convert their glycogen into pyruvate or lactate when stimulated: liver by glucagon or adrenaline, muscle by adrenaline. The fact that the glycogen in liver was of normal structure but was grossly elevated indicates that the glycogenesis pathway was active. The key piece of information is the ability of the liver sample to convert carbons from alanine into glycogen but not into glucose. This implies that the reaction catalysed by glucose 6-phosphatase was abnormal. This is the finding in glycogen storage disease type I, also known as von Gierke's disease. If you had such a patient, their abdomen would be abnormal owing to great liver enlargement and they would suffer from frequent occurrences of hypoglycaemia. Recall that glucose 6-phosphatase is required for glucose production by the liver from both the glycogenolytic and gluconeogenic pathways!

Protein and amino acid metabolism

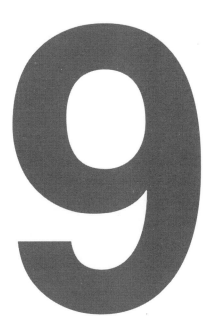

9.1 General aspects

Amino acids are required for the synthesis of proteins and many other vital body components (Fig. 76). Some can be made in the body from by-products of carbohydrate and fat metabolism but other amino acids must be obtained from the diet. The amino acid pool in the body not only reflects those obtained from the diet but also the continuous breakdown of endogenous proteins. Utilisation of amino acids for the synthesis of protein and other nitrogenous constituents of the organism depletes the amino acid pool. Any excess of supply over demand is oxidised to glucose and fatty acid precursors as well as ATP. The carbon skeletons of amino acids are processed by unique pathways leading to the formation of acetyl-CoA and various TCA cycle intermediates.

Ammonia. Amino acids present a special metabolic problem in that they have the potential to form ammonia, which is very toxic, and mechanisms must exist to solve that problem.

Dietary proteins

Dietary proteins vary according to the diet of the individual. The important nutritional issue is that there should be sufficient protein in the diet to replace the amino acids that are degraded (Chapter 19).

Protein digestion involves endo- and exopeptidases

Dietary proteins are broken down to their constituent amino acids by the action of a series of proteolytic enzymes that catalyse the hydrolysis of peptide bonds. Small peptides are produced from larger peptides by the action of *endopeptidases*, which catalyse the hydrolysis of peptide bonds *within* proteins. The endopeptidases are relatively specific in the peptide bonds that they

attack. *Exopeptidases* catalyse the hydrolysis of *terminal* peptide bonds in peptides, thus producing free amino acids as products. Most of the peptidases are secreted as inactive zymogens that have to be activated for them to be effective in protein digestion (see Figs 29, 30). The logic of this arrangement must be obvious since, otherwise, these proteolytic enzymes would destroy their cells of origin!

Pepsin is the key protease in the stomach

Protein is hydrolysed by *pepsin*, an endopeptidase that has an optimum pH of about 1.0. When food enters the stomach the production of hydrochloric acid converts pepsinogen to pepsin and creates the optimal (pH) environment for pepsin action. HCl also denatures dietary protein, with the result that peptide bonds that had been within globular proteins are now more accessible to proteolytic enzymes.

Trypsin, chymotrypsin from the pancreas function in the duodenum

Proteins are completely converted to small peptides in the duodenum by the action of other endopeptidases that originate in the pancreas: *trypsin, chymotrypsin* and *elastase*. These enzymes are produced as inactive zymogens. Trypsinogen is activated to trypsin by the action of *enteropeptidase* secreted from mucosal cells when food enters the small intestine. Trypsin is then able to convert additional trypsinogen to trypsin (i.e. it is autocatalytic), chymotrypsinogen to chymotrypsin, proelastase to elastase and pancreatic *procarboxy-peptidases A* and *B* to their active forms (Fig. 30).

Amino acids and small peptides are produced in the brush border and within intestinal mucosal cells

Exopeptidases – *dipeptidases, carboxypeptidases* and *aminopeptidases* – complete the hydrolysis of the small peptides formed by endopeptidase action. The combined effect of peptidases is to produce mainly free amino acids, but also some dipeptides and tripeptides.

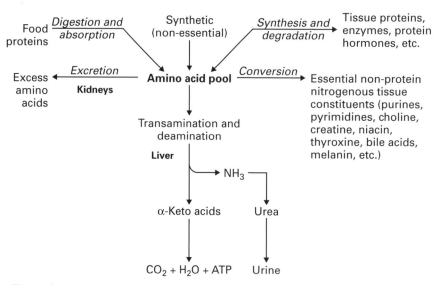

Fig. 76 General aspects of amino acid metabolism.

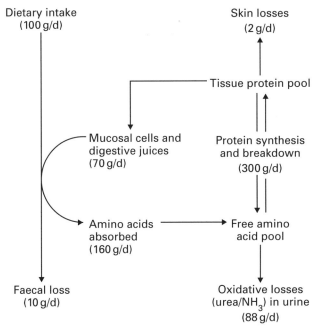

Fig. 77 Whole body protein turnover with data for one individual.

Absorption of amino acids is by secondary active transport

Free amino acids plus dipeptides and tripeptides utilise a group of specific transporters that are in the brush border of mucosal cells. Both sodium-dependent and facilitated transport are involved.

Protein turnover

If one measures the nitrogen excretion from the body one would have an inaccurate impression of the total daily turnover of protein that occurs in humans. The data shown in Figure 77 can be analysed to reveal whole body protein metabolism in a normal 70 kg adult man consuming 100 g protein per day.

Nitrogen balance. This is calculated by measuring skin losses, faecal losses plus the excretion of urea and ammonia in urine (conversion factor: 1 g urinary N = 6.25 g protein). Since excretion of nitrogen balances intake the subject is in 'nitrogen balance'.

Whole body protein metabolism. This is calculated by using tracer amino acids. The data shown in Figure 77 is for an individual where it is clear that whole body protein metabolism averages 300 g/day, which is much greater than the dietary protein intake of 100 g/day. About 23% of the protein turnover represents the production of digestive enzymes and the rapid degradation of mucosal cells in the gut. Proteolysis of these in the gut generates amino acids that are returned to the free amino acid pool. About 77% of daily protein turnover is more obscure including turnover of muscle protein.

9.2 **Protein disposal**

Protein catabolism involves:

- protein breakdown to amino acids (some will be reused and not degraded further)
- nitrogen removal from amino acids: transamination/deamination to give ammonia and keto acids
- urea cycle to dispose of ammonia
- keto acid metabolism via TCA cycle.

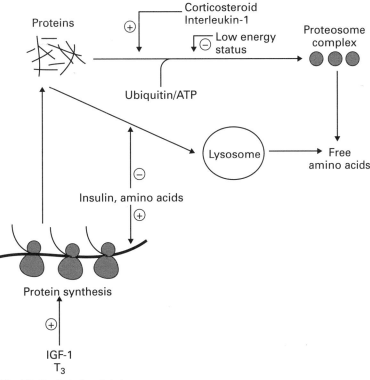

Fig. 78 Control of protein turnover.

Protein breakdown involves lysosomal and non-lysosomal pathways

The pathways for protein breakdown are shown in Figure 78.

The lysosomal pathway
Lysosomes contain an array of proteolytic enzymes that are mainly involved in the breakdown of three classes of protein: extracellular, membrane-associated and some intracellular proteins with long half-lives. This pathway is ATP independent and is inhibited by insulin and amino acids. Coupled with the action of insulin and amino acids to increase protein synthesis, this explains the positive nitrogen balance that can occur in the fed state especially in growing children.

The non-lysosomal pathway
The major non-lysosomal pathway involves *ubiquitin*, is ATP dependent and processes abnormal proteins and normal proteins with short half-lives, as well as the proteins of the muscular apparatus (actin and myosin). Ubiquitin is a small, highly conserved protein that is found in all cells. In the ubiquitin pathway, proteins are covalently linked to ubiquitin. Corticosteroids and the cytokine interleukin-1 activate the ubiquitin pathway.

Nitrogen disposal from amino acids

For the majority of the amino acids found in the body (exceptions are threonine and lysine) the amino group is transferred to α-ketoglutarate forming glutamate and the keto acid corresponding to the amino acid (Fig. 79).

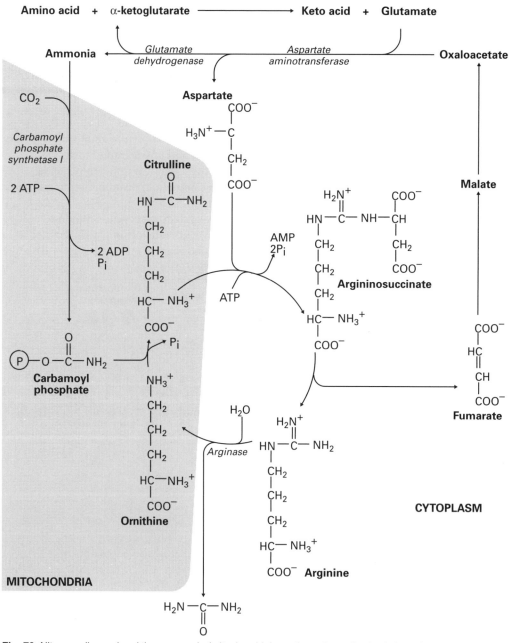

Fig. 79 Nitrogen disposal and the urea cycle (mitochondrial reactions shown in shaded area).

The biological advantage of such an arrangement is that the subsequent steps are common, since it is only the glutamate nitrogen which has to be handled. Glutamate is deaminated and the ammonia produced is converted to urea.

Transamination. The enzymes catalysing the transamination reactions are *aminotransferases* (transaminases), which have pyridoxal phosphate (PLP) as coenzyme. Liver, kidney, muscle, and brain contain appreciable amounts of these enzymes.

Deamination. The glutamate formed is then subjected to oxidative deamination by *glutamic dehydrogenase*, with ammonium as a product and α-ketoglutarate regenerated (Fig. 79). Glutamate dehydrogenase activity will affect the rate of ammonia production as well as the availability of carbon skeletons for the TCA cycle. GDP and ADP are allosteric activators. Hence, a lower energy charge accelerates the entry of carbon skeletons into the TCA cycle for conversion to substrates that can be oxidised to carbon dioxide, with the eventual production of ATP.

The urea cycle detoxifies ammonia

Ammonia is toxic if the concentration goes above 4×10^{-5} M in blood. Therefore, it is vital to deal efficiently with the ammonia generated.

Extra-hepatic tissues. Ammonia generated is converted to glutamine by *glutamine synthetase*:

$$\text{Glutamate} + NH_3 + ATP \rightarrow \text{Glutamine} + ADP + P_i$$

The glutamine formed is transported to the gut, kidney and liver.

Liver. The liver has a high capacity to catabolise amino acids; ammonia is disposed of by conversion to urea; this is a non-toxic compound that can be transported in the blood to the kidneys and excreted in the urine. The pathway used is the urea cycle (Fig. 79), also discovered by Krebs.

Carbamoyl phosphate is synthesised from ammonia and carbon dioxide in a reaction catalysed by *carbamoyl phosphate synthetase I* (CPSI). CPSI is stimulated by *N*-acetylglutamate and NH_4^+ (formed from glutamine by the action of *glutaminase*). Both of these are positively correlated with amino acid turnover in the body. The interaction of carbamoyl phosphate and ornithine generates citrulline, which then acquires another nitrogen from aspartate to form argininosuccinate, which is then converted to arginine and a molecule of fumarate (processing of fumarate in the TCA cycle generates oxaloacetate, which is used once more to form the required aspartate). The hydrolysis of arginine, catalysed by *arginase*, yields urea plus ornithine. Urea has two nitrogen atoms; one arises from ammonia and the other is derived from aspartate. Other important points include:

- in order to ensure that ammonia is removed efficiently, there is high expenditure of ATP in the

formation of carbamoyl phosphate and in the synthesis of argininosuccinate

- the first two reactions are mitochondrial in location, the other reactions are in the cytosol. The localisation of CPSI to the mitochondria in hepatocytes is important since a second enzyme (CPSII) is involved in carbamoyl phosphate synthesis required for pyrimidine nucleotide biosynthesis (Chapter 12) and is localised to the cytosol
- ornithine is used in the first reaction, where ammonia enters the cycle as carbamoyl phosphate, and is regenerated in the last reaction of the cycle
- entry of ornithine and exit of citrulline (across the inner mitochondrial membrane) utilises transport systems.

The metabolism of amino acid carbons

Following the removal of amino acid nitrogen, the resultant keto acids are metabolised to TCA cycle intermediates. Thus, carbons from amino acids can all eventually be converted to acetyl-CoA, which can undergo complete oxidation in the TCA cycle or serve as a precursor for fatty acid biosynthesis. Although many of the amino acids share common types of reaction in terms of their catabolism, more often than not each of the amino acids undergoes a complicated series of unique steps. This can be simplified to some extent as the carbon skeletons appear in six major metabolites (Fig. 80).

The entry points for amino acid carbons into the TCA cycle are:

- oxaloacetate
- fumarate
- succinyl-CoA
- α-ketoglutarate
- acetyl-CoA.

Other keto acids produce pyruvate, which is readily converted to oxaloacetate.

Glucogenic amino acids. Amino acids for which the carbon atoms are metabolised to intermediates of the TCA cycle other than acetyl-CoA are glucogenic. To determine whether or not an amino acid is glucogenic, use Figure 80 and observe whether or not the metabolism of the amino acid metabolite will result in an increase in the level of oxaloacetate. If the answer is **yes**, the amino acid is glucogenic. If the answer is **no**, the amino acid is ketogenic.

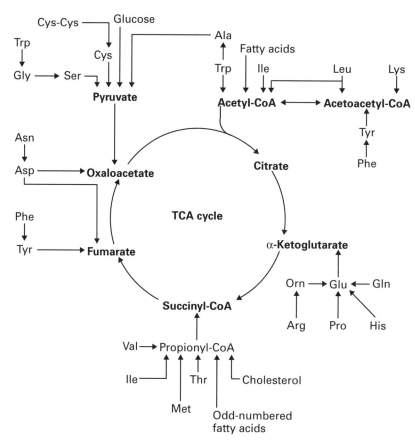

Fig. 80 Entry points for amino acid carbons into the TCA cycle.

Ketogenic amino acids. Those amino acids that are metabolised to acetyl-CoA are ketogenic. Some amino acids are both glucogenic and ketogenic, e.g. phenylalanine, tyrosine and isoleucine. Only lysine and leucine are purely ketogenic!

9.3 The synthesis and roles of individual amino acids

Those amino acids that cannot be synthesised in the body are termed essential amino acids (Table 6). The requirement for amino acids varies with species and with the state of the organism. For example, eight of the twenty amino acids used for protein synthesis are essential for adults with an additional two (histidine and arginine) being essential in growing children.

Specific amino acids

Because of the unique pathways for the metabolism of the 20 common amino acids, this is a huge topic; we will concentrate on the truly important information on each. Several of the amino acids are involved in the synthesis of vital body constituents.

Table 6 Amino acid requirements for an adult

Essential amino acids	Non-essential amino acids	Conditionally essential amino acids[a]
Phe[b]	Gly	Cys (synthesised from Met)
Trp	Ser	Tyr (synthesised from Phe)
Val	Ala	Gln (synthesised from Glu, for which requirements are high in illness)
Ile	Tyr	His (synthesised from Glu; required in diet in babies)
Leu	Asp	Arg (formed in urea cycle; required in growing children)
Met[c]	Asn	
Lys	Glu	
Thr	Gln	
	Cys	
	Pro	
	Arg	
	His	

[a]Amino acids that can be synthesised in the body but this may at times be inadequate, leading to a dietary requirement.
[b]Tyr in diet spares the requirement for Phe.
[c]Cys in diet spares the requirement for Met.

Small amino acids

Glycine

- δ-aminolaevulinic acid, a key intermediate in *haem* synthesis is made from glycine and succinyl-CoA
- required for detoxification reactions in the liver
- principal inhibitory transmitter in the brain stem and spinal cord.

Alanine

- most important glucogenic amino acid; it is exported from muscle during fasting and exercise.

Aromatic amino acids: phenylalanine, tyrosine, tryptophan, histidine

Phenylalanine

- precursor of tyrosine; the enzyme catalysing this reaction, *phenylalanine hydroxylase*, defective in phenylketonuria (pp. 265–266).

Tyrosine

- precursor of *melanin* in melanocytes
- precursor of *thyroid hormones* in the thyroid gland
- precursor of catecholamines such as *adrenaline, noradrenaline* and *dopamine* (important neurotransmitters)
- phosphorylation of tyrosine in some proteins by *tyrosine kinases* controls metabolic reactions
- insulin receptor has tyrosine kinase activity.

Tryptophan

- precursor of the neurotransmitter *serotonin* (5-hydroxytryptamine)
- precursor of nicotinamide (p. 244).

Histidine

- precursor of one-carbon unit (formimino-FH_4)
- is decarboxylated to *histamine*, a biologic amine that stimulates gastric acid secretion by effects on H_2 receptors and also causes contraction of smooth muscle through actions on H_1 receptors.

Branched-chain amino acids: valine, isoleucine, leucine

All branched-chain amino acids

- catabolised via a branched-chain ketoacid dehydrogenase (BCKADH) system, which is similar to the PDC (p. 79).
- BCKADH is the enzyme defective in *maple syrup urine disease*.

Leucine

- metabolism requires biotin.

Basic amino acids: arginine, lysine

Arginine
- precursor of creatine
- synthesised in urea cycle from ornithine.
- precursor of nitric oxide (p. 232)

Lysine
- lysine residue interacts with a glutamine when Factor XIIIa converts a low-tensile strength fibrin polymer into a high-tensile strength clot (p. 254).

Sulphur-containing amino acids: cysteine, methionine

Cysteine
- provides the functional SH group of glutathione, acyl carrier protein and coenzyme A.

Methionine
- activated as S-adenosyl-methionine is a methyl donor in methylation reactions, e.g. noradrenaline to adrenaline
- provides sulphur for cysteine biosynthesis.

Hydroxy amino acids: serine, threonine

Serine
- provides carbons for cysteine synthesis
- part of phospholipid, phosphatidyl serine
- required for synthesis of sphingolipids
- principal source of 1-carbon units in the body
- phosphorylation of serine residues in some proteins by *serine kinases* controls the function of the proteins.

Threonine
- phosphorylation of threonine by protein kinases occurs in some signal transduction mechanisms.

Acidic amino acids and their amides: glutamate and glutamine, aspartate and asparagine

Glutamate
- participates in transamination reactions in nitrogen disposal
- component of *glutathione* and *tetrahydrofolate*
- most abundant excitatory neurotransmitter in brain
- decarboxylated to γ-aminobutyric acid (GABA) in neurons.

Glutamine
- transports ammonia from extra-hepatic tissues to the liver and splanchnic bed
- participates in purine nucleotide biosynthesis
- participates in GMP biosynthesis
- participates in pyrimidine nucleotide biosynthesis
- generates ammonium ions through action of glutaminase in the renal response to acidosis

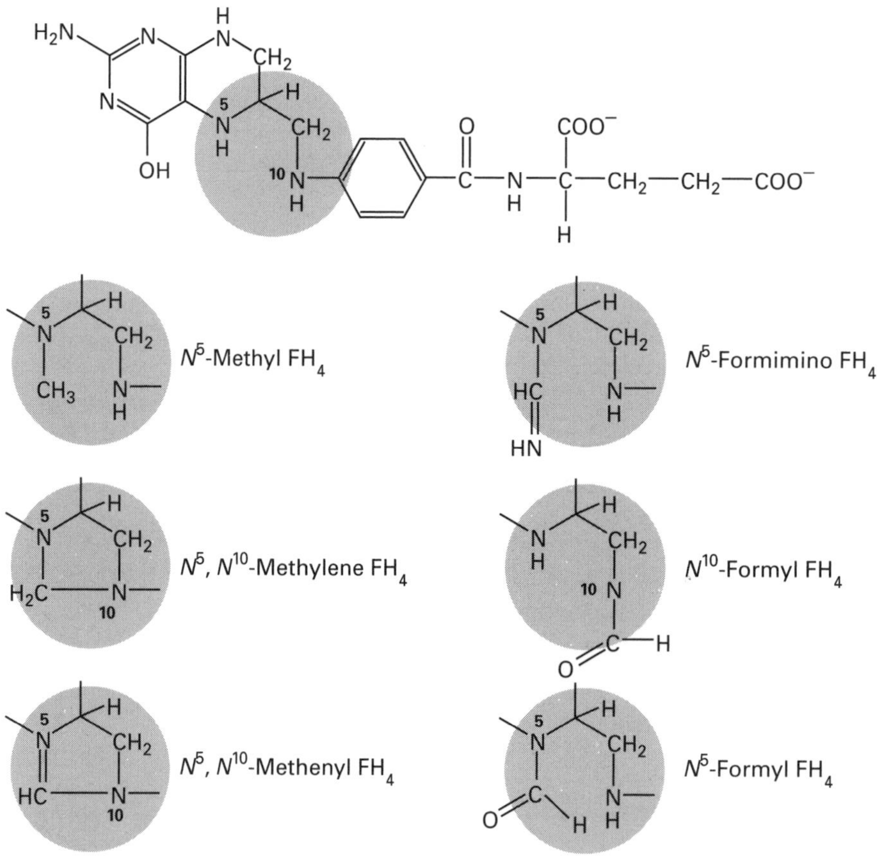

Fig. 81 Derivatives of tetrahydrofolate (FH$_4$). Various one-carbon units can be attached to N^5 and/or N^{10} of FH$_4$.

- detoxification reactions in the liver
- precursor for glutamate in neurons
- fuel for enterocytes (p. 145).

Aspartate
- biosynthesis of urea
- purine nucleotide biosynthesis
- AMP biosynthesis
- pyrimidine nucleotide biosynthesis
- acts as a neurotransmitter.

Asparagine
- N-linked diogosaccharide synthesis.

9.4 One-carbon metabolism

The utilisation or formation of carbon dioxide by carboxylation and decarboxylation reactions are common and require cofactors:

- carboxylation: biotin
- decarboxylations: thyamine pyrophosphate (TPP), pyridoxal phosphate.

'One-carbon metabolism' refers to sources of carbon in a more reduced form than carbon dioxide. These one-carbon units participate in several reactions related to the biosynthesis of key components of cells. They are carried on two carriers: *tetrahydrofolate* (FH$_4$; a derivative of folic acid, a vitamin) and *S-adenosyl-methionine* (SAM; an essential amino acid, methionine, activated by the adenosyl moiety).

Sources of one-carbon units

- carried by FH$_4$: serine, glycine, histidine
- carried by SAM: methyl-FH$_4$.

Uses of one-carbon units

- carried by FH$_4$: purine and pyrimidine nucleotide synthesis
- carried by SAM: biosynthesis of creatine, adrenaline and phosphatidylcholine.

Tetrahydrofolate carries one-carbon units

FH$_4$ is a reduced pteridine (Fig. 81), which is derived from folate, a water-soluble vitamin present in the diet. Animals and humans depend on plants for their principal supply. FH$_4$ is formed in the intestinal mucosa and is converted at that site to N^5-methyl-FH$_4$. This 'traps' the FH$_4$, making it unavailable for the production of the critical one-carbon derivatives used for purine and pyrimidine nucleotide synthesis. The solution to this problem is the reaction where

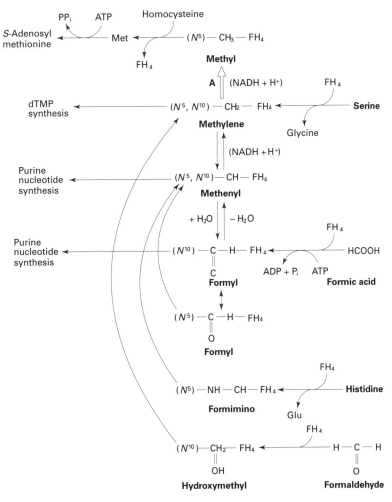

Fig. 82 Metabolism of tetrahydrofolate. The methylated derivative of FH_4 is a 'trap' for FH_4 because reaction A is irreversible.

methionine is regenerated from homocysteine, catalysed by homocysteine-N^5-methyl-FH_4 transferase:

N^5-methyl-FH_4 + Homocysteine → Methionine + FH_4

This reaction involves a vitamin B_{12} coenzyme, methyl-cobalamin, which participates in the reaction. Obviously, the regeneration of methionine has two biological advantages. One is to produce more methionine. The other is to untrap FH_4. The reduction of N^5, N^{10}-methylene FH_4 is irreversible! In an individual with a B_{12} deficiency, the reaction is defective and N^5-methyl-FH_4 accumulates. In addition, there is increased excretion of formiminoglutamate, formate, and 4(5) amino-5(4)-imidazole carboximide, an intermediate in the synthesis of purine nucleotide synthesis. These metabolites all require folate cofactors for further conversion. Hence, it is thought that the importance of the transmethylation reaction lies not so much in the synthesis of methionine, but in the regeneration of FH_4.

The one-carbon units carried by FH_4 are described in Figure 81 and can be interconverted as shown schematically in Figure 82. The primary source of one-carbon units derives from serine in the reaction catalysed by *serine hydroxymethyltransferase*.

S-Adenosylmethionine is a source of methyl groups

Methionine contains a methyl group that can be transferred to other molecules after the methionine has been 'activated' by interaction with ATP to form SAM. SAM then interacts with acceptor molecules by a process known as *transmethylation*. Examples of transmethylation using SAM include:

- adrenaline from noradrenaline (p. 221)
- phosphatidylcholine from phosphatidylethanolamine (addition of three methyl groups)
- creatine synthesis: the last step is an N-methylation

  Glycine + Arginine → Guanidinoacetate → creatine

9.5 Haem synthesis

Haem proteins such as haemoglobin and the cytochromes have critical functions in the body in oxygen transport and biological oxidation, respectively. Other haem proteins include myoglobin, catalase and tryptophan

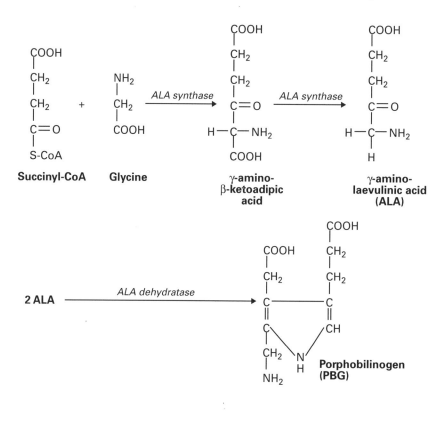

Fig. 83 The structure of haem. Haem consists of a porphyrin ring that is coordinated with an atom of iron. The porphyrin ring has four pyrrole rings. There are two side chains on each of the pyrroles, propionyl (P; CH_2CH_2COOH), methyl (M; CH_3) and vinyl (V; $CH=CH_2$). In haem, the clockwise order of these groups is M, V, M, V, M, P, P, M.

pyrrolase. Cytochrome oxidase is the terminal carrier of the electron transport chain. Cytochromes P-450 are involved in xenobiotic metabolism in the liver and also in steroid hormone biosynthesis. The structure of haem is shown in Figure 83.

Haem synthesis starts with glycine and succinyl-CoA

The initial and final steps of haem synthesis occur in the mitochondria. The reaction of succinyl-CoA with glycine is the starting point for the synthesis of the porphyrin ring. Condensation of these two compounds yields δ-aminolaevulinic acid (ALA), catalysed by *ALA synthase* (Fig. 84), an enzyme that requires pyridoxal phosphate. Condensation of two ALA molecules gives a pyrrole, porphobilinogen (PBG); this is catalysed by *ALA dehydratase*, an enzyme that contains zinc and is

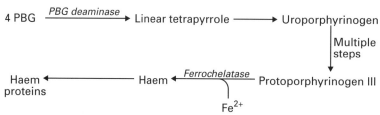

Fig. 84 The synthesis of porphobilinogen and haem.

inactivated by lead. The association of four PBG molecules, catalysed by *PBG deaminase*, gives a straight-chain tetrapyrrole, which is cyclised to form a porphyrinogen. Multiple steps yield the precursor of haem, protoporphyrin III, which incorporates ferrous iron, catalysed by *ferrochelatase*, to yield haem. Ferrochelatase also contains zinc and is inactivated by lead.

Regulation of haem synthesis

Haem regulates its formation by several actions on ALA synthase. They include feedback inhibition, interference with the transport of the enzyme into mitochondria (its site of action), and repression of transcription of the ALA synthase gene. The last effect is profound given the short half-life (about 60 minutes) of ALA synthase. In summary, in the liver haem synthesis increases when haem levels are low and vice versa. In contrast, erythrocyte haem synthesis is an 'all or none' phenomenon that follows inevitably erythroid cell differentiation.

BOX 9.2
Clinical note: Porphyrias

Porphyrias are disorders where there are partial deficiencies in haem biosynthetic pathway enzymes, leading to the accumulation of haem precursors. Acute intermittent porphyria is the most common hepatic porphyria; the defect here is in PBG deaminase. Neurological symptoms are present (e.g. the periodic madness of George III of Britain). Several drugs (e.g. barbiturates) when administered to patients increase the synthesis of cytochromes P-450; this places demands upon the haem pool and more haem is synthesised through induction of ALA synthase. If a patient has a deficiency in PBG deaminase, this will lead to even greater accumulation of intermediates and exacerbation of symptoms. Interestingly, exacerbation of symptoms also occurs in patients who reduce their calorie intake (diet) and, in contrast, a high glucose intake suppresses haem synthesis and relieves symptoms.

Self-assessment: questions

Multiple choice questions

1. Pyridoxal phosphate:
   a. Is the coenzyme for transamination reactions
   b. Is a fat-soluble vitamin
   c. Is a coenzyme of the pyruvate dehydrogenase complex
   d. Is the coenzyme for amino acid decarboxylation reactions

2. Negative nitrogen balance is produced in humans by the removal from the diet of which of the following amino acids?
   a. Leucine
   b. Methionine
   c. Serine
   d. Lysine
   e. Glutamate

3. The urea cycle:
   a. Includes a reaction where arginine is hydrolysed to urea
   b. Is a cyclic process where ornithine acts like a catalyst or regenerating substrate
   c. Is a pathway where ATP is produced
   d. Has enzymes distributed between the nucleus and cytosol in liver
   e. Is a major pathway for the production of ammonia in the body

4. Glucogenic amino acids:
   a. Include leucine
   b. When metabolised will increase the net production of oxaloacetate
   c. Include valine
   d. Are of particular importance in the fed state
   e. Include alanine and glutamine

5. Which of the following amino acids are both essential and ketogenic?
   a. Valine
   b. Lysine
   c. Aspartate
   d. Leucine
   e. Serine

6. Tetrahydrofolate (FH_4):
   a. Is derived from one of the water-soluble vitamins
   b. In the gut is converted to N^5-methyl-FH_4
   c. Is a coenzyme involved in fatty acid oxidation
   d. Is produced in a reaction that regenerates methionine

   e. Carries methyl groups used directly for the synthesis of adrenaline from noradrenaline

7. The methyl group in creatine can be derived from the following, directly or indirectly:
   a. N^5-methyl-FH_4
   b. N^5,N^{10}-methylene-FH_4
   c. S-Adenosylmethionine
   d. Serine
   e. Creatinine

8. Phenylalanine:
   a. Is an aromatic amino acid
   b. Is a purely ketogenic amino acid
   c. Accumulates in the blood of subjects with phenylketonuria (PKU)
   d. Is the precursor of tyrosine
   e. Is a non-essential amino acid

9. Transamination of an amino acid:
   a. Involves an enzyme that has NAD^+ as coenzyme
   b. Is important for our ability to synthesise proteins
   c. Requires ATP
   d. Only occurs in muscle
   e. Is a reaction that produces ammonia

10. With regard to nitrogen disposal in humans:
    a. Glutamic dehydrogenase catalyses an irreversible reaction
    b. Carbamoyl phosphate synthetase I (CPSI) is a cytosolic enzyme
    c. The urea cycle is a cyclic process in which ornithine acts as a catalyst or regenerating substrate
    d. The urea cycle is an efficient pathway for ATP synthesis
    e. The small intestine has the highest overall urea cycle activity in the body

11. Identify correct statements about haem metabolism:
    a. Haem is only found in the body in haemoglobin and cytochrome oxidase
    b. Succinyl-CoA and glycine are the starting substrates for haem synthesis
    c. Haem synthesis occurs entirely in the mitochondria
    d. A rate-controlling enzyme in haem synthesis is δ-aminolaevulinic acid synthase
    e. Haem synthesis increases in the liver when cytochrome P-450 synthesis is induced

True/false questions

Are the following statements true or false?

1. Ferrochelatase is inhibited by lead.
2. Serine is the principal source of one-carbon units in the body.
3. Our dietary protein only contains essential amino acids, with the non-essential amino acids being formed from them in the body.
4. Glutamine formation and secretion from muscle has an important role to play in nitrogen disposal from muscle.
5. Leucine is the principal glucogenic amino acid in the body.
6. Amino acids which have carbons that are converted to succinyl-CoA are potentially glucogenic.
7. Tyrosine is the precursor of adrenaline, noradrenaline and thyroid hormones.
8. Alanine is the principal ketogenic amino acid in the body.

Short essay questions

1. Describe connections between the urea cycle and the TCA cycle (both discovered by Krebs).
2. Describe how, as humans, we deal with the potential problem of ammonia toxicity.
3. Explain the term 'conditionally essential amino acid' and give as many examples as you can.

Self-assessment: answers

Multiple choice answers

1. a. **True.** Pyridoxal phosphate is the coenzyme for many reactions of amino acid catabolism.
   b. **False.** Pyridoxal is one of the water-soluble group of B vitamins.
   c. **False.** It is not one of the five coenzymes of that complex.
   d. **True.** These reactions can result in the formation of important biological amines such as dopamine.

2. a. **True.** All of the branched-chain amino acids are essential.
   b. **True.** Although it can be regenerated from homocysteine plus N^5-methyl-FH_4, some is required to replace that which is broken down in the body.
   c. **False.** Serine's carbons can be derived from glucose and the amino group from glutamate.
   d. **True.** Lysine is an essential amino acid.
   e. **False.** Glutamate is readily synthesised, associated with the transamination of any amino acid. Its carbons are derived from α-ketoglutarate.

3. a. **True.** The other product is ornithine.
   b. **True.** The other name for the urea cycle is Krebs' ornithine cycle.
   c. **False.** Several ATPs are required.
   d. **False.** The enzymes occur in mitochondria and cytosol.
   e. **False.** This is the pathway for converting potentially toxic ammonia to urea.

4. a. **False.** Leucine is the archetypical ketogenic amino acid since HMG-CoA (the precursor of acetoacetate) is an intermediate in its catabolism.
   b. **True.** This is a definition of a glucogenic amino acid.
   c. **True.** Its carbons produce succinyl-CoA.
   d. **False.** They are important in the fasted state when one has to synthesise glucose.
   e. **True.** Alanine is the most important glucogenic amino acid in the fasted stated and glutamine also leaves muscle at that time and is glucogenic via glutamate.

5. a. **False.** Valine is essential but its metabolism yields succinyl-CoA and hence it is entirely glucogenic.
   b. **True.** Lysine is essential and its metabolism gives acetoacetyl-CoA, which is an intermediate in ketone body production in the liver.
   c. **False.** Aspartate is easily converted to oxaloacetate by transamination and oxaloacetate

is an intermediate in the gluconeogenic pathway.
   d. **True.** Leucine is essential and its catabolism yields HMG-CoA, the immediate precursor of acetoacetate.
   e. **False.** Serine is converted to pyruvate, which is a starting point for gluconeogenesis in the liver.

6. a. **True.** The vitamin is folate.
   b. **True.** This traps the tetrahydrofolate and requires that the methyl group be transferred to homocysteine to free the FH_4.
   c. **False.** FAD and NAD^+ are involved in fatty acid oxidation.
   d. **True.** See answer to 6b.
   e. **False.** S-Adenosylmethionine (SAM) supplies the methyl group for adrenaline synthesis.

7. a. **True.** The methyl is transferred to homocysteine forming methionine, which is then converted to SAM; this interacts with guanidinoacetate to give creatine.
   b. **True.** This compound can be reduced to N^5-methyl FH_4.
   c. **True.** see 'a'.
   d. **True.** Via N^5,N^{10}-methylene-FH_4.
   e. **False.** Creatinine is a methyl group 'sink'.

8. a. **True.** There are three aromatic amino acids: phenylalanine, tyrosine and tryptophan.
   b. **False.** It is both ketogenic and glucogenic.
   c. **True.** Newborns are screened for PKU by analysis of their blood phenylalanine.
   d. **True.** Hydroxylation yields tyrosine. This is the system that is deficient in PKU.
   e. **False.** It is essential (tyrosine is not).

9. a. **False.** The coenzyme is pyridoxal phosphate.
   b. **True.** Transamination is required to make sure there is synthesis of enough non-essential amino acids from their keto acid precursors.
   c. **False.** There is no direct participation of ATP in transamination.
   d. **False.** Although important in muscle, transamination occurs in any tissue where there is significant amino acid catabolism.
   e. **False.** An amino group is transferred to α-ketoglutarate. This reaction generates glutamate and it is its oxidative deamination that yields ammonia.

10. a. **False.** Glutamate can be formed from ammonia and α-ketoglutarate, catalysed by glutamate dehydrogenase and driven by NADH or NADPH.

b. **False.** CPSI is located in liver mitochondria. CPSII, involved in pyrimidine nucleotide biosynthesis (Chapter 12), is in the cytosol.

c. **True.** It behaves in an similar fashion to oxaloacetate in the TCA cycle.

d. **False.** There is a considerable utilisation of ATP in the urea cycle, no doubt ensuring efficient removal of ammonia.

e. **False.** The small intestine has activity of some of the urea cycle enzymes but lacks the complete cycle. The cycle is restricted to the liver.

11. a. **False.** Several other cytochromes including cytochrome *b* and *c* and cytochromes P-450 are haem proteins.

b. **True.** Succinyl-CoA is an intermediate in the TCA cycle.

c. **False.** Haem synthesis starts in the mitochondria but later steps occur in the cytosol.

d. **True.** There is feedback control by haem, which decreases synthesis of the enzyme.

e. **True.** Since cytochromes P-450 are haem proteins, when they are induced (as they are by many drugs; Chapter 17) haem synthesis increases.

True/false answers

1. **True.** This is part of the known toxicity of lead, e.g. for children.

2. **True.** It generates the important one-carbon intermediate, $N^{5,10}$-methylene FH_4 in a reaction that also produces glycine.

3. **False.** Both types of amino acid are present in the diet. The key point is that one has to have sufficient essential amino acids in our diet whereas deficiencies in the non-essential amino acids can be made good by metabolic processes.

4. **True.** Glutamine is formed by the amidation of glutamate; this allows for nitrogen disposal.

5. **False.** HMG-CoA, the immediate precursor of acetoacetate, is an intermediate in the catabolism of leucine.

6. **True.** The succinyl-CoA is converted to oxaloacetate via the TCA cycle and oxaloacetate is glucogenic.

7. **True.** Tyrosine has a very important role in the biosynthesis of several biologically active molecules.

8. **False.** Alanine is converted to pyruvate and hence is glucogenic. It is a major source of glucose in the fasted state.

Short essay answers

1. It is important to recognise that only one of the two nitrogens in the urea formed by the urea cycle is derived directly from ammonia. Carbamoyl phosphate is produced by the interaction of ammonia, carbon dioxide and ATP, catalysed by carbamoyl phosphate synthetase I. The carbamoyl phosphate then interacts with ornithine to give citrulline. The next reaction is the production of argininosuccinate by the interaction between citrulline and aspartate, catalysed by argininosuccinate synthase. In the next step, argininosuccinate is converted to arginine with the other product being fumarate. Arginine is hydrolysed to give urea and regenerates ornithine for continued operation of the cycle.

The fumarate formed from argininosuccinate is an intermediate in the TCA cycle, being converted to malate and then oxaloacetate by the action of fumarase and malate dehydrogenase, respectively. Oxaloacetate can be transaminated to give aspartate and thus maintain the production of the intermediate that supplies one of the nitrogens that ends up in urea.

N.B. It is important to understand the fundamental role of cycles in intermediary metabolism. The urea cycle is a classic example where one has to consider how the cycle is sustained.

2. The catabolism of amino acids raises the problem of dealing with the disposal of their nitrogen. The initial reaction for most amino acids when they are catabolised is transamination with α-ketoglutarate, yielding the keto acid corresponding to the amino acid plus glutamate. To continue the process, the glutamate has to be converted back to α-ketoglutarate. A major way for this to occur is by the action of glutamate dehydrogenase, with the other product being ammonia. Ammonia is toxic at a blood concentration above 4×10^{-5} M so the body has to have efficient ways of dealing with it.

Ammonia formed in extra-hepatic tissues is not allowed to enter blood and circulate (with the potential to affect brain function). Ammonia is incorporated into glutamine by the action of glutamine synthase. Glutamine is not toxic and can be transferred safely in the blood to be metabolised in the splanchnic bed and also in the liver. Ammonia formed from glutamine or any other amino acid in the liver is not a problem because that organ is the sole site of the urea cycle, which is our major way of dealing with potentially toxic ammonia.

The urea cycle involves converting the ammonia along with bicarbonate into carbamoyl phosphate; this combines with ornithine to form citrulline. Further processing of citrulline yields argininosuccinate through an interaction with aspartate (this disposes of a second nitrogen) and then arginine. Arginine is then converted to the non-toxic product urea, and ornithine is regenerated, thus completing the cycle.

3. Conditionally essential amino acids are those that are non-essential under some circumstances but

become essential under other situations. The body has the ability to make them but in some cases, the ability is not developed, is insufficient or is lost. This can be the situation in the neonate and in individuals with specific inborn errors of metabolism affecting amino acids.

Cysteine is one such amino acid. It is obtained from many dietary proteins but can also be synthesised by a pathway where the sulphur is derived from methionine and the carbons from serine. If this pathway has low activity, as occurs in neonates, then cysteine becomes essential and it is important to ensure that there are adequate levels in dietary protein.

Tyrosine is non-essential in that it is in many dietary proteins, but most of our requirements come from its production from phenylalanine, catalysed by phenylalanine hydroxylase. In individuals with phenylketonuria (PKU), where the phenylalanine hydroxylase system is defective, tyrosine becomes an essential amino acid.

Other examples are *glutamine*, the requirements for which are increased in severe illness, *histidine*, required to be sufficient in the diet of babies, and *arginine*, required in increased amounts in growing children.

Lipid synthesis and transport

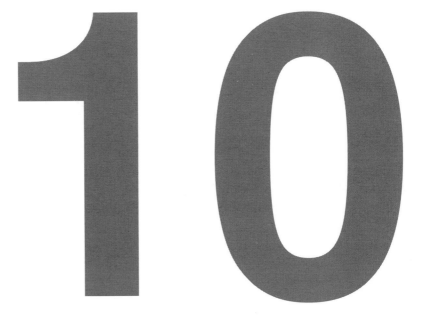

10.1 Fatty acid and triacylglycerol biosynthesis

Fatty acids occur in most of the complex lipids that are so critical to membrane function. In addition, it is advantageous for the body to have the ability to synthesise from carbohydrate or amino acids long-chain (high potential energy) fatty acids, which are incorporated into triacylglycerols and then stored in adipose tissue for use in times of fasting and during long-term exercise. The potential for biosynthesis of fatty acids occurs principally in adipose tissue, mammary glands, and liver.

Fatty acid biosynthesis

In summary, the fatty acid synthesis pathway utilises 8 acetyl-CoA molecules and ends with the synthesis of palmitic acid (C_{16}) (Fig. 85). The process requires that malonyl-CoA be formed from the acetyl-CoA and this is the principal rate-controlling step. A fatty acid synthetase (FAS) multienzyme protein catalyses fatty acid chain growth by 2 carbons each cycle. The FAS also enables carbonyl groups to be reduced to methylenes so there is a requirement for NADPH. Palmitic acid can be elongated to give larger fatty acids such as stearate (C_{18}). Fatty acids can also be unsaturated in the body to produce, for example, oleate ($C_{18:1}$). Odd-numbered fatty acids can also be synthesised. Important features of fatty acid biosynthesis include:

- acetyl-CoA for fatty acid synthesis needs to be transferred to the cytosol from mitochondria but it cannot cross the inner mitochondrial membrane. This problem is overcome by synthesising citrate

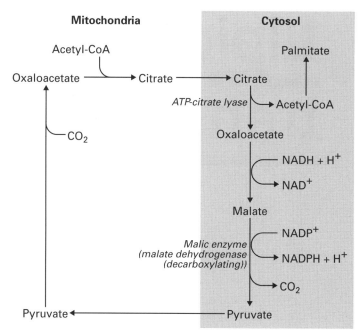

Fig. 86 The citrate-malate-pyruvate cycle.

from acetyl-CoA and the citrate can then exit the mitochondria (Fig. 86)

- malonyl-CoA formation is catalysed by *acetyl-CoA carboxylase*. The enzyme contains biotin to act as a CO_2 carrier. Bicarbonate stimulates fatty acid synthesis

$$CH_3.CO.SCoA + HCO_3^- + ATP \rightarrow$$
$$HOOC-CH_2.CO.SCoA + ADP + P_i$$

- long-term regulation of acetyl-CoA carboxylase is at the level of the gene transcription, whereas short-term regulation is achieved by allosteric and covalent mechanisms. Citrate activates the enzyme but the dependence on citrate varies with the state of phosphorylation. The enzyme can be polymerised from an octomer into large aggregates of 1000 kDa. Polymerisation is associated with activation irrespective of the activating ligand. The addition of citrate or dephosphorylation of the less active form of the enzyme results in polymerisation to the active form. Palmitoyl-CoA, the end-product of fatty acid synthase, is an effective inhibitor of the enzyme. It has been shown in vitro that activation by citrate precedes polymerisation, suggesting that polymerisation is an in vitro event. When the energy charge is low ([AMP]) is high), an AMP-activated kinase phosphorylates acetyl-CoA carboxylase to an inactive form

- the carbonyl group formed in the initial reaction of fatty acid synthesis is reduced to a methylene group by the following series of reactions; reduction, dehydration, reduction, with NADPH providing the reducing power. This sequence is the opposite of that found in fatty acid beta-oxidation

- FAS, isolated from animals, is a multi-enzyme complex with seven enzyme activities and an acyl carrier protein (ACP) in a single polypeptide chain.

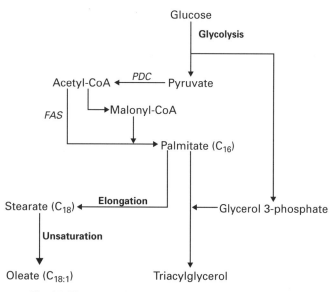

Fig. 85 The conversion of glucose to fatty acids and triacylglycerols.

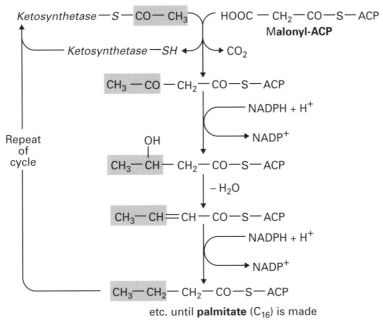

Fig. 87 Fatty acid synthesis.

Acyl groups are attached to ACP during the reactions catalysed by FAS. The FAS monomer cannot carry out the condensation reaction that initiates the production of palmitate since the ketosynthetase (KS) and ACP are too far apart. Hence the requirement for the dimeric form of the enzyme complex arranged head to tail. Two important sulphydryl (SH) groups are involved in fatty acid synthesis. One on KS can carry an acyl group and the other is on ACP, which initially carries a malonyl group (Fig. 87). When both SH sites are charged, condensation occurs leaving a larger ketoacyl group on the ACP. Reduction, dehydration followed by reduction produces an acyl group now two carbons longer. The carbon dioxide incorporated into malonyl-CoA is lost at the condensation step. The cycle shown in Figure 87 is repeated until the acyl group has 16 carbons. A thioesterase (deacylase) removes the completed fatty acid from the ACP. Highest activity of the thioesterase is exhibited with palmitoyl-CoA, and to a lesser extent with stearoyl-CoA (C_{18}) and myristoyl-CoA (C_{14}). In the lactating mammary gland, a different thioesterase is present, *thioesterase II*. This enzyme preferentially hydrolyses fatty acyl-CoA derivatives of chain length C_8 and C_{12} and plays a role in determining the fatty acid content of triacylglycerols in milk

- synthesis of odd-numbered fatty acids uses the same pathway as is used for even-numbered except that the primer molecule is propionyl-CoA (with a 3-carbon acyl group) rather than acetyl-CoA with its 2-carbon acyl group
- synthesis of unsaturated fatty acids requires *fatty acid desaturases* located in the endoplasmic reticulum. *Cis* double bonds are introduced no farther in the fatty acid chain than the C_9 to C_{10}

position of palmitic acid, i.e. must be seven or more carbon atoms from the ω end. Mammalian systems can desaturate various chain lengths at Δ^4, Δ^5, Δ^6, and Δ^9 positions. The desaturase complex contains cytochrome b_5, NADH-cytochrome b_5 reductase and the desaturase. The overall reaction is:
Palmityl CoA (C_{16}) + NADH + H$^+$ + O$_2$ →
Palmitoleyl CoA ($C_{16:1}$) + NAD$^+$ + 2 H$_2$O

- the body is capable of synthesising many unsaturated fatty acids and these have a special role in the lipids found in membranes. It is important to note, however, that some unsaturated fatty acids cannot be synthesized; linoleic acid (18:2;9,12) and γ-linolenic acid (18:3;9,12,15) are considered to be *essential fatty acids*
- fatty acid elongation enzymes are located in mitochondria and on the endoplasmic reticulum. *Elongases* on the endoplasmic reticulum add two carbon units via malonyl-CoA. The sequence of reactions is the same as those outlined for the synthesis of palmitate except the intermediates are CoA derivatives rather than ACP-derivatives. NADPH is the reductant. Elongases present in the mitochondrion add acetyl units in a reverse of beta-oxidation with the exception that the final reduction is carried out with NADPH.

Triacylglycerol biosynthesis

Free fatty acids are not found in significant quantities in tissues but are present largely as esters. Synthesis of triacylglycerols occurs primarily in adipose tissue and liver. Two fatty acyl-CoA molecules interact with glycerol 3-phosphate to produce phosphatidic acid (Fig. 88). The reaction proceeds preferentially with C_{16} and C_{18} saturated and unsaturated fatty acyl-CoA

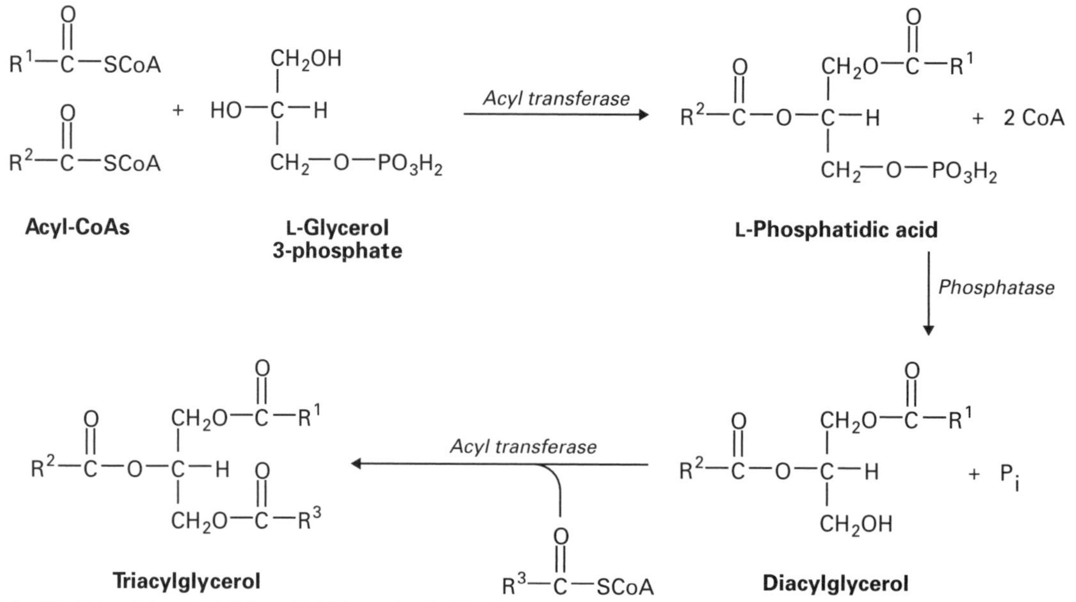

Fig. 88 Triacylglycerol (triglyceride) biosynthesis. This is the pathway that is used in adipose tissue and the liver.

Table 7 Composition of plasma lipoproteins

	Chylomicrons	VLDL	LDL	HDL
Density	<0.95	0.95–1.006	1.019–1.063	1.063–1.21
Protein (%)	1–2	10	25	45–55
Triacylglycerol (%)	80–95	55–65	10	3
Phospholipid (%)	3–6	15–20	22	30
Cholesterol (%)	1–3	10	8	33
Cholesteryl ester (%)	2–4	5	37	15

derivatives. The glycerol 3-phosphate is derived from the glycolytic intermediate dihydroxyacetone phosphate. Phosphatidic acid is dephosphorylated to yield diacylglycerol (DAG) which is then acylated to form a triacylglycerol.

In the liver, triacylglycerols are incorporated into very low density lipoprotein (VLDL) for transport to adipose tissue where fat is stored (p. 142).

10.2 Triacylglycerol transport

The important issues vis-à-vis fat transport are:

- how is fat transported from the gut to storage sites?
- how is fat transported from the liver to storage sites?

Since fats are hydrophobic they have to be packaged in a way that allows them to be transported in an aqueous medium. The packaging involves the formation of *lipoproteins* consisting of aggregates of apolipoproteins, triacylglycerols, cholesteryl esters and phospholipids in various proportions. The core of the particle contains hydrophobic lipids and the apolipoproteins and the phospholipid head groups are on the outside. The major classes of lipoprotein are shown in Table 7 and their functions are given in Table 8.

Table 8 Major functions of lipoproteins

	Apoprotein	Functions
Chylomicrons	Apo-As, Apo-B-48, Apo-CII, Apo-E	Triacylglycerols from gut
VLDL	Apo-B100, Apo-CII, Apo-E	Triacylglycerols from liver to adipose tissue
LDL	Apo-B100	Enriched in cholesteryl esters; deliver cholesterol to extra-hepatic tissues
HDL	Apo-As, Apo-Cs, Apo-E	Scavenges for cholesterol as it circulates in blood

Fat is transported in chylomicrons from the gut to storage sites

During digestion, dietary triacylglycerols are hydrolysed to fatty acids and monoglycerides, which are absorbed into the intestinal mucosal cells in micelles (p. 76). Triacylglycerols are reformed in mucosal cells using a pathway that involves monoglyceride (Fig. 89); they are then incorporated into *chylomicrons*. The chylomicrons are secreted into the lymphatic system, entering blood at the level of the thoracic duct. In blood, other apoproteins are transferred from HDL to chylomicrons: these include apoproteins ApoE and ApoCII. HDL, the so-called 'good cholesterol', removes cholesterol from the plasma membranes of extrahepatic

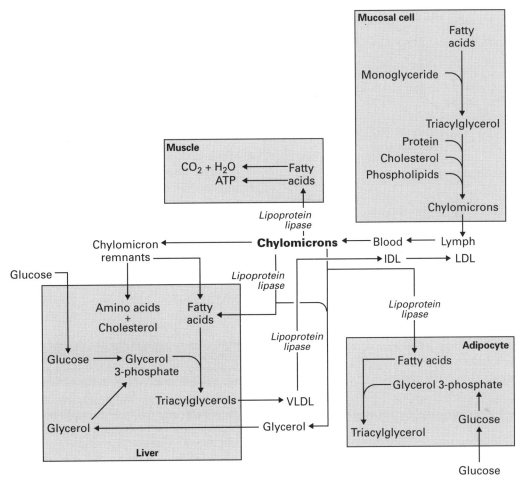

Fig. 89 Inter-organ fat metabolism in the fed state.

cells and helps in the removal of cholesterol from the body.

Fat is transported in VLDL from the liver to storage sites

Fatty acids synthesised in the liver, or delivered to the liver from chylomicrons, are converted to triacyl-glycerols using a pathway that involves phosphatidate (p. 123); they are incorporated into VLDL (Fig. 89) and also acquire ApoCII from circulating HDL.

Lipoprotein lipase clears fatty acids from chylomicrons and VLDL

Chylomicrons and VLDL are cleared of their triacylglycerols by the action of *lipoprotein lipase* (LPL), an enzyme that is attached to endothelial cells lining capillary walls. LPL is produced in adipocytes, cardiac muscle, other muscle cells and also in the mammary gland. Its level is increased by insulin action. The ApoCII component of chylomicrons and VLDL activates LPL. The products of LPL action on the lipoprotein-associated triacylglycerol are glycerol and fatty acids. LPL action on VLDL leaves intermediate density lipoproteins (IDL), the precursors of LDL.

Adipose tissue. Fatty acids taken up into adipocytes are converted to and stored as triacylglycerols, by the pathways described above (p. 123).

BOX 10.1
Clinical note: Defective LPL

Subjects with defective LPL will have hyper-triglyceridaemia after a meal because of their impaired ability to clear chylomicrons. High speed centrifugation of their blood will show chylomicrons floating on the surface.

Muscle. In muscle cells, the fatty acids serve as fuels, being completely oxidised for ATP synthesis. Some triacylglycerols are stored here too.

Chylomicron clearance. LPL depletes chylomicrons of their triacylglycerols, resulting in a remnant particle that is metabolised by the liver since receptors in that tissue recognise their ApoE component.

10.3 Cholesterol and bile acids

Cholesterol

Cholesterol is the most commonly occurring steroid: it is present in nearly all living organisms but not in plants. It contains the common steroid ring system (Fig. 90). Cholesterol has a number of roles:

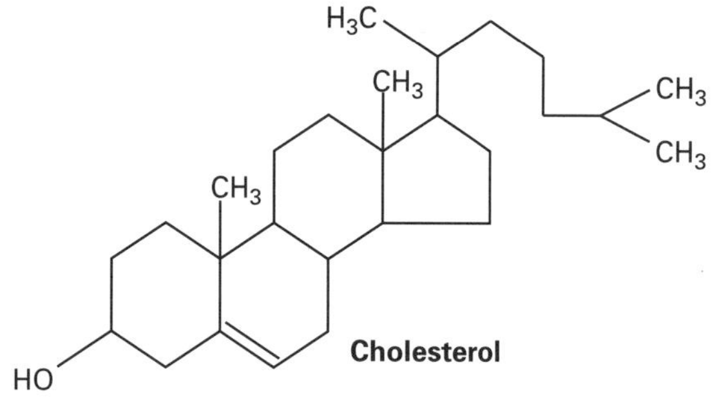

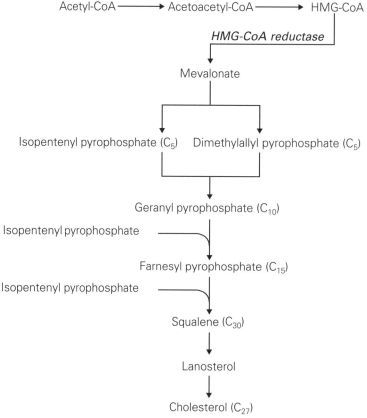

Fig. 90 Structure of cholesterol.

- structural component of membranes
- an important component of plasma lipoproteins
- a precursor of bile acids
- a precursor of steroid hormones.

There is great interest in cholesterol metabolism because of its association with cardiovascular disease. In Western societies, the cholesterol intake in the diet per day is 600–1200 mg, of which 300–400 mg are absorbed. Above average levels can be found in skin and egg yolk. Cholesterol and cholesteryl esters in the diet are absorbed along with other fats (p. 76).

Cholesterol is synthesised from acetyl-CoA

In addition to dietary sources, cholesterol can be synthesised in the body, with the liver and the intestinal mucosal cells being the principal sites. Cholesterol in the diet controls to some extent the amount of cholesterol synthesised in that there is feedback inhibition of liver cholesterol synthesis (but not of synthesis in mucosal cells). Mucosal cell synthesis of cholesterol is directly affected by bile acids, with high levels being inhibitory. The biosynthetic pathway is outlined in Figure 91. The key points are:

- all of the carbons are derived from acetate (acetyl-CoA)
- HMG-CoA is an intermediate; its conversion to mevalonate is the key rate-controlling step
- from mevalonate, active C_5 compounds are formed and these condense to yield intermediates with 10, 15 and, finally, 30 carbons; the last compound is *squalene*
- cyclisation yields the parent steroid *lanosterol*, from which cholesterol is formed
- this pathway occurs in the cytosol and requires NADPH.

BOX 10.2
Clinical note: Inhibitors of HMG-CoA reductase in treatment of hypercholesterolaemia

Compactin, isolated from cultures of a species of *Penicillium*, and mevinolin, isolated from *Aspergillus*, are competitive inhibitors of HMG-CoA reductase and, therefore, lower plasma cholesterol. This is an important therapy for some patients with elevated cholesterol levels.

Acetyl-CoA ⟶ Acetoacetyl-CoA ⟶ HMG-CoA

HMG-CoA reductase

Mevalonate

Isopentenyl pyrophosphate (C_5)   Dimethylallyl pyrophosphate (C_5)

Geranyl pyrophosphate (C_{10})

Isopentenyl pyrophosphate ⟶

Farnesyl pyrophosphate (C_{15})

Isopentenyl pyrophosphate ⟶

Squalene (C_{30})

Lanosterol

Cholesterol (C_{27})

Fig. 91 Cholesterol biosynthesis.

HMG-CoA reductase is the important control step in cholesterol biosynthesis

There is evidence that a diurnal variation in HMG-CoA reductase activity occurs in humans, with a maximum activity between midnight and 4:00 a.m. HMG-CoA reductase activity changes in response to dietary cholesterol and hormonal status. Regulation includes inhibition of HMG-CoA reductase gene expression by cholesterol as well as phosphorylation of the enzyme. The expression of HMG-CoA reductase is only inhibited 90% by treatment with compounds such as compactin (see Box 10.2) but there is also feedback inhibition by cholesterol itself on the enzyme catalysing squalene synthesis. This means that where HMG-CoA reductase inhibitors are used clinically there is enough farnesyl pyrophosphate to allow for the synthesis of important non-sterol isoprenoids such as farnesylated proteins. The control of HMG-CoA reductase and LDL receptor transcription (see Fig. 92) involves the interaction between a sterol regulatory element (SRE) and a SRE binding protein. High cholesterol inhibits the formation of SRE binding protein.

Cholesterol is transported to extrahepatic tissues as LDL

Most extra-hepatic tissues, although having a requirement for cholesterol, have low activity of the cholesterol biosynthetic pathway. Their cholesterol requirements are supplied by LDL, which is internalised by receptor-mediated endocytosis. This process is depicted in Figure 92 and the following are the key features.

1. 'high-affinity' LDL receptors are present to which the apoprotein B-100 of LDL binds; there is then internalisation of the receptor–LDL complex and processing of this complex leads to the provision of cholesterol for the cell in question
2. internalisation occurs at special parts of the plasma membrane surface termed *coated pits*, which are depressions in the cell surface with a specific protein, *clathrin*, bound to the cytoplasmic surface giving it a 'coated' appearance (Fig. 38)
3. coated pits then 'pinch' off from the surface to form coated vesicles
4. coated vesicles lose their coat after endocytosis to become *endosomes* (smooth surface vesicles)
5. the receptors in the endosome then return to the cell surface and the LDL in the endosomes fuses with lysosomes where the LDL proteins and cholesteryl esters are hydrolysed
6. the free cholesterol formed down-regulates LDL receptor synthesis in the cell and also controls endogenous cholesterol synthesis by repression of HMG-CoA reductase
7. cholesterol is stored as cholesteryl esters, formed by the action of acyl-CoA:cholesterol acyltransferase (ACAT).

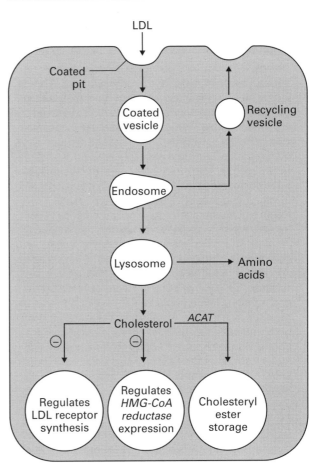

Fig. 92 Receptor-mediated endocytosis for cholesterol delivery to cells. ACAT, acyl-CoA:cholesterol acyltransferase.

Bile acids

Compared to other steroids of biological significance, bile acids have hydroxyl groups at position 7 in the B ring (Fig. 93). Two series of bile acids are synthesised: one yields cholic acid and the other chenodeoxycholic acid. In the cholic acid series, there are hydroxyl groups at positions 3, 7 and 12 in the steroid nucleus. In the chenodeoxycholic acid series, the hydroxyls are only at the 3 and 7 positions. Both function in fat digestion and absorption (Chapter 7). *Bile salts* are conjugates of the bile acids and are very effective as detergents since they are amphiphiles containing a polar region (in the side chain) and a non-polar region, the steroid nucleus.

Bile acids are synthesised from cholesterol

Bile acids are produced in the liver (Fig. 94). The initial step involves 7α-hydroxylation of cholesterol and then there are further hydroxylations and limited side chain cleavage to yield a C_{24} steroid with a carboxyl at carbon-24 in the side chain. 7α-hydroxylation is controlled. Cholic acid can form an amide with the amino groups of taurine ($H_2NCH_2CH_2SO_3H$) or glycine (H_2NCH_2COOH) to form *taurocholic acid* and *glycocholic acid*, respectively. It is these two compounds that are the major bile salts secreted in the bile. Similar conjugates are formed with chenodeoxycholic acid.

BOX 10.3
Clinical note: Defective LDL receptors

Defects in the LDL receptor system results in *hypercholesterolaemia* and *arteriosclerosis*. There are numerous disorders of lipoprotein metabolism but *familial hypercholesterolaemia* (FH) has been the most studied. FH is inherited as an autosomal dominant trait with a gene dosage effect, i.e. homozygotes are more severely affected than are heterozygotes. Heterozygotes number about 1 in 500 persons. They have twofold elevations in plasma cholesterol (range 7.8–12 mmol/litre). Homozygotes number 1 in 1 million persons. They have severe hypercholesterolaemia (as high as 20 mmol/litre). Coronary heart disease begins in childhood and frequently causes death before age 20. The primary defect in FH is a mutation in the receptor for plasma LDL. FH heterozygotes have one normal allele and one mutant allele at the LDL receptor locus; as a result, their cells are able to bind and take up LDL at approximately half the normal rate. Phenotypic homozygotes possess two mutant alleles at the LDL receptor locus; their cells show a total or near-total inability to bind or take up LDL. Subjects with defective LDL receptors have absent or reduced receptor-mediated endocytosis in the liver and extra-hepatic tissues. This results in increased cholesterol biosynthesis in extra-hepatic tissues but, more important, IDL clearance by the liver is impaired and more LDL will then be formed. Treatment for heterozygotes and homozygotes involves lowering the plasma level of LDL. In heterozygotes, the best strategy is to stimulate the single normal gene to produce more LDL receptor mRNA.

Conversion of bile acids to non-absorbable forms by intestinal bacteria is a major route of excretion of cholesterol. There is a significant enterohepatic circulation involving bile acids.

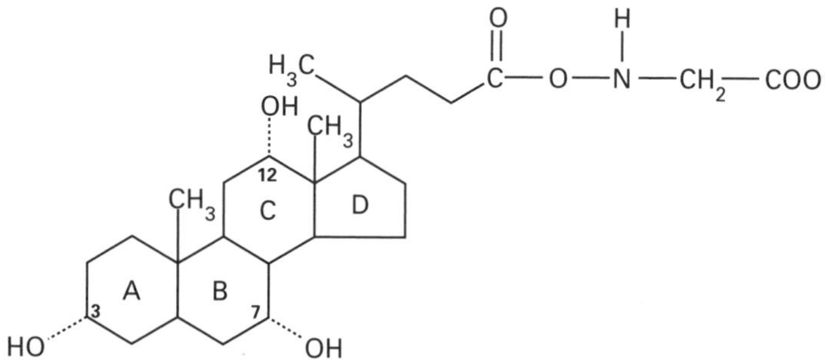

Fig. 93 Structure of the bile acid glycocholic acid.

BOX 10.4
Clinical note: Bile acid binders in treatment of hypercholesterolaemia

Cholestyramine, an anion exchange resin, binds bile acids in the gut and prevents their reabsorption. Cholestyramine has been utilised therapeutically, along with inhibitors of HMG-CoA reductase, to control cholesterol levels in hypercholesterolaemic subjects.

Steroid hormones are derived from cholesterol

In the adrenal cortex, gonads and placenta, cholesterol is the precursor of active steroid hormones made by these tissues, including cortisol, aldosterone, testosterone, oestradiol and progesterone (Chapter 18). 7-Dehydrocholesterol is the precursor of vitamin D, which can be made in skin under the influence of ultraviolet light (pp. 226–227).

10.4 Complex lipids

Phospholipids

Phosphoglycerides are amphiphiles having both polar and non-polar groups. Some, such as phosphatidyl-

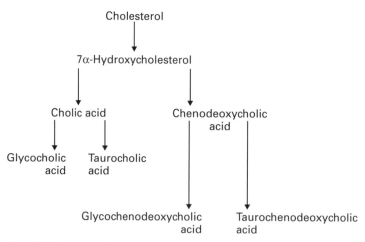

Fig. 94 Bile acid synthesis.

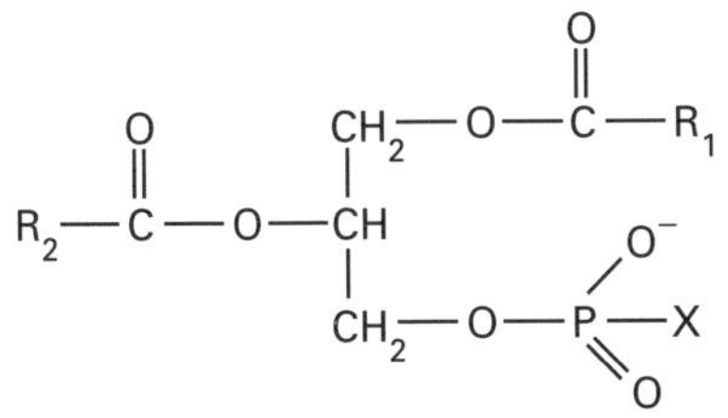

Fig. 95 General formula for a glycerophospholipid. X = choline (PC), ethanolamine (PE), serine (PS), glycerol (PG), inositol (PI).

choline (PC), are dipolar ions. They are all important constituents of cell membranes (see also Box 5.1).

This class of complex lipids includes PC, phosphatidylethanolamine (PE), phosphatidylglycerol (PG), phosphatidylinositol (PI) and phosphatidylserine (PS). The general formula for the phosphoglycerides is given in Figure 95.

CTP is involved in phospholipid biosynthesis

The major pathways involved in phospholipid bio-synthesis are outlined in Figure 96. Phosphatidate (diacylglycerol 3-phosphate) is an intermediate in the synthesis of phospholipids as it is in the synthesis of triacylglycerols. Depending upon the particular phospholipid, activated intermediates are formed using the pyrimidine nucleotide CTP.

- CDP-diacylglycerol is an intermediate in the major pathways for PS, PI and PG formation
- CDP-choline and CDP-ethanolamine are intermediates in PC and PE synthesis with phosphorylcholine and phosphorylethanolamine being precursors.

In another important pathway, decarboxylation of PS yields PE, which can then be converted to PC by three

successive methylations involving *S*-adenosyl-methionine (SAM). In the liver, PS can be formed from PE by the enzyme-catalysed transfer of serine for the ethanolamine moiety of the phospholipid. Cardiolipin (diphosphatidylglycerol), a phospholipid mainly found in mitochondria, is formed from PG by interacting with CDP-diacylglycerol.

Sphingolipids

Sphingolipids are important in the nervous system and abnormal levels are found in several diseases affecting that system. Gangliosides play a special role in plasma membrane receptors for hormones, viruses, etc. They contain, in addition to sugar residues, the compound *N*-acetylneuraminic acid (NANA), otherwise known as *sialic acid*.

Ceramide is a key intermediate in sphingolipid synthesis

Sphingolipid biosynthesis is outlined in Figure 97. All sphingolipids are based on sphinganine, which is formed from serine and palmitoyl-CoA. The addition of choline to ceramide gives *sphingomyelin*; the addition of sugars gives *cerebrosides*, *globosides* and *gangliosides*.

The sphingolipidoses

The sphingolipidoses are inherited disorders of sphingo-lipid metabolism and most of them are autosomal recessive. In several of these disorders, homozygotes show progressive mental and motor deterioration, with onset in childhood and fatal outcomes. One current interest in the sphingolipidoses stems from the finding

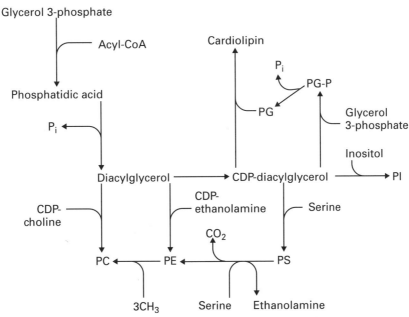

Fig. 96 The biosynthesis of phospholipids. CDP derivatives participate in the two major pathways.

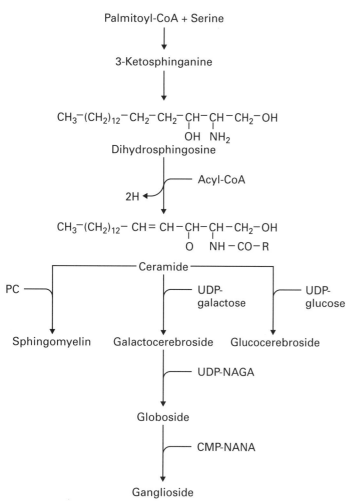

Fig. 97 The biosynthesis of sphingolipids. NANA, N-acetylneuraminic acid (sialic acid).

that these diseases are amenable to heterozygote detection and prenatal diagnosis, since most are autosomal recessive. The sphingolipidoses are *lipid storage diseases* and in each of them the defect is in an enzyme of the degradative pathway occurring in lysosomes.

Tay–Sachs disease (TSD)

TSD is the most common ganglioside storage disease. The heterozygote frequency for TSD mutation among Ashkenazi Jews is 1 in 27; it is 1 in 125 for non-Jews. Heterozygotes can be reliably determined by a serum assay of the deficient enzyme, *hexosaminidase A*. This was the first example of a genetic disease where the birth of an affected child has been prevented by mass screening for heterozygotes in at-risk populations.

Other sphingolipidoses

- Niemann-Pick disease, where sphingomyelin accumulates
- Gaucher's disease, where glucocerebroside accumulates
- Fabry's disease (X-linked inheritance), where a globoside accumulates
- Krabbe's disease, affecting galactocerebroside metabolism.

10.5 Prostaglandins and related compounds

Eicosanoids

The eicosanoids form a group of 'local' hormones and are produced in most tissues of the body. They are participants in the inflammatory response that follows injury or infection. They include *prostaglandins*, *thromboxanes*, *prostacyclin* and *leukotrienes* and are derived from *arachidonate*, a polyunsaturated fatty acid that is synthesised from the essential fatty acid linoleate. Eicosanoids act through receptors in the plasma membranes of target cells, where they influence either protein kinase A or intracellular calcium levels.

Biosynthesis

Arachidonate is normally present at the *sn*-2 position of phospholipids and is released when phospholipase A_2 is activated by various stimuli (Fig. 98).

The cyclooxygenase pathway. This pathway forms prostaglandins (including PGE_2, $PGF_{2\alpha}$ and PGD_2), prostacyclin (PGI_2) and thromboxane A_2. Arachidonate is converted by the cyclooxygenase complex to PGG_2, which contains a five-membered ring and hydroperoxy group. The latter is reduced to a hydroxyl in the formation of PGH_2. Prostacyclin is derived from PGH_2 by the action of PGI synthase in endothelial cells. Thromboxane A_2 is formed from PGH_2 by the action of thromboxane synthase an enzyme present in platelets.

The lipoxygenase pathway. This pathway forms leukotrienes in mast cells and leucocytes. Lipoxygenases catalyse hydroperoxidations at various positions in arachidonate to give 5-, 12- and 15-HPETEs (hydroperoxyeicosatetraenoic acids) from which a variety of HETEs (hydroeicosatetranoic acids) are formed. 5-HPETE is also the precursor of leukotriene LTA_4, which in turn is converted to LTB_4 and LTC_4. LTC_4 is formed from LTA_4 by the addition of reduced glutathione and is then processed to yield in turn LTD_4 and LTE_4. Leukotrienes have many biological actions including increasing vascular permeability and being potent bronchoconstrictors.

Aspirin acts as an anti-inflammatory agent by inhibiting cyclooxygenase

Aspirin (acetylsalicylate) acetylates and irreversibly inactivates cyclooxygenase. Levels of the active enzyme in platelets are especially susceptible because these cells do not have nuclei and cannot regenerate cyclooxygenase. Cyclooxygenase in endothelial cells is also affected but the enzyme at that site is restored to normal within a few hours. If subjects are treated with low-dose aspirin, there is a large fall in thromboxane A_2 relative to PGI_2 and platelet aggregation is inhibited. Low-dose aspirin therapy is used effectively to prevent myocardial infarction and is also used in patients to prevent recurrence of a heart attack. Other non-

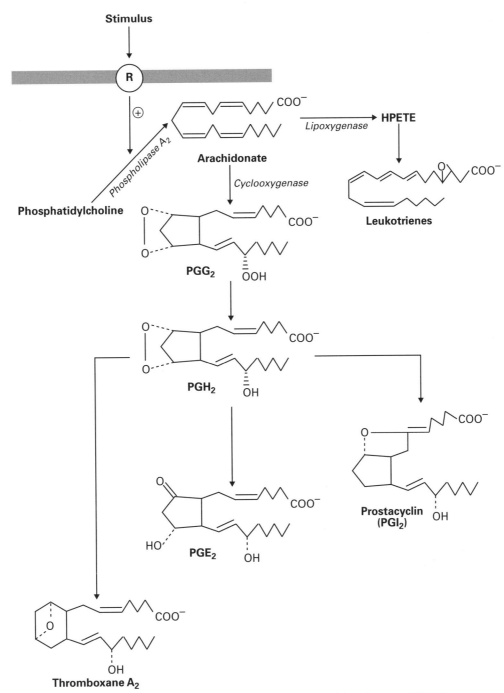

Fig. 98 Conversion of arachidonate to prostaglandins, leukotrienes and thromboxanes. HPETE, hydroperoxyeicosatetraenoic acid.

steroidal anti-inflammatory drugs (NSAIDs) such as ibuprofen and acetaminophen are reversible inhibitors of cyclooxygenase.

Glucocorticoids act as anti-inflammatory agents by inhibiting phospholipase A$_2$

Glucocorticoids are potent anti-inflammatory agents that are used extensively in clinical practice for conditions such as chronic obstructive lung disease. They increase the production of proteins called lipocortins, which inhibit phospholipase A$_2$. As can be seen from Figure 98, inhibition of phospholipase A$_2$ will reduce the synthesis of prostaglandins, leukotrienes and thromboxane.

Self-assessment: questions

Multiple choice questions

1. The following statements describe cholesterol metabolism in normal subjects:
   a. In most extra-hepatic tissues cholesterol biosynthesis occurs at lower rates than in the liver
   b. Vitamin D can be produced by the action of ultraviolet light on 7-dehydrocholesterol
   c. HMG-CoA, mevalonate, geranyl pyrophosphate and squalene are all intermediates in cholesterol biosynthesis
   d. HMG-CoA reductase gene expression is increased when cholesterol intake in the diet is high
   e. Cholesterol metabolism to bile acids will be decreased in the liver if there is reduced bile acid recycling through the enterohepatic circulation

2. HMG-CoA reductase:
   a. Catalyses the rate-limiting step in cholesterol biosynthesis
   b. Is located in the cytosol
   c. Can be inhibited by several drugs that benefit patients with hypercholesterolaemia
   d. Requires NADH
   e. Is in both the cholesterol and ketone body synthetic pathways

3. Lipoprotein lipase (LPL):
   a. Catalyses the hydrolysis of triacylglycerols in adipocytes
   b. Is activated by apoprotein CII
   c. Catalyses the hydrolysis of triacylglycerols in both VLDL and chylomicrons
   d. Has its synthesis inhibited by insulin
   e. Is required for triacylglycerol digestion in the gut

4. The following statements describe LDL:
   a. IDL is a precursor of LDL
   b. LDL contributes to the build-up of atherosclerotic plaque
   c. The surface of LDL consists of cholesteryl esters and triacylglycerol
   d. The defect in familial hypercholesterolaemia involves LDL receptors
   e. Cholesterol from LDL regulates HMG-CoA reductase in the liver and extra-hepatic tissues

5. The LDL receptor:
   a. Is not found on hepatocytes
   b. Recognises apoprotein CII on the LDL
   c. Number is increased in heterozygotes of familial hypercholesterolaemia
   d. Is required for the clearance of IDL by the liver
   e. Is concentrated in coated pits of cells

6. The following statements describe phospholipid biosynthesis in the body:
   a. PC can be made from PS
   b. CDP-diacylglycerol is an intermediate in the synthesis of several phospholipids
   c. Phospholipids have to be supplied in the diet
   d. Phospholipids do not contain any unsaturated fatty acids
   e. Cardiolipin is the major phospholipid found in plasma membranes

7. Bile acids are:
   a. Synthesised mainly in mucosal cells of the small intestine
   b. Inhibitors of cholesterol biosynthesis
   c. Amphipathic compounds
   d. Conjugated with glycine or taurine
   e. The major metabolites of cholesterol in the body

8. In fatty acid biosynthesis:
   a. The intermediates in the conversion of the β-ketoacyl chain into the saturated acyl chain are covalently linked to acyl carrier protein (ACP)
   b. One of the products is NADPH
   c. Unsaturation can result in oleate synthesis but not linoleate
   d. Carbon dioxide is incorporated into palmitate
   e. Citrate enables acetyl-CoA to be transported to the cytosol where fatty acid synthesis takes place

9. Acetyl-CoA carboxylase:
   a. Requires biotin for the fixation of carbon dioxide
   b. Is activated by citrate
   c. Catalyses the production of malonyl-CoA for fatty acid biosynthesis
   d. Is located in the mitochondria of cells synthesising fatty acids
   e. Catalyses a rate-controlling step in fatty acid biosynthesis

10. The following statements describe fatty acid synthesis:
    a. Oleate cannot be synthesised in the body
    b. De novo fatty acid synthesis occurs in mitochondria
    c. The ACP component of the fatty acid synthetase (FAS) multi-enzyme complex contains the B vitamin pantothenate
    d. Palmitate can be elongated to produce fatty acids with 18 or 20 carbons
    e. Arachidonic acid can be synthesised in the body provided we take linoleic acid in our diet

11. In the pathway for triacylglycerol synthesis in the liver:
   a. Diacylglycerol (DAG) is an intermediate
   b. Fatty acyl-CoAs are required
   c. A phosphatidic acid is an intermediate
   d. Glycerol is the direct precursor of the glycerol 3-phosphate required for triglyceride synthesis in adipocytes
   e. Only saturated fatty acids can be incorporated into triacylglycerols

12. Phospholipase A_2:
   a. Is indirectly involved in the synthesis of prostaglandins, thromboxanes and leukotrienes
   b. Is inhibited by aspirin
   c. When activated, results in the release of arachidonic acid from phospholipids
   d. Is only involved in the digestion of phospholipids

13. Steroid anti-inflammatory agents inhibit:
   a. Indirectly the formation of prostaglandins, thromboxanes and leukotrienes
   b. The cyclooxygenase component of the multi-enzyme complex which is involved in the synthesis of prostaglandins
   c. The release of arachidonic acid from phospholipids by phospholipase A_2
   d. The lipoxygenase which converts arachidonic acid to 5-HPETE

True/false questions

Are the following statements true or false?

1. Clathrin is concentrated in the Golgi apparatus in extra-hepatic tissues.

2. The LDL receptor recognises apoprotein B-48 in LDL.
3. Atheromatous plaques recovered from a patient who has died from a coronary contain high concentrations of cholesterol and its esters.
4. Chylomicrons and VLDL both contain apoprotein CII.
5. Extra-hepatic tissues derive cholesterol from a circulating lipoprotein by a process that involves receptor-mediated endocytosis.
6. Cholesterol 7α-hydroxylase is a rate-controlling step in bile acid synthesis in the liver.
7. The synthesis of PC from PE requires S-adenosyl-methionine.
8. Gangliosides are unique from other sphingolipids in their content of N-acetylgalactosamine.
9. The action of acetyl-CoA carboxylase generates an intermediate in fatty acid biosynthesis that is also an inhibitor of fatty acid utilisation.
10. Mammalian fatty acid synthetase (FAS) is active as a dimer.
11. Dipalmitoylphosphatidylcholine is the principal phospholipid in surfactant.

Short essay questions

1. Discuss cholesterol metabolism in the body in the context of the pathogenesis of familial hypercholesterolaemia.
2. Compare and contrast the roles of pancreatic lipase, lipoprotein lipase (LPL) and 'hormone-sensitive' lipase (HSL) in the body.
3. Construct a table that contrasts fatty acid oxidation with fatty acid synthesis.
4. Explain the essential role played by a product of glucose metabolism in the synthesis of triacylglycerols from fatty acids in the body.

Self-assessment: answers

Multiple choice answers

1. a. **True.** Extra-hepatic tissues receive their cholesterol from plasma LDL by receptor-mediated endocytosis.
   b. **True.** This is an important source of vitamin D. Smog and industrial pollution lower the ability to make vitamin D in the skin.
   c. **True.** Acetyl-CoA is the starting point for their synthesis.
   d. **False.** High cholesterol in the diet suppresses the expression of HMG-CoA reductase.
   e. **False.** Because of the need to synthesise more bile acids, cholesterol metabolism to bile acids in the liver will increase under these circumstances.

2. a. **True.** The product is mevalonate.
   b. **True.** HMG-CoA reductase is located in the cytosol.
   c. **True.** These drugs include lovostatin.
   d. **False.** The coenzyme is NADPH.
   e. **False.** HMG-CoA reductase is not involved in ketone body production.

3. a. **False.** This lipase is attached to endothelial cells and hydrolyses triacylglycerol in VLDL and chylomicrons.
   b. **True.** Apo-CII is present in both VLDL and chylomicrons.
   c. **True.** That is implied by its name, since no specific lipoprotein is specified.
   d. **False.** Insulin increases LPL expression and this is consistent with the fed state where more fat is being stored.
   e. **False.** The lipase involved in fat digestion is pancreatic lipase.

4. a. **True.** IDL is produced when VLDL is 'cleared' of triacylglycerols by the action of lipoprotein lipase and is then converted to LDL by interactions with lipoproteins such as HDL.
   b. **True.** Cholesterol of elevated LDL is incorporated into these plaques.
   c. **False.** These lipids are in the interior of the LDL particle.
   d. **True.** There are many molecular defects in the various types of FH but each lead to a defective LDL receptor system.
   e. **True.** Cholesterol represses the expression of the HMG-CoA reductase gene.

5. a. **False.** The LDL receptor in hepatocytes is involved with LDL and IDL metabolism.
   b. **False.** It recognises apoprotein B-100 on LDL and IDL.

c. **False.** Is half the normal level in FH heterozygotes.
   d. **True.** An important point in the pathogenesis of FH, since elevated IDL levels will lead to increased LDL levels.
   e. **True.** This facilitates efficient endocytosis of LDL particles.

6. a. **True.** PS can be decarboxylated to PE, which by the addition of three methyl groups produces PC.
   b. **True.** Specifically, it is involved in PS, PI and PG synthesis.
   c. **False.** Phospholipids are synthesised in most tissues.
   d. **False.** Most often, the fatty acid at the 2 position in phospholipids is unsaturated.
   e. **False.** Cardiolipin is mainly found in the mitochondrial inner membrane.

7. a. **False.** They are synthesised in the liver.
   b. **True.** High levels of bile acids lower HMG-CoA reductase synthesis.
   c. **True.** They have hydrophobic and hydrophilic components. Hence, they act as detergents.
   d. **True.** The bile salts are formed: glycocholate, taurocholate, glycochenodeoxycholate and taurochenodeoxycholate.
   e. **True.** Other compounds such as steroid hormones are synthesised from cholesterol but, on a mass basis, bile acids are by far the major metabolites.

8. a. **True.** The ketoacyl group being attached to the long side chain of ACP allows for interaction with the enzymes catalysing reduction of the ketone.
   b. **False.** NADPH is used in the two reductase-catalysed steps in FAS.
   c. **True.** Linoleate is an essential fatty acid.
   d. **False.** The carbon dioxide used to form malonyl-CoA from acetyl-CoA is lost in the reaction catalysed by the ketosynthetase of FAS.
   e. **True.** The inner mitochondrial membrane is impermeable to acetyl-CoA; this is overcome by making citrate from oxaloacetate and acetyl-CoA within the mitochondria and then cleaving it in the cytosol to yield acetyl-CoA and oxaloacetate.

9. a. **True.** Biotin is the coenzyme for carboxylations in intermediary metabolism. Carboxybiotinyl-enzyme is an intermediate in the reaction.
   b. **True.** Most books imply that citrate does so by polymerising the enzyme but, in fact, the activation precedes any polymerisation.

c. **True.** Seven malonyl-CoA molecules are required for each palmitate synthesised.

d. **False.** The enzyme is in the cytosol, as is FAS.

e. **True.** The enzyme is activated by citrate and its activity is affected by phosphorylation.

10. a. **False.** Oleate ($C_{18:1}$) is produced by the unsaturation of stearate (C_{18}) catalysed by fatty acid desaturase located in the smooth endoplasmic reticulum.

b. **False.** The reactions occur in the cytosol.

c. **True.** Pantothenate is also found in coenzyme A.

d. **True.** This process can occur in mitochondria where acetyl-CoA is used, or in the cytosol where malonyl-CoA is used.

e. **True.** Linoleic acid is an essential fatty acid required for the production of arachidonate and, therefore, prostaglandins, leukotrienes, thromboxane and prostacyclin.

11. a. **True.** It is formed by the dephosphorylation of phosphatidic acid.

b. **True.** Acylation of glycerol 3-phosphate utilises fatty acyl-CoAs.

c. **True.** Phosphatidic acid is the product of acylation of glycerol 3-phosphate.

d. **False.** The glycerol 3-phosphate is derived from the metabolism of glucose in the adipocyte. Glycerol kinase is not present in adipocytes.

e. **False.** Triacylglycerols stored in adipocytes contain both saturated and unsaturated fatty acids.

12. a. **True.** Its action on phospholipids generates arachidonate, the precursor of these eicosanoids.

b. **False.** Aspirin inhibits cyclooxygenase and, therefore, specifically thromboxane and prostaglandin synthesis.

c. **True.**

d. **False.** Although A_2 is involved in phospholipid digestion, it is also involved in eicosanoid synthesis.

13. a. **True.** Due to the fact that they inhibit phospholipase A_2.

b. **False.** It is aspirin that does so, not steroid anti-inflammatory agents.

c. **True.** See a.

d. **False.** Their action is on phospholipase A_2.

True/false answers

1. **False.** It is concentrated in 'coated pits'.

2. **False.** It is apoprotein B-100 that binds to the LDL receptor.

3. **True.** This is part of the evidence relating cholesterol with coronary artery disease.

4. **True.** They are both acted upon by LPL and apo-CII activates that enzyme.

5. **True.** The lipoprotein is LDL.

6. **True.** Following 7α-hydroxylation, other hydroxyls are added and side-chain cleavage occurs to give the C_{24} bile acids.

7. **True.** *S*-adenosylmethionine provides the methyl groups for many important methylations involved in the synthesis of key compounds in the body.

8. **False.** Gangliosides differ from other sphingolipids in containing sialic acid, also called *N*-acetylneuraminic acid.

9. **True.** Malonyl-CoA is required for fatty acid biosynthesis but it is also an inhibitor of carnitine acyltransferase I, the rate-limiting step in fatty acid utilisation.

10. **True.** It is the monomer that is inactive.

11. **True.** It is not the only component but it is very important.

Short essay answers

1. It is now clear that there is a correlation between elevated levels of circulating cholesterol and the pathogenesis of coronary heart disease (CHD). However, it is complicated in that CHD is multi-factorial.

   There is a very clear relationship between elevated cholesterol and CHD in the case of familial hypercholesterolaemia (FH), an autosomal dominant disorder affecting the receptor-mediated endocytosis pathway for LDL metabolism in the body. Homozygotes for this disorder have defective or absent LDL receptor in the liver and extra-hepatic tissues. The consequence is that the handling of both IDL and LDL is grossly impaired. IDL is usually cleared by the liver, a process involving the LDL receptor. IDL is also the precursor of LDL and since IDL is not being cleared by the liver, LDL production will increase, contributing to the increase in LDL levels.

   The defective LDL receptor-mediated endocytosis pathway in extra-hepatic tissues results in these tissues turning on their endogenous cholesterol biosynthetic pathways. The combination of these two alterations to normal metabolism contributes in a major way to the enormous increase in LDL found in FH. It seems clear that the very high LDL levels increases the potential for the LDL to be oxidised and then picked up by scavenger cells and other cell types leading to the production of xanthomas and artheromas.

   FH homozygotes unless treated heroically to reduce their cholesterol levels (or given a liver transplant) die in their teens or early twenties. Heterozygotes also have very high cholesterol levels and they die in their 30s or 40s.

2. It is important to recognise that these three lipases function in three different anatomical sites.

   Pancreatic lipase is secreted from the pancreas, ending up in the small intestine where it catalyses

Table 8 A comparison of fatty acid oxidation and synthesis

Parameter	Fatty acid oxidation	Fatty acid synthesis
Location in cells	Mitochondria	Cytosol
Transport	Carnitine	Acetate as citrate
Carrier	Coenzyme A	Acyl carrier protein
Addition or removal of C_2 units	Acetyl-CoA	Malonyl-CoA
Oxidation/reduction of keto $\rightleftharpoons$ hydroxyl	$NAD^+/NADH + H^+$	$NADPH + H^+/NADP^+$
Oxidation/reduction of crotonyl $\rightleftharpoons$ butyryl	$FAD/FADH_2$	$NADPH + H^+/NADP^+$

the hydrolysis of triacylglycerol derived from the diet. The products are 2-monoacylglycerol plus two fatty acid molecules (partial hydrolysis). This process is facilitated by the fact that the dietary triacylglycerol has been emulsified by the action of bile acids and salts, which are also secreted into the small intestine in association with the digestion of a meal. Both bile release from the gallbladder and pancreatic lipase secretion from the pancreas are under the control of cholecystokinin, a gastrointestinal hormone whose secretion is particularly high when fat is in the diet. Co-lipase, also secreted from the pancreas, has a key role to play in helping overcome the inhibition of pancreatic lipase action by bile salts.

Lipoprotein lipase (LPL) is an enzyme attached to endothelial cells that catalyses the hydrolysis of triacylglycerols carried in chylomicrons and VLDL. The fatty acids released can either be stored in adipose tissue or used as fuels in, for example, muscle. LPL is activated by apoprotein CII, which is a component of both VLDL and chylomicrons. LPL is synthesised in adipose tissue cells stimulated by insulin and is then translocated to the endothelial cells. The fact that insulin has this action is consistent with its role in fuel storage.

Hormone-sensitive lipase (HSL) is a triacylglycerol lipase found within adipocytes; it catalyses the first step in the complete hydrolysis of stored triacylglycerols to glycerol and three fatty acid molecules. It is the key enzyme in lipid mobilisation and is activated by a series of regulatory hormones that counteract the inhibitory action of insulin. Lipid mobilisation is increased in the fasting state to provide an alternative fuel to glucose for tissues such as muscle and liver. Activation of HSL by hormones such as glucagon involves phosphorylation, brought about by cyclic AMP-dependent protein kinase.

3. Table 8 contrasts fatty acid oxidation and synthesis.

4. In tissues other than the intestinal mucosa, triacylglycerol is synthesised by adding two fatty acyl groups from acyl-CoA to glycerol 3-phosphate to yield phosphatidic acid. This is followed by removal of the phosphate and then the addition of a third acyl group from acyl-CoA. In tissues other than the liver (e.g. adipose tissue), the source of the glycerol 3-phosphate is dihydroxyacetone phosphate, an intermediate in glycolysis. In the liver some glycerol 3-phosphate can be derived by the direct phosphorylation of glycerol but that kinase is absent in adipose tissue. Therefore, adipose tissue is dependent upon glucose uptake and metabolism to generate the glycerol 3-phosphate required for the triacylglycerol synthesis that occurs there following a meal.

Integration of metabolism

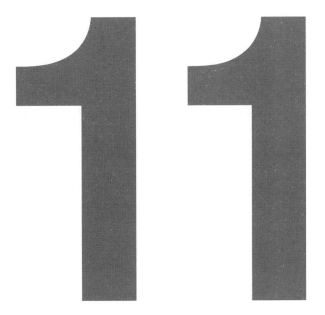

11

11.1 The fed and fasted states

The strategy of metabolism is to store fuel when food is available and to mobilise these stores when necessary.

Regulation of body weight

Many individuals are able to maintain exquisite control of their metabolism, as is evidenced by the fact that over periods of many years they show quite small fluctuations in body weight despite consuming a staggering number of calories in the form of carbohydrates, protein and fat. Also, when individuals through dieting achieve weight loss they usually regain the weight over time. This is suggestive of regulatory mechanisms being involved to control the amount of energy (triacylglycerols) stored in adipose tissue. From studies on obese mice, it has been shown that adipose tissue produces a polypeptide hormone, *leptin*, that is involved in controlling food intake. Leptin deficiency and/or leptin resistance leads to obesity. Insulin, the hormone of the fed state, also appears to act in the negative feedback control of adiposity. It is thought that both insulin and leptin through interactions in the hypothalamus control food intake and energy expenditure. What follows is an account of how the storage of fuels is achieved and how fuels are mobilised for the various tissues of the body. Familiarity with the contents of Chapters 7–10 will assist the reader in understanding the control of metabolism.

The fed state

It is interesting to examine the amount of the various fuels that are stored in normal subjects (Table 9). Many people tend to believe that glucose and glycogen are the most significant fuels in humans, but it is quite clear that in terms of total stored fuel triacylglycerols are prodigious by comparison.

How does one measure control of metabolism in the fed state?

This is done routinely using a *glucose tolerance test* in which a subject fasts overnight, a fasting blood sample is taken and a glucose drink is swallowed. Blood glucose is measured at 30 minute intervals for up to 150 minutes. On average, normal subjects show a blood glucose concentration rise from 90 mg/100 ml (5 mM) to about 140 mg/100 ml (7.8 mM). The effectiveness of control measures glucose concentrations and is illustrated by considering the fate of 50 g glucose which is completely

absorbed into a person with 5 litre blood volume or 15 litre extracellular fluid (ECF) volume. Clearly, the glucose concentration would rise to over 1000 mg/100 ml if the glucose was confined to the blood and to 333 mg/100 ml in the ECF and yet in normal individuals blood levels rarely exceed 180 mg/100 ml after a carbohydrate meal. The important question is 'Why does the blood glucose not reach very high (unphysiological) values?' An answer is revealed by the study of subjects with diabetes mellitus. Their blood glucose levels reach much higher levels (greater than 10 mM) following a challenge with oral glucose. These patients either make little or no insulin or they have insulin resistance. Clearly, insulin is vital to the ability to control blood glucose in the fed state.

Insulin

It is the hormone of the fed state and important points about it are:

- it is a small protein hormone with 51 amino acid residues consisting of two peptide chains (A and B) linked by two disulphide bonds; it is synthesised in pancreatic beta cells
- insulin secretagogues are factors that increase insulin secretion. The principal one is glucose. High blood glucose levels lead to increased glucose metabolism in beta cells, depolarisation of the cell, calcium entry and insulin release (Fig. 99)
- the major sites for insulin action in the body are the liver, muscle and adipose tissue (Fig. 100 and Table 10)
- the most common endocrine disorder in the global sense is *diabetes mellitus*. There are two major forms of diabetes mellitus: insulin-dependent diabetes mellitus (IDDM) and non-insulin-dependent diabetes mellitus (NIDDM). The most common findings in diabetes mellitus are hyperglycaemia, glucosuria, decreased glycogenesis, decreased fatty acid synthesis, increased lipolysis, increased fatty acids in blood, ketonaemia, ketonuria, metabolic acidosis and negative nitrogen balance. All of these are easily explained given our knowledge of the actions of insulin on target tissues. Ketonaemia is usually restricted to IDDM.

The fasted state

The regulation of blood glucose concentration in the fasted state is of prime importance to those tissues in the body (e.g. brain) that cannot utilise other fuels such as fatty acids. The liver plays the major role, but muscle protein turnover also contributes inasmuch as alanine and glutamine, the amino acids leaving muscle in the fasted state, are glucogenic. Hormone-stimulated enzyme induction may also play an important role. The key hormone of the fasted state is *glucagon* with several others, including growth hormone, adrenocorticotropic hormone (ACTH), cortisol, adrenaline, and thyroid

Table 9 Distribution of stored fuels in a 70 kg man

Storage fuel	Weight (kg)	Energy (kjoules)
Glucose: extracellular	0.02	334
Glycogen: liver	0.07	1 170
muscle	0.12	2 000
Triacylglycerol: adipose	9	564 000
Protein: muscle	6	100 300

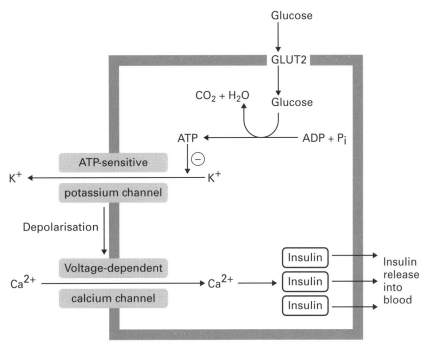

Fig. 99 Control of insulin secretion by glucose.

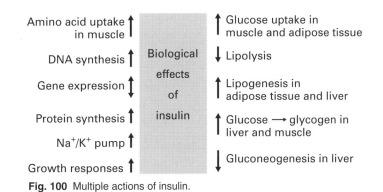

Fig. 100 Multiple actions of insulin.

Table 10 Effect of insulin in target tissues

Tissue	Activation	Inhibition
Liver	Glycogenesis Lipogenesis	Gluconeogenesis Ketogenesis
Adipose tissue	Glucose uptake Lipogenesis	Lipolysis
Muscle	Glycogenesis Glucose uptake Amino acid uptake	Protein degradation

hormone having important roles; as a group they are referred to as *counter-regulatory hormones*.

How does one measure a subject's response to hypoglycaemia?

A subject fasts overnight, a fasting blood sample is taken and insulin is administered; the amount of insulin injected depends upon weight of the subject. Blood samples are taken and glucose is measured to determine that hypoglycaemia was produced (usually within 30 minutes). In normal subjects glucagon, growth hormone, cortisol and ACTH levels will be high at the 90-minute time period and fasting glucose levels restored.

Counter-regulatory hormones

The following is a summary of key points related to each of these hormones. Chapter 18 contains additional details concerning hormone biosynthesis, transport, metabolism and signal transduction mechanisms.

Glucagon
- it is a small peptide with 29 amino acid residues made in the pancreatic alpha cells
- its secretion is increased when the blood glucose falls to less than 5 mM. Glucagon secretion is also increased following a protein meal and in response to prolonged exercise.
- the main sites for glucagon action are the liver and adipose tissue (Table 11) where it brings about mobilisation of fuels for use in other tissues in the body. Muscle lacks glucagon receptors so there is no effect on that tissue.

Table 11 Effect of glucagon in target tissues

Tissue	Activation
Liver	Glycogenolysis
	Gluconeogenesis
	Ketogenesis
	Amino acid catabolism
	Urea synthesis
Adipose tissue	Lipolysis
Muscle	No effect

Growth hormone

- human growth hormone (hGH) is a single chain polypeptide of 191 amino acid residues with two disulphide bridges made in the somatotrophs of the anterior pituitary
- the control of hGH secretion is complex. There is a pronounced circadian rhythm, with secretion being elevated during the sleep period. hGH is controlled positively by growth hormone-releasing hormone (GHRH) and negatively by somatostatin (GHIF), both produced in the hypothalamus
- growth hormone action on growth is mediated by insulin-like growth factor 1 (IGF-1), i.e. hGH's action on growth is mainly indirect
- direct actions of hGH include increasing fatty acid release from adipose tissue and serving as an insulin antagonist.

Adrenocorticotrophic hormone (ACTH; corticotropin)

- it is a peptide of 39 amino acid residues formed from its precursor, pro-opiomelanocortin (POMC), in the corticotrophs of the anterior pituitary
- ACTH secretion is stimulated by pulses of corticotropin releasing hormone (CRH) from the hypothalamus and suppressed by negative feedback by cortisol. Increased secretion of ACTH occurs in stress.
- its principal role is to control cortisol production by the adrenal cortex
- it also has important effects on intermediary metabolism, including stimulation of adipocyte triacylglycerol lipase, resulting in fat mobilisation.

Cortisol

- it is a steroid hormone formed from cholesterol in the zona fasciculata cells of the adrenal cortex
- its production is controlled by ACTH; blood levels are high during stress
- it has a pronounced circadian rhythm
- cortisol can cross the plasma membrane of cells and has the potential to influence the properties of cells provided that they possess glucocorticoid receptors
- cortisol increases protein turnover and gluconeogenesis; long-term treatment with high doses of glucocorticoid can cause diabetes mellitus.

Thyroxine

- thyroid hormones are iodinated amino acids, thyroxine (T_4) and tri-iodothyronine (T_3) synthesised in the follicular epithelial cells of the thyroid gland
- T_4 secretion is controlled by the circulating level of thyroid stimulating hormone (TSH), which influences all metabolic steps in thyroidal follicular cells including iodide uptake, iodination and processing of thyroglobulin
- thyroid hormones have effects on almost every cell in the body. T_4 is a prohormone that is deiodinated in target tissues to the active hormone T_3
- actions of thyroid hormones include enhancement of cellular intermediary metabolism (they increase the basal metabolism rate (BMR)); they sustain brain growth and development and are required for normal growth hormone secretion to occur. They increase lipid mobilisation from adipose tissue.

Adrenaline

- adrenaline is a catecholamine made primarily in chromaffin cells of the adrenal medulla, part of the sympathetic nervous system
- adrenaline secretion results when acetylcholine stimulates an influx of calcium from the extracellular fluid into the cytosol of chromaffin cells
- metabolic effects include stimulation of liver and muscle glycogenolysis and lipid mobilisation from adipose tissue
- adrenaline inhibits insulin release from the pancreas; this action contributes to the normalisation of blood glucose during hypoglycaemia.

Starvation is a special situation

During the first week or so of starvation, the individual makes glucose from protein in order to satisfy the fuel needs of the brain. This is the *gluconeogenic phase*. If starvation is prolonged, the individual enters the *protein conservation phase* (or he/she will die!). There is increased ketone body production coupled with decreased utilisation of ketone bodies in muscle (probably because of decreased OAA levels). The result is a large increase in circulating ketone bodies, which achieve concentrations that enable them to compete with glucose as the fuel for the brain. The individual develops a significant metabolic acidosis but survives for a longer period. Fatty acids per se cannot be utilised directly as fuels by the brain because they cannot cross the blood–brain barrier.

11.2 Metabolic support and control in tissues

The major tissues of the body work together in order to maintain a constant supply of oxidisable fuels to all cells. In this chapter we focus on the major metabolic pathways related to fuel metabolism in brain, liver, muscle and adipose tissue. What is presented is a very

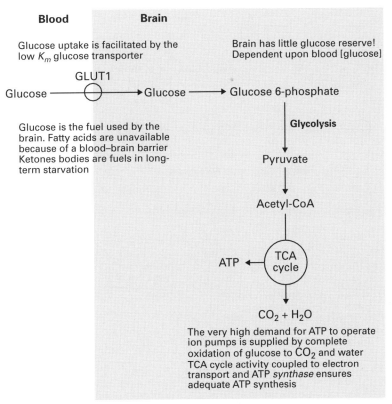

Fig. 101 Control of metabolism in the brain in the fed or fasted state.

general treatment of the subject but if you review the major points that follow on these tissues and consult the figures, you should have a clear picture of the important concepts of integrated metabolism in the body.

The brain uses glucose as its fuel and cannot use fatty acids

Much of the brain's ATP production is used to generate and maintain the concentration gradients of Na^+, K^+ and Ca^{2+} across the plasma membrane of neurones and of H^+ across vesicular membranes. Na^+/K^+-ATPase is the major user of ATP. Under non-starving conditions, glucose is the fuel used by the brain (Fig. 101). The brain requires a *steady* supply of glucose (from blood) in order to function normally. Levels of blood glucose less than 2.5 mM lead to brain dysfunction. The brain has low levels of stored glycogen – about 1% of the concentration found in the liver – and so temporary anaerobic metabolism is very limited. It is important to recognise that the brain cannot utilise fatty acids as fuel because they cannot cross the blood–brain barrier. Also, the brain seems unable to use as fuels the high concentrations of glutamate and aspartate present.

Normal conditions. Although the brain constitutes only 2% of the body weight of adults, 20% of the total resting oxygen consumption of the body occurs there.

Starvation. The brain uses *ketone bodies* as an exceptional fuel to conserve body protein in prolonged starvation (see above).

Liver stores glycogen in the fed state and releases it in the fasted state

The liver is ideally placed in the body to serve as a metabolic clearing house. It has the major role to play in controlling the levels of blood glucose in that it responds to both insulin and glucagon, the principal hormones of the fed and fasted states, respectively. The critical functions possessed by the liver that relate to fuel metabolism are as follows.

In the fed state (Fig. 102). Liver takes up large quantities of glucose most of which is converted to glycogen. Some triacylglycerol is also formed. Insulin controls these processes. Glucose metabolism provides the glycerol 3-phosphate required for triacylglycerol synthesis. Fatty acids are converted to triacylglycerols, which are carried in VLDL for storage as fat elsewhere in the body.

In the fasted state (Fig. 103). Liver glycogen serves as a reservoir of glucose; glycogenolysis ensures that the blood glucose concentration is sufficient to supply fuel to the brain and other glucose-dependent tissues. Glucose can also be produced by gluconeogenesis. Oxidation of fatty acids in liver in the fasted state provides the ATP required for gluconeogenesis and for the other biosynthetic reactions occurring there. Some of the fatty acids are converted to ketone bodies, which are exported for use by muscles.

Integrated control of liver metabolism. Glycogenolysis, gluconeogenesis and glycogenesis are controlled chiefly by the ratio of glucagon to insulin in blood.

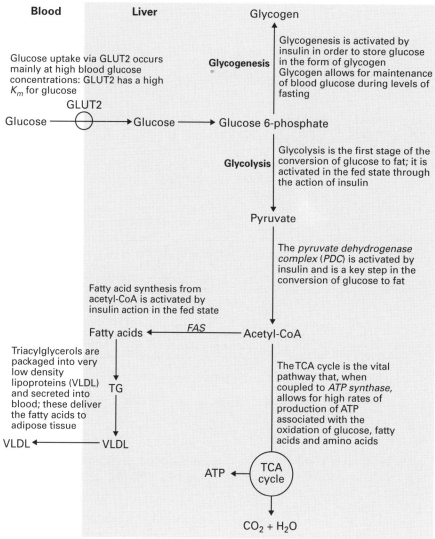

Fig. 102 Liver metabolism in the fed state.

Adipose tissue stores triacylglycerols in the fed state and releases fatty acids and glycerol in the fasted state

As can be seen from Table 9, adipose tissue contains by far the major store of energy in the body, in the form of triacylglycerols. It is a 'fuel buffer', which the body can call upon during lengthy periods of fasting or exercise. Healthy fat individuals survive starvation for a longer period than non-obese subjects. The major points related to fuel metabolism are as follows.

In the fed state (Fig. 104). Fatty acids and glucose are taken up by adipose tissue. The fatty acids come from VLDL and chylomicrons by the action of endothelial lipoprotein lipase (LPL) (Chapter 10). Glucose metabolism provides the glycerol 3-phosphate required for triacylglycerol synthesis. Insulin is the key hormone of storage in that it increases glucose uptake through recruitment of GLUT4 to the plasma membrane. It also induces LPL synthesis and translocation to endothelial cells and inhibits hormone-sensitive lipase (HSL).

In the fasted state and during exercise (Fig. 105). Insulin levels fall, counter regulatory hormones rise and

HSL is activated, leading to fatty acid production from triacylglycerols.

HSL action produces free fatty acids, which are released into blood, bound to albumin and transported to liver, skeletal and cardiac muscle etc. to serve as fuel. Glycerol is also produced and it goes to the liver where it can be converted into glucose.

Muscle also stores glycogen in the fed state and can utilise fatty acids

Muscle can use a variety of different fuels, including glucose (glycogen), fatty acids and ketone bodies. They can be completely oxidised to carbon dioxide and water. The initial pathway of glucose metabolism in muscle is glycolysis. *Phosphofructokinase-1* is the key control step of glycolysis (p. 77). A potential end-point of glycolysis is *lactic acid*, the formation of which allows for increased ATP production in muscle during high-intensity physical exercise. Muscle contains stores of glycogen that are metabolised to provide ATP and this is very important in support of short bursts of activity. Long-term exercise requires fatty acid use. The tendency is to focus

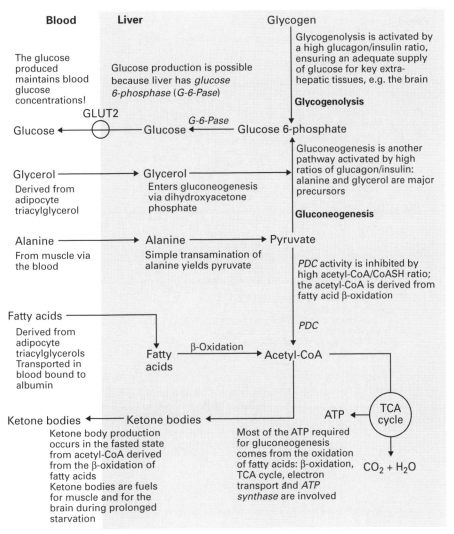

Fig. 103 Liver metabolism in the fasted state.

upon glucose metabolism in muscle but the following points are critical.

In the fed state (Fig. 106). Glucose uptake and glycogen storage are stimulated by insulin.

In the fasted state (Fig. 107). Under fasted conditions (e.g. overnight) the respiratory quotient (RQ) of muscle is approximately 0.7. This indicates that the fuel being used is long-chain fatty acids (the RQ for glucose is 1.0). Muscle cannot export glucose to contribute to glucose homeostasis in the fasted state since it does not contain glucose 6-phosphatase. For the same reason, muscle does not participate in gluconeogenesis. However, in the fasted state, muscle degrades some of its protein to alanine, which is a glucogenic substrate in the liver; thus, indirectly, muscle contributes to glucose homeostasis.

Metabolic support for the heart, kidney, intestine and skin

Cardiac muscle utilises all fuels and especially fatty acids

The heart needs to produce ATP constantly and at a high rate. In order to accomplish this it has the ability to oxidise all fuels and has a higher content of mitochondria than most other tissues. At rest, the heart has a much higher rate of oxygen consumption per kilogram compared with skeletal muscle. Heart is one of the major contributors to the basal metabolic rate, again much more important than skeletal muscle. Fuels used by heart muscle include:

Glycogen is stored in the heart in the fed state but is not a major contributor to the fuel needs of the heart. It is available for use when oxygen supply to heart muscle is impaired.

Glucose is transported via (insulin-dependent) GLUT4. Its utilisation is greatest immediately following meals containing carbohydrate. Insulin action activates cardiac muscle PFK-1.

Lactate is produced by anaerobic glucose metabolism in skeletal muscle (during vigorous exercise) and can be readily used by heart muscle because its high oxidative capacity results in lactate/pyruvate and $NAD^+/NADH$ ratios that favour the oxidation of lactate to pyruvate. The major form of lactate dehydrogenase in heart is LD_1 (H_4).

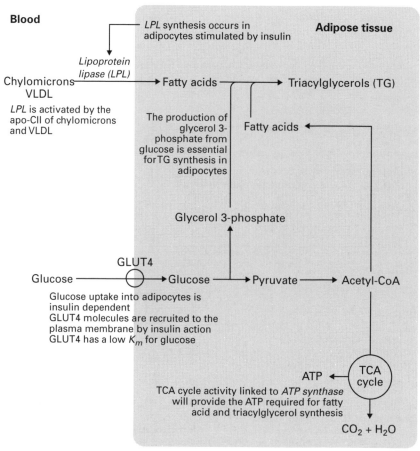

Fig. 104 Adipose tissue metabolism in the fed state.

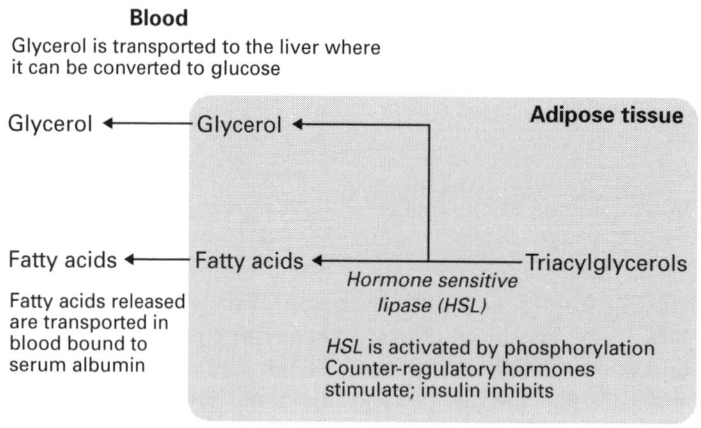

Blood

Glycerol is transported to the liver where it can be converted to glucose

Fig. 105 Adipose tissue metabolism in the fasted state.

Fatty acids are quantitatively the most important fuels for heart muscle. This is consistent with their role as the major storage form of energy in the body (as triacylglycerols) and the fact that they have higher potential to generate ATP compared with glucose. Exercise increases fatty acid release from adipose tissue, providing more fuel to support the increased work required to increase cardiac output. The heart preferentially uses fatty acids over glucose.

Ketone bodies are very well catabolised in the heart. Consistent with this ability, the heart has a high level of β-hydroxybutyrate dehydrogenase.

Creatine kinase

The heart has a high content of creatine kinase, the enzyme catalysing the formation of ATP from CP plus ADP. The major isoforms of creatine kinase in heart muscle are MM and MB with the latter being 30 times higher than in skeletal muscle.

The kidney

The renal medulla is apparently restricted to glucose as the fuel that it uses to generate ATP. The renal cortex utilises glucose, fatty acids and ketone bodies as fuels.

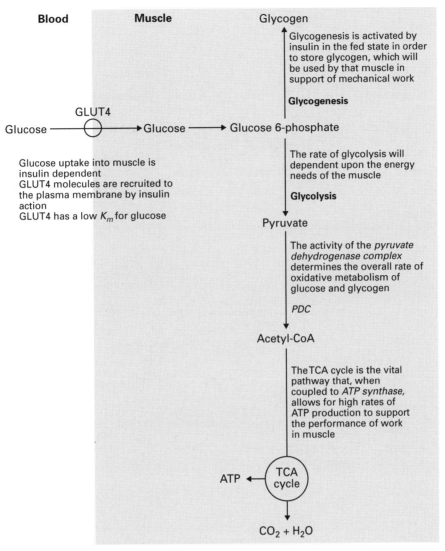

Fig. 106 Muscle metabolism in the fed state.

The intestine

The colon and the small intestine have different fuel preferences.

- Glucose, glutamine, glutamate, asparagine and aspartate are metabolised by *enterocytes* to provide ATP. Enterocytes have very active glutaminases and use glutamine derived from the circulation. The amino acids are oxidised to carbon dioxide or converted to alanine and lactate. During an overnight fast, these amino acids are in short supply in the lumen and most of the glutamine is obtained from the bloodstream. Under these conditions, glutamine and ketone bodies provide almost all of the fuel for the small intestine. In critically ill patients, most of the glutamine for enterocytes arises from increased protein breakdown in skeletal muscle.
- Bacteria in the lumen of the colon use undigested starch and non-starch polysaccharides (also known

as dietary fibre) as fuel. One of their fermentation products is *butyrate*, a short-chain fatty acid, that is the major fuel for *colonocytes*. This may be part of the explanation of why diets high in starch and non-starch polysaccharides protect against colonic cancer. They cause colonocyte proliferation and stimulate mucosal growth. Butyrate is beta-oxidised to yield acetyl-CoA, which enters the TCA cycle leading to ATP synthesis. Butyrate is not a product of metabolism in other cells of the body which means that colonocyte function can be impaired by antibiotic therapy and can result in mucosal barrier breakdown.

The skin

Skin derives most of the required ATP by anaerobic glycolysis, with lactate being one of the constituents of sweat. Lactic acid in sweat is considered to be bactericidal.

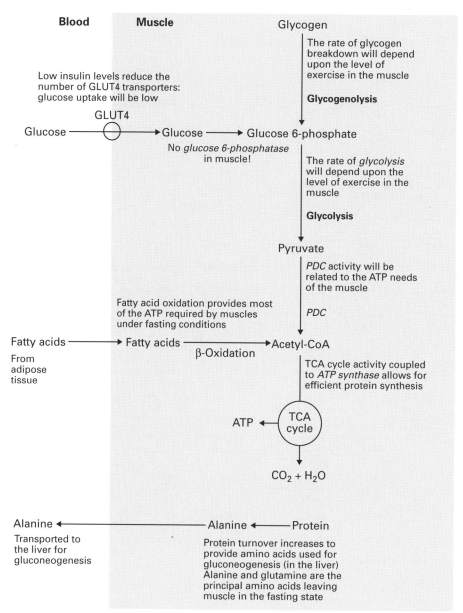

Blood   **Muscle**

Fig. 107 Muscle metabolism in the fasted state.

11.3 **Use of fuels during exercise**

Skeletal muscle fuel use depends on level of activity

Metabolic pathways of muscle include oxidative metabolism of carbohydrate, fats and amino acids and formation of lactate from carbohydrate. Under certain circumstances muscular work is also supported by protein catabolism. Oxidative capacity is limited by mitochondrial numbers as these contain the enzymes of the TCA cycle, the electron transport chain and ATP synthase and beta-oxidation of fatty acids. Fast twitch muscle cells have few mitochondria; slow twitch muscle cells have many mitochondria and the number can be increased by training.

> **BOX 11.1**
> **Clinical note: Heart attack**
>
> Leakage of enzymes unique to the heart into the blood as a consequence of a myocardial infarction provides an indicator of damaged cardiac muscle. The LDH isozyme (LDH-1) of heart and creatine kinase (it is usually not necessary to measure the CK-MB isozyme) are elevated in blood following a heart attack.

Metabolism during exercise. During exercise energy expenditure in muscle increases greatly. Skeletal muscle, because of its large mass, accounts for a large proportion of the body's energy expenditure at rest despite having a low metabolic rate per unit mass. What is special about muscle cells is that their metabolic rate can vary over a wide range, increasing more than 200–1000 times

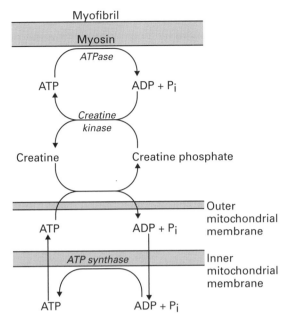

Fig. 108 The creatine phosphate (CP) shuttle.

from rest to maximal exercise. The immediate available substrates are in muscle itself. They are creatine phosphate (CP) and glycogen which can be utilised without delay when energy output must increase. Creatine phosphate acts as an energy buffer that maintains ATP levels in muscle cells (Fig. 108). CP and glycogen are in close contact with the contractile machinery within muscle. CP is spontaneously converted to *creatinine* in muscle. Creatinine is excreted in urine and its production is relatively constant from day to day in normal individuals. N.B. Because SAM is involved in its synthesis, (p. 113) creatinine excretion represents a 'sink' for methyl groups.

The following is a summary of fuel metabolism in exercise where sprinting, middle distance running and marathon running are compared.

High-power exertion (e.g. sprinting) is supported by anaerobic glycolysis

The controlling event in a working muscle is the hydrolysis of ATP to ADP + P_i by muscular contraction. The resultant increase in ADP concentration will cause

CP to be used to reform ATP (catalysed by creatine kinase) in order to support continued muscular contraction. For continued high exertion, metabolism of glycogen to lactate has to be switched on (and is). In summary, for a 100 metre sprint, muscles are using:

- available ATP
- ATP formed from CP
- ATP formed by anaerobic metabolism of glycogen; oxidative metabolism is too slow!

For a 1000 metre run oxidative metabolism can be used

A longer exercise is powered by anaerobic glycolysis plus oxidative metabolism, mainly of glycogen and glucose. The rate is slower so overall velocity is slower. The increase in glycogen metabolism is controlled by:

- AMP levels increase, which activate glycogen phosphorylase and PFK-1
- adrenaline secretion increases and activates glycogen phosphorylase via activation of cyclic AMP-dependent protein kinase A (p. 229).

Marathon running requires use of increasing amounts of fatty acids

The runner must use lots of fat since there are not enough glycogen stores even if 'carbohydrate loading' is attempted to increase the stores.

- overall velocity will be lower since fat oxidation is slower
- in a run lasting several hours, stored triacylglycerols and glycogen are used for 98% of the energy production and only 2% come from use of protein
- the evidence for a switch to the utilisation of fat comes from the observation that the respiratory quotient (RQ = CO_2/O_2) declines throughout
- blood glucose falls significantly during a marathon and about 90% of the total liver glycogen is used
- blood insulin levels gradually fall and there is an increase in glucagon levels
- the increase in glucagon coupled with the fall in insulin allows for efficient fat mobilisation from adipose tissue since hormone sensitive lipase will be active.

Self-assessment: questions

Multiple choice questions

1. The following occur in cardiac muscle but not in the brain, even in the fasted state:
   a. Glucose uptake via a glucose transporter
   b. Fatty acid oxidation
   c. Glycolysis
   d. The reaction in which glucose is converted to glucose 6-phosphate
   e. The TCA cycle

2. In a normal subject in the fasted state one would find:
   a. A high ratio of glucagon to insulin in blood
   b. Oxidation of fatty acids to acetyl-CoA in liver and processing of the latter to acetoacetic acid and other ketone bodies
   c. Production of glycerol and fatty acids from triacylglycerols in adipose tissue
   d. High activity of phosphofructokinase 1 in the liver
   e. RQ of about 0.7 in muscle, provided that the subject was at rest

3. A high ratio of insulin to glucagon in blood will result in:
   a. Activation of muscle and liver glycogen synthase
   b. Inhibition of glucose transport into muscle and adipose tissue
   c. Inhibition of liver gluconeogenesis
   d. Inhibition of fatty acid mobilisation
   e. Activation of ketogenesis in the liver

4. A high ratio of glucagon to insulin in blood will result in:
   a. Increased glucose release from liver
   b. Increased release of alanine from muscle
   c. Decreased activity of hormone-sensitive lipase (HSL) in adipose tissue
   d. A fall in the levels of phosphoenolpyruvate carboxykinase (PEPCK) in liver
   e. Activation of muscle glycogenolysis

5. Insulin action in normal subjects includes:
   a. Recruitment of GLUT4 molecules to the plasma membrane in muscle
   b. Activation of pyruvate dehydrogenase in liver
   c. Activation of hormone-sensitive lipase in adipocytes
   d. Stimulation of a series of reactions leading to the activation of glycogen phosphorylase in both liver and muscle
   e. Induction of glucokinase synthesis in the liver

6. The following statements describe insulin secretion:
   a. Adrenaline action (directly) on the pancreatic beta cell, via interaction with the $\alpha 2$-adrenoceptor, results in decreased insulin secretion
   b. Hyperglycaemia is the major stimulus for increased insulin secretion
   c. Glucose metabolism in beta cells causes a decrease in ATP levels
   d. Changes in potassium levels in beta cells leads to depolarisation of the cells, calcium entry and increased insulin secretion
   e. GLUT2 is the glucose transporter most important for glucose uptake into beta cells in the fed state

7. The following compounds within skeletal muscle can directly or indirectly support muscle contraction:
   a. ADP
   b. AMP
   c. ATP
   d. Creatine phosphate
   e. Creatinine

8. Energy metabolism of the brain:
   a. Is dependent upon uptake of fatty acids from blood
   b. Is dependent upon glutamate as an energy source
   c. Is dependent upon the blood glucose concentration
   d. Can be supported by the catabolism of acetoacetate and β-hydroxybutyrate
   e. In the resting state utilises a high percentage of the oxygen utilised in the body

9. Cardiac muscle can use the following as fuels:
   a. Stearate
   b. Glucose
   c. Acetoacetate
   d. Lactate
   e. All of the above

True/false questions

Are the following statements true or false?

1. Both glucose and fatty acids are efficient fuels for muscle, with the latter requiring an active carnitine palmitoyltransferase-I (CPTI) system.
2. Blood glucose levels greater than 20 mM following a carbohydrate load are consistent with a subject making insufficient insulin.
3. In brain ATP production is mainly through anaerobic glycolysis.

4. An RQ of 1.0 in skeletal muscle indicates that the major fuels being oxidised are fatty acids.
5. Muscle is not able to produce and excrete glucose.
6. Hormones made in corticotrophs, somatotrophs and the zona fasciculata are all 'counter regulatory' hormones.
7. Glucose is the principal fuel of colonocytes.
8. Marathon runners show a gradual decrease in circulating levels of insulin and a gradual decrease in RQ of skeletal muscle during the race.

Short essay questions

1. Prepare a table that summarises the mechanisms that are involved in preventing hyperglycaemia in the fed state and allows for lipid storage. You are not required to differentiate between enzyme activation and enzyme induction.
2. Prepare a table that summarises the mechanisms that are involved in preventing hypoglycaemia in the fasted state and allows for lipid mobilisation. You are not required to differentiate between enzyme activation and enzyme induction.
3. Prepare a table that indicates the fuels used by the intestine, renal medulla, renal cortex, cardiac muscle, liver and the skeletal and nervous systems.
4. Compare and contrast fuel metabolism in skeletal muscles during (a) a 100 metre sprint and (b) a marathon.

Self-assessment: answers

Multiple choice answers

1. a. **False.** Glucose uptake into all cells occurs via glucose transporters.
   b. **True.** There is a blood–brain barrier to the uptake of fatty acid, which means that fatty acids cannot be fuels for the brain.
   c. **False.** Both the brain and cardiac muscle use glucose as a fuel and glycolysis is involved.
   d. **False.** This is the first step in glucose metabolism in both tissues.
   e. **False.** Again, both tissues are capable of oxidative metabolism of glucose and the TCA cycle has a vital role in that process.

2. a. **True.** Low glucose levels in fasting stimulate glucagon release from the pancreas.
   b. **True.** Fatty acids are mobilised from adipose tissue and ketone bodies are by-products of their metabolism in the liver.
   c. **True.** Glucagon activates hormone-sensitive lipase of adipose tissue.
   d. **False.** Gluconeogenesis is activated and PFK-1 activity will be low.
   e. **True.** In the fasting state, muscle uses fatty acids as fuel and that preserves more glucose for brain use.

3. a. **True.** Insulin action activates glycogen synthase in both tissues.
   b. **False.** GLUT4 molecules are recruited to the plasma membranes of both tissues by insulin action.
   c. **True.** Insulin promotes glycolysis rather than gluconeogenesis in the liver.
   d. **True.** Lipogenesis is increased and less fatty acids are released from adipose tissue.
   e. **False.** Since fatty acid mobilisation is inhibited, there is less fatty acid oxidation in liver and, therefore, less ketone body synthesis.

4. a. **True.** Both glycogenolysis and gluconeogenesis are activated, resulting in increased production of glucose 6-phosphate; since the liver possesses glucose 6-phosphatase, glucose is produced and released by transport involving GLUT2.
   b. **True.** Protein turnover in muscle is increased and alanine is formed and excreted to serve as a gluconeogenic precursor in the liver.
   c. **False.** HSL is activated under these conditions, allowing for fatty acid production and release from adipose tissue.
   d. **False.** In fact, PEPCK is induced, with this enzyme catalysing a key step in gluconeogenesis.

   e. **False.** Glucagon does not activate muscle glycogenolysis.

5. a. **True.** This accounts for the increased rate of uptake of glucose that occurs.
   b. **True.** This is important for those individuals with a high rate of fatty acid synthesis from glucose.
   c. **False.** Insulin inhibits fatty acid mobilisation from adipose tissue.
   d. **False.** Glycogen phosphorylase is inhibited; it is glycogen synthase that is activated.
   e. **True.** This allows for efficient entry of glucose into the glycogenesis pathway.

6. a. **True.** Adrenaline, by inhibiting insulin secretion, assists in the response to hypoglycaemia.
   b. **True.** By so doing, insulin increases and this directs glucose into its storage forms.
   c. **False.** ATP increases leading to increased insulin secretion.
   d. **True.** Increased ATP inhibits a potassium-sensitive channel, causes depolarisation, calcium entry and insulin secretion.
   e. **True.** Its high K_m fits well with the need for insulin secretion when glucose levels are high.

7. a. **True.** Catalysed by adenylate kinase, 2ADP are converted to ATP + AMP, with the former being available to support muscle contraction.
   b. **False.** It can only be converted to ATP by using ATP. (An increase in AMP levels activates glycolysis and glycogenolysis.)
   c. **True.** It is the substrate used in the contraction cycle.
   d. **True.** It acts as a buffer replenishing ATP from ADP.
   e. **False.** It is a metabolite of creatine phosphate produced spontaneously and excreted in urine.

8. a. **False.** There is barrier to the uptake of fatty acids into brain from blood.
   b. **False.** Despite being present at high concentration, the brain does not utilise glutamate and other amino acid neurotransmitters as fuels.
   c. **True.** This is because other fuels are not usable and glycogen levels in brain tissue are very low.
   d. **True.** This only occurs to a significant extent during long-term starvation, when these fatty acid metabolites achieve levels that can compete with blood glucose.
   e. **True.** Under these conditions about 20% of the body's total oxygen utilisation occurs in the brain.

Table 12 Glucose homeostasis in the fed state

Organ	Pathway activated	System activated	Pathway inhibited	System inhibited
Liver	Glycogenesis	Glycogen synthase	Glycogenolysis	Phosphorylase
	Glycolysis	PFK-1, pyruvate kinase	Gluconeogenesis	F-1,6-BPase, PEPCK
Skeletal muscle	Glycogenesis	Glycogen synthase	Glycogenolysis	Phosphorylase
	Glucose uptake	GLUT4		
	Glycolysis	PFK-1, pyruvate kinase		
Adipose tissue	Glucose uptake	GLUT4	Fat mobilisation	HSL
	Glycolysis	PFK-1		
	Fat storage	LPL		

See text for abbreviations.

Table 13 Glucose homeostasis in the fasted state

Organ	Pathway activated	System activated	Pathway inhibited	System inhibited
Liver	Glycogenolysis	Phosphorylase	Glycogenesis	Glycogen synthase
	Gluconeogenesis	F-1, 6-BPase, PEPCK, pyruvate carboxylase	Glycolysis	PFK-1, pyruvate kinase
Skeletal muscle	Protein degradation	Ubiquitin pathway	Glycogenesis	Glycogen synthase
Adipose tissue	Fat mobilisation	HSL	Fat storage	LPL
			Glucose uptake	GLUT4
			Glycolysis	PFK-1

See text for abbreviations.

9. a. **True.** Fatty acids are the principal fuels.
    b. **True.** Glucose is also used (remember you need some glucose to oxidise fatty acids completely to CO_2 and water).
    c. **True.** Excellent fuel for the heart. Easily enters the TCA cycle.
    d. **True.** Another excellent fuel, readily converted to pyruvate. Links exercising skeletal muscle and increased cardiac output.
    e. **True.**

True/false answers

1. **True.** Other than in short sprints, muscle uses fatty acids and glycogen (or glucose) as fuels.
2. **True.** This is an abnormally high glucose level and consistent with diabetes mellitus. Insufficient insulin means that glucose is less efficiently stored in liver and muscle.
3. **False.** The fact that under quiescent (non-exercise) conditions the brain uses about 20% of the total oxygen being used by an individual points to the fact that aerobic metabolism (of glucose) is what is happening.
4. **False.** An RQ of 1.0 indicates that glucose (or glycogen) is the fuel being used. With long-chain fatty acids as fuel, the RQ is close to 0.7.
5. **True.** This is because muscle does not contain glucose 6-phosphatase.
6. **True.** They are ACTH, growth hormone and cortisol.
7. **False.** Short-chain fatty acids produced by colonic bacteria are the fuels for colonocytes.

8. **True.** The decrease in insulin allows fat mobilisation to increase from adipose tissue. The greater use of fatty acids as fuel is reflected in a significant decrease in RQ in muscle.

Short essay answers

1. Table 12 summarises the mechanisms that prevent hyperglycaemia in the fed state and allow storage of energy as lipid.
2. Table 13 summarises the mechanisms that prevent hypoglycaemia in the fasted state and allow mobilisation of energy stored as lipids.
3. Table 14 lists the fuels used by the tissues in question and the relevant pathways.

Table 14 The fuels used by various tissues

Tissue	Fuel used	Pathway
Intestine		
Enterocytes	Glutamine	TCA cycle
Colonocytes	Short-chain fatty acids	Beta-oxidation plus TCA cycle
Kidney		
Medulla	Glucose	Glycolysis
Cortex	Glucose, fatty acids	Oxidative metabolism, TCA cycle, etc.
Muscle		
Cardiac muscle	Fatty acids, glucose, lactate, ketone bodies	Oxidative metabolism, TCA cycle, etc.
Skeletal muscle	Glycogen, ketone bodies, fatty acids, glucose	Glycolysis, oxidative metabolism, TCA cycle, etc.
Liver	Fatty acids, glucose, lactate, amino acids	Oxidative metabolism, TCA cycle, etc.

4. **High-power exertion (e.g. sprinting).** ATP, creatine phosphate and then anaerobic metabolism of glycogen (glucose) occurs. Control of glucose metabolism occurs through activation of glycogenenolysis and glycolysis at the level of phosphorylase and PFK-1.

In a marathon. Fatty acids and glucose are utilised with the proportion of fatty acids used increasing, the longer the run (RQ gradually falls). Fatty acids are released in increasing amounts from adipose tissue through activation of hormone-sensitive lipase, brought about by a decrease in insulin and an increase in glucagon.

Purine and pyrimidine nucleotides

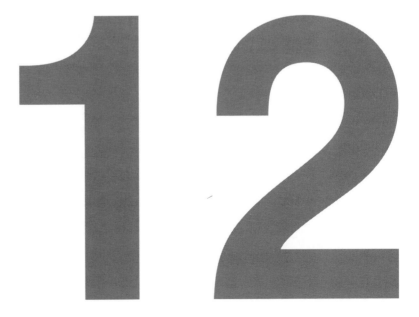

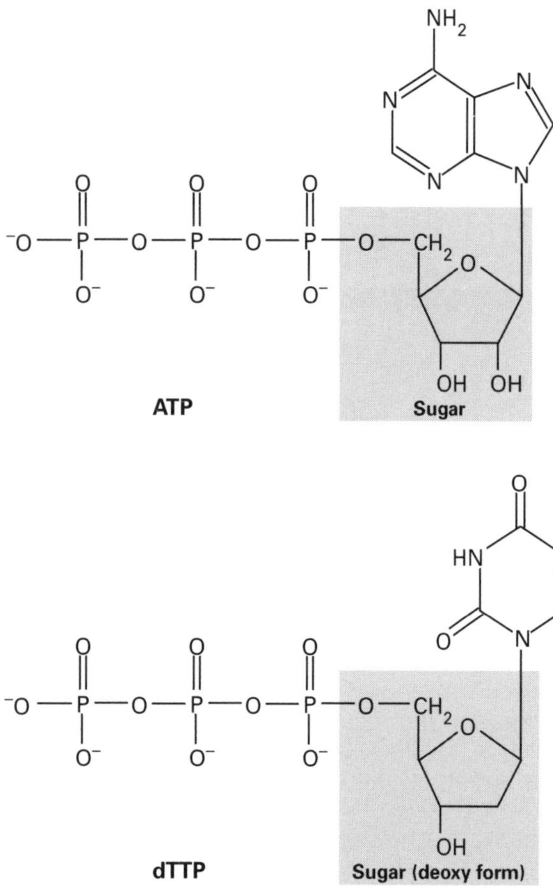

Table 15 Purine and pyrimidine nucleotide nomenclature

Base	Abbreviation	Type	Nucleoside	Nucleotide[a]
Adenine	A	Purine	Adenosine	Adenylate
Guanine	G	Purine	Guanosine	Guanylate
Cytosine	C	Pyrimidine	Cytidine	Cytidylate
Thymine	T	Pyrimidine	Thymidine	Thymidylate
Uracil	U	Pyrimidine	Uridine	Uridylate

[a]Nucleotides are named by adding the position and number of phosphate groups to the name of the nucleoside, e.g. adenosine 5'-triphosphate (ATP). Ribonucleotides are assumed unless the prefix d- or deoxy is used.

ATP

dTTP

Sugar

Sugar (deoxy form)

Fig. 109 The structures of a purine ribonucleotide (ATP) and a pyrimidine deoxyribonucleotide (dTTP). The corresponding nucleosides would only have base and sugar.

The general structures of nucleotides and nucleosides are shown in Figure 109 and the nomenclature in Table 15. A nucleotide consists of a purine or pyrimidine base, a sugar (D-ribose or 2-deoxy-D-ribose) and one or

more phosphates. Nucleosides lack the phosphates. Note that purine (smaller name) bases are larger molecules than pyrimidine (larger name) bases. Nucleoside triphosphates (NTP) are required for RNA synthesis and dNTP for DNA synthesis (Chapters 13 and 14).

As shown in Table 16, purine and pyrimidine nucleotides have a wide variety of metabolic roles in addition to being constituents of DNA and RNA.

12.1 Synthesis of purines and pyrimidines

Purine nucleotide synthesis

Purine nucleotides are synthesised by two pathways:

- the *de novo pathway*, which uses simple intermediates, is found in most tissues of the body (Fig. 110)
- the *salvage pathway*, which allows free purine bases produced by the degradation of nucleic acids or purine nucleotides to be reclaimed.

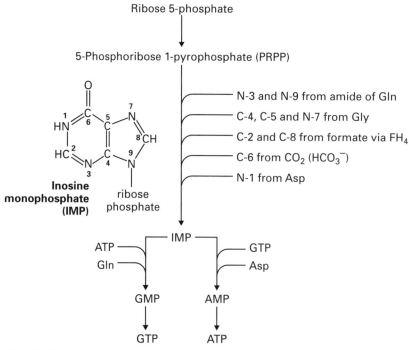

Ribose 5-phosphate

5-Phosphoribose 1-pyrophosphate (PRPP)

N-3 and N-9 from amide of Gln
C-4, C-5 and N-7 from Gly
C-2 and C-8 from formate via FH$_4$
C-6 from CO$_2$ (HCO$_3^-$)
N-1 from Asp

Inosine monophosphate (IMP)

ribose phosphate

ATP
Gln

IMP

GTP
Asp

GMP

AMP

GTP

ATP

Fig. 110 The de novo pathway of purine nucleotide biosynthesis.

Table 16 The roles of purine and pyrimidine nucleotides and nucleosides

Nucleic acid biosynthesis	NTP and dNTP
Energy metabolism	ATP, GTP
Allosteric modifiers	ATP, ADP, AMP, NADH
Cell signalling	Cyclic AMP, cyclic GMP, GTP
Coenzymes	$NAD^+/NADH^+$, $NADP^+/NADPH$, FAD, S-adenosyl-methionine, adenosyl-vitamin B_{12}, coenzyme A
Carbohydrate, glycoprotein and glycolipid biosynthesis	UDP-glucose, UDP-NAGA, UDP-galactose, GDP-mannose
Ganglioside biosynthesis	CMP-NANA
Phospholipid biosynthesis	CDP-choline, CDP-ethanolamine, CDP-diacylglycerol
Bile pigment metabolism and xenobiotic metabolism	UDP-glucuronate
Transmethylation reactions	S-Adenosyl-methionine

The de novo pathway starts with PRPP

This pathway is complex and the following describe the essential features:

1. The starting point for the de novo synthesis of a purine nucleotide is an activated ribose phosphate, phosphoribosylpyrophosphate (PRPP) which is synthesised by transfer of a pyrophosphate group from ATP to the carbon-1 of ribose 5-phosphate.
2. The committed step in purine biosynthesis is the formation of 5-phosphoribosylamine from PRPP and glutamine. The reaction is driven forward by the hydrolysis of pyrophosphate.
3. Additional carbon and nitrogen atoms are added until the parent purine nucleotide is formed. Nitrogens are provided by the amide group of glutamine, aspartate and glycine. Carbons are derived from glycine, bicarbonate, as well as two tetrahydrofolate derivatives (Fig. 110).
4. Altogether, 10 reactions lead to the synthesis of IMP, which is not a component of the nucleotide pool or a constituent of the nucleic acids. The purine base of inosinate is called hypoxanthine.
5. IMP is the precursor of AMP and GMP. AMP is synthesised by the substitution of an amino group for the carbonyl group at carbon-6; this is accomplished by the addition of aspartate followed by elimination of fumarate (as in the urea cycle). GTP is required in the synthesis of AMP. Guanylate (GMP) is synthesised by the NAD^+-dependent

oxidation of IMP to xanthylate (XMP) followed by the transfer of an amino group from the amide of glutamine. ATP is required for GMP synthesis.

In the salvage pathway PRPP is added to purine bases

Free purine bases formed by degradation of nucleic acids are recycled by transfer of a 5′-phosphoribosyl group from PRPP to the base. This is more efficient and economical than de novo synthesis. The salvage pathway is outlined in Figure 111. The relevance of the salvage pathway is indicated in the inherited disorder Lesch–Nyhan syndrome, where *hypoxanthine–guanine phosphoribosyl transferase* (HGPRTase) is absent.

'Product inhibition' is a feature of the control of purine nucleotide biosynthesis

The initial steps catalysed by PRPP synthetase and PRPP amidotransferase are inhibited by the purine nucleotide products AMP, GMP and IMP acting synergistically (Fig. 112). In contrast, PRPP has a positive effect, causing the PRPP amidotransferase (for which it is substrate) to shift to the active form. There is also regulation at the branch point at IMP, with AMP inhibiting the conversion of IMP into adenylosuccinate, which is its precursor, and GMP inhibiting the conversion of IMP into XMP, its precursor (Fig. 112). GTP serves as an energy source for the adenylosuccinate synthase reaction while AMP is a competitive inhibitor of this step. Similarly, ATP is the energy source in the conversion of XMP to GMP while GMP is an inhibitor of XMP formation. These controls serve to balance the synthesis of adenine and guanine nucleotides. For example, an excess of GTP favours the conversion of IMP to adenylosuccinate, which is the immediate precursor of AMP. In the salvage pathways, the product of the phosphoribosyltransferase reactions are feedback inhibitors.

Pyrimidine nucleotide biosynthesis

The de novo pathway for pyrimidine nucleotide biosynthesis contrasts with that for purines in that the sugar and phosphate are added from PRPP after the pyrimidine ring has been formed. This pathway involves two complexes that are multi-enzyme polypeptides. A salvage pathway also exists for pyrimidine nucleotides.

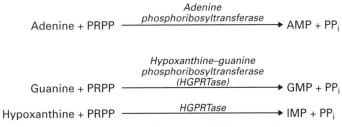

Fig. 111 The salvage pathway of purine nucleotide synthesis.

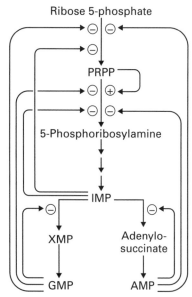

Fig. 112 The control of purine nucleotide synthesis.

The de novo pathway

This pathway is complex and involves two multifunctional enzymes. Key points about this pathway are:

1. Carbamoyl phosphate is required and is produced in a reaction that involves glutamine (not ammonia) and the enzyme, *carbamoyl phosphate synthetase II* (CPSII), is in the cytosol.
2. The second step in pyrimidine biosynthesis is the formation of *N*-carbamoylaspartate (Fig. 113) from aspartate and carbamoyl phosphate; this reaction is catalysed by aspartate transcarbamoylase (ATCase). Dihydroorotase (DHOase) catalyses the cyclisation of *N*-carbamoylaspartate to dihydroorotate.
3. In higher eukaryotes or mammals, **C**PSII, **A**TCase and **D**HOase are covalently linked to form a single chain, 240 kDa multi-functional enzyme called **CAD**.

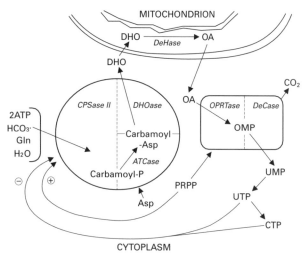

Fig. 113 Pyrimidine nucleotide biosynthesis. (Based upon M.E. Jones (1980) *Annual Review of Biochemistry*, **49**, 253–279.)

4. Dihydroorotate is oxidised to orotate in an NAD⁺-dependent reaction then orotate phosphoribosyl transferase (OPRTase) transfers a ribose phosphate group from PRPP to orotate to form the pyrimidine nucleotide orotidylate (OMP). Decarboxylation of OMP catalysed by orotidine-5′-monophosphate decarboxylase (DeCase) yields the parent pyrimidine nucleotide uridylate (UMP).
5. Again, in eukaryotes, OPRTase and DeCase are associated in a single 52 kDa protein. CTP is derived from UTP, a reaction catalysed by CTP synthetase (Fig. 113). The carbonyl oxygen at carbon-4 of UTP is replaced by an amino group donated by the amide group of glutamine.

In the salvage pathway PRPP is added to pyrimidine bases

Pyrimidine bases can be 'salvaged' by conversion to the nucleotides via pyrimidine phosphoribosyltransferase.

$$\text{Pyrimidine} + \text{PRPP} \rightarrow$$
$$\text{Pyrimidine nucleoside monophosphate} + \text{PP}_i$$

Orotate, uracil and thymine are substrates but cytosine is not.

'Product inhibition' is a feature of the control of pyrimidine nucleotide biosynthesis

The main control of pyrimidine nucleotide synthesis in mammals is exerted at the level of CPSII; the enzyme is inhibited by UTP and CTP (Fig. 113). In addition, UMP and, to a lesser extent, CMP inhibit DeCase. CTP synthetase is inhibited by CTP to prevent all of the UTP from being converted to CTP. Also, since pyrimidine nucleotide synthesis is dependent upon a supply of PRPP, the activity of PRPP synthetase is a factor in determining flux through the pathway.

Synthesis of trinucleotides

To convert both purine and pyrimidine mononucleotides to trinucleotides (e.g. AMP to ATP and GMP to GTP), two additional kinases are required. These kinases are not specific for the base involved.

BOX 12.1
Clinical note: Orotic aciduria

In a clinical condition called orotic aciduria, excessive amounts of orotic acid are produced because of deficiencies in either OPRTase or DeCase, the enzymes in the second multi-enzyme protein. Orotic aciduria can also result from a deficiency of ornithine transcarbamoylase in the urea cycle. Can you reason why?

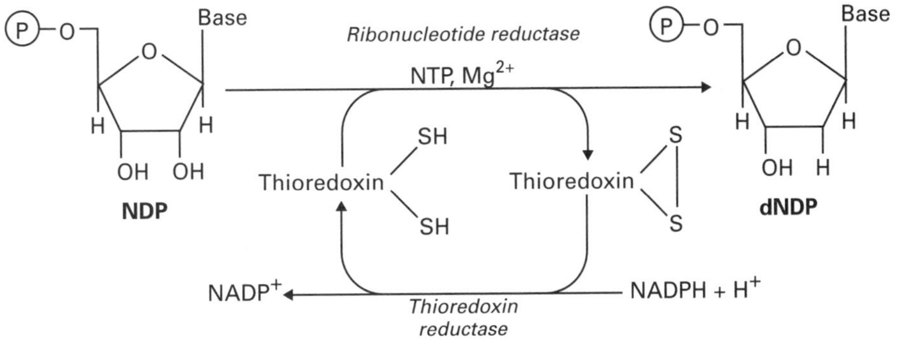

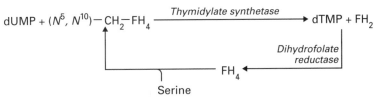

Fig. 114 The synthesis of deoxyribonucleotides catalysed by ribonucleotide reductase.

$$dUMP + (N^5, N^{10}) - CH_2 - FH_4 \xrightarrow{\text{Thymidylate synthetase}} dTMP + FH_2$$

Dihydrofolate reductase

FH_4

Serine

Fig. 115 The synthesis of deoxythymidine (dTMP).

12.2 Deoxyribonucleotide synthesis

During DNA replication (S phase), deoxyribonucleotides are required to support DNA synthesis. The deoxyribonucleotides are formed by reduction of the 2' hydroxyl of the corresponding ribonucleotide (Fig. 114). Thioredoxin, a small protein (12 kDa), is oxidised at the same time and is regenerated finally by NADPH. The reduction of a specific NDP requires a specific NTP as a positive modulator of ribonucleotide reductase; the enzyme is also regulated by other NTPs.

Control of deoxyribonucleotide synthesis is vital to survival of an organism

An organism must synthesise the four dNTPs in amounts that will allow for DNA synthesis. One potential consequence of imbalance in dNTP synthesis is *mutagenesis*. The pathways are controlled by feedback inhibition. From studies of *Escherichia coli* ribonucleotide reductase, we know that there are two allosteric sites.

- the overall activity of ribonucleotide reductase is controlled by ATP binding to one of these sites (the *activity site*). Binding of dATP at the activity site inhibits the enzyme's activity towards all substrates, so abnormally high levels of dATP are toxic!
- the final activity is controlled by the level of modulators at the second site (the *specificity site*).

The synthesis of deoxythymidine is a target for anti-cancer drugs

DNA contains thymine (T), the methylated analogue of uracil (U) (Chapter 13) and deoxythymidine is required for DNA synthesis (Chapter 13).

A rapidly growing tumour is going to require a high rate of DNA synthesis. *Thymidylate synthetase* catalyses the transfer of a one-carbon unit to dUMP and in the process reduces the one-carbon to a methyl group. In addition to serving as a one-carbon donor, N^5,N^{10}-methylene FH_4 acts as the reducing agent (Fig. 115). For

---

BOX 12.2
Clinical note: Anti-cancer drugs

Analogues of FH_4, such as *aminopterin* and *methotrexate*, are potent inhibitors of dihydrofolate reductase and, as such, are most toxic to proliferating cells because they block recycling of FH_2. Methotrexate binds so tightly to dihydrofolate reductase that it is classified as a pseudoirreversible inhibitor. When tumour cells are treated with methotrexate, the cells die. Although a valuable drug in the treatment of rapidly growing tumours, such as acute leukaemia and choriocarcinoma, it is quite toxic as it also kills rapidly growing non-malignant cells.

5-Fluorouracil (5-FU), another anti-cancer drug, is converted into fluorouridylate (F-dUMP). F-dUMP is a substrate for thymidylate synthase but catalysis results in a covalent complex formed by F-dUMP, methylene-FH_4 and the sulphydryl of thymidylate synthase. This is another example of suicide inhibition. 5-FU and methotrexate can be used as a cocktail in chemotherapy.

There are several other groups of drugs that have been synthesised or isolated from natural products and are involved in inhibition of nucleotide synthesis or interconversions which are useful as anti-tumour agents. These include 6-mercaptopurine, 8-azaguanine, 6-azauracil, 5-iodouracil and 5-fluorooratate. Of current interest is 3'-azido-3'-deoxythymidine (AZT), which inhibits reverse transcriptase of retroviruses such as HIV, the cause of AIDS.

this reason, it is dihydrofolate (FH_2) that is produced in this reaction. FH_2 must be reduced to FH_4 by *dihydrofolate reductase* using NADPH, since it is FH_4 that participates in one-carbon transfers (p. 112).

12.3 Synthesis of nucleotide coenzymes

Many nucleotide coenzymes function in the principal pathways of intermediary metabolism and, clearly, they have to be synthesised in cells. Examples include:

- NAD⁺ (nicotinamide adenine dinucleotide) which can be synthesised from dietary nicotinate and also from nicotinate made in the body from tryptophan
- FAD (flavin adenine dinucleotide) which is synthesised from riboflavin and ATP
- Coenzyme A, synthesised from pantothenate, cysteine and ATP
- *S*-adenosylmethionine, formed from methionine and ATP by the transfer of an adenine and ribose from ATP.

The biosynthesis of NAD⁺, FAD and Coenzyme A all involve the transfer of AMP from ATP to the phosphoryl group of a phosphorylated intermediate, resulting in the formation of PP_i; cleavage of PP_i to $2P_i$ has a large negative ΔG which drives the reaction.

12.4 Purine and pyrimidine catabolism

Purines are catabolised to uric acid

Hydrolytic reactions of purine nucleotides result in the formation of purine mononucleotides (AMP, GMP, IMP). These are further degraded via a nucleotidase, which removes the phosphate. The nucleoside is then converted to the free base and either ribose 1-phosphate or deoxyribose 1-phosphate by nucleoside phosphorylase. AMP is deaminated by AMP deaminase and the product, IMP, is hydrolysed to the nucleoside inosine by a nucleotidase. Inosine can be converted to hypoxanthine via nucleoside phosphorylase.

The purine bases hypoxanthine, adenine, and guanine are oxidised in the liver to uric acid (Fig. 116), which is excreted via the kidneys. Uric acid is not very water-soluble and the mean concentration in adult males is close to the limit of solubility. An increase in uric acid levels for whatever reason can lead to crystallisation out of uric acid crystals in various sites in the body, resulting in gouty arthritis and kidney damage (stones). Xanthine oxidase (which contains molybdenum) is the target for drugs (e.g. allopurinol) used to treat patients with gout.

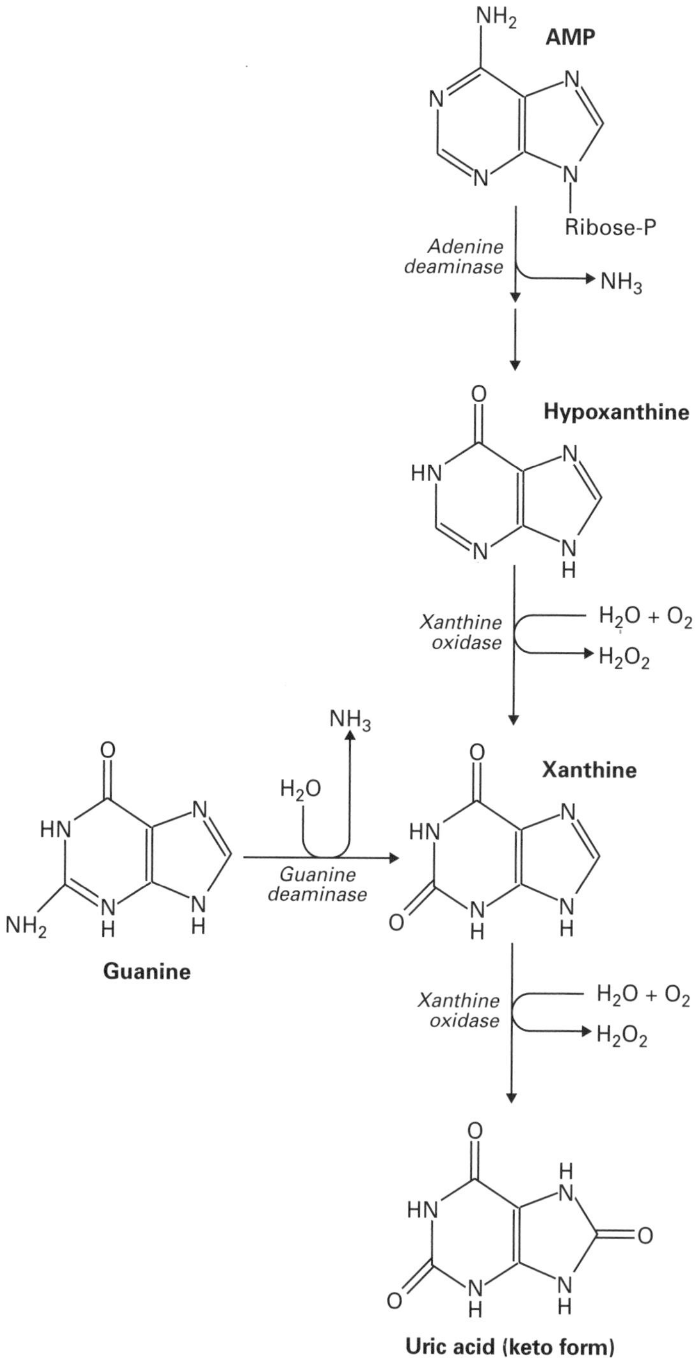

Fig. 116 Purine catabolism to uric acid.

> **BOX 12.3**
> **Clinical note: Lesch–Nyhan syndrome**
>
> A severe or complete deficiency of HGPRTase activity results in Lesch–Nyhan syndrome, which is characterised by mental retardation and, in the most severe cases, self-mutilation. Lack of HGPRTase precludes the salvage of hypoxanthine and guanine, leading to decreased levels of IMP or GMP and increased levels of PRPP. Both these factors increase the de novo pathway of purine biosynthesis as the pathway is no longer subject to proper regulation (Fig. 112). The disease is characterised by excessive uric acid production and hyperuricaemia.

Pyrimidine metabolites including β-alanine

Degradation of the pyrimidine nucleotides, primarily UMP, CMP and TMP, involves hydrolysis to their respective bases in reactions comparable to those for purine nucleotides. Degradation of the pyrimidine bases generates ammonia, malonyl-CoA, β-alanine and methylmalonyl-CoA, all very water soluble. An intermediate in the catabolism of cytosine and uracil, β-alanine, is required for Coenzyme A biosynthesis.

Self-assessment: questions

Multiple choice questions

1. The conversion of dUMP to dTMP:
   a. Uses N^{10}-formyl-FH$_4$ as the direct methyl donor
   b. Is directly inhibited by methotrexate
   c. Is directly inhibited by 5'-fluoro-UMP
   d. Yields NADH as a product
   e. Yields dihydrofolate as a product

2. The direct source of the sugar phosphate incorporated in the de novo synthesis of purine nucleotides is:
   a. GMP
   b. Ribulose 5-phosphate
   c. UTP
   d. Glucose 6-phosphate
   e. 5-Phosphoribosyl 1-pyrophosphate (PRPP)

3. In the synthesis of GMP and AMP from IMP:
   a. AMP synthesis involves a deamination
   b. GMP synthesis requires ATP
   c. The NH$_2$ group in GMP is derived from glutamine and that in AMP is derived from aspartate
   d. GTP is required for AMP synthesis
   e. AMP synthesis occurs via 3'-5'-cyclic AMP

4. Gout and/or increased uric acid production:
   a. May be caused by impaired excretion of uric acid by the kidneys
   b. May result from a partial deficiency of hypoxanthine-guanine phosphoribosyltransferase (HGPRTase)
   c. May result from overproduction of 5-phosphoribosyl 1-pyrophosphate (PRPP)
   d. Can be treated with allopurinol, which inhibits xanthine oxidase and results in excretion of hypoxanthine and xanthine

5. The following statements describe pyrimidine biosynthesis in mammals:
   a. The rate of UMP synthesis is regulated by UTP, which inhibits carbamoyl phosphate synthetase II (CPSII)
   b. Pyrimidines can be 'salvaged' by conversion to the nucleotides in a reaction using PRPP and catalysed by pyrimidine phosphoribosyltransferase
   c. CTP synthetase is inhibited by CTP, which prevents all of the UTP from being converted to CTP
   d. In the de novo pathway, the first three reactions occur in a multi-enzyme complex
   e. CPSII utilises glutamine as the source of an amino group

6. Methotrexate:
   a. Is an intermediate in dTMP synthesis
   b. Inhibits thymidylate synthetase
   c. Is an activator of dihydrofolate reductase
   d. When combined with 5-fluorouracil (5-FU) inhibits dTMP synthesis
   e. Is an analogue of folate

True/false questions

Are the following statements true or false?
1. The ribose in purine but not in pyrimidine nucleotides is supplied by 5-phosphoribosyl 1-pyrophosphate (PRPP).
2. Tetrahydrofolate donates single-carbon units at several stages in the biosynthesis of purines.
3. Biosynthesis of purine and pyrimidine nucleotides is closely regulated through feedback inhibition by end-products of the respective pathways.
4. Ribonucleotide reductase is closely regulated through feedback inhibition by several different nucleotides.
5. Gout is caused by low levels of uric acid, resulting from defects in either catabolism or biosynthesis of purines.
6. Many potential anti-cancer drugs are inhibitors of nucleotide biosynthesis.

Short essay questions

1. Discuss the roles of glutamine and aspartate in supplying nitrogens (amino groups) in the biosynthesis of purine and pyrimidine nucleotides in the body.
2. Discuss the importance of the reaction catalysed by thymidylate synthase and its relevance to cancer chemotherapy.

Self-assessment: answers

Multiple choice answers

1. a. **False.** The source of the methyl group is N^5, N^{10}-methylene-FH_4.
   b. **False.** The effect of methotrexate is secondary through inhibition of dihydrofolate reductase.
   c. **True.** 5′-Fluorouracil is administered and is converted to 5′-fluoro-UMP, which is an inhibitor of thymidylate synthase; this catalyses the conversion of dUMP to dTMP.
   d. **False.** The other product is dihydrofolate.
   e. **True.**

2. a. **False.** GMP is one of the products of purine nucleotide synthesis.
   b. **False.** Ribulose 5-phosphate is the precursor of ribose 5-phosphate but is not directly involved in purine and pyrimidine nucleotide synthesis.
   c. **False.** UTP is a pyrimidine nucleotide important in glycogen synthesis but does not supply the ribose phosphate for purine nucleotide synthesis.
   d. **False.** Glucose 6-phosphate is a precursor of ribose phosphate but not directly involved in nucleotide synthesis.
   e. **True.** Formed in a reaction involving ribose 5-phosphate and ATP, catalysed by PRPP synthase.

3. a. **False.** AMP synthesis from IMP requires an amidation.
   b. **True.** This contributes to the 'balance' between adenine and guanine nucleotides.
   c. **True.** Aspartate and glutamine are often used to supply amino groups in the biosynthesis of key compounds.
   d. **True.** Again, this contributes to 'balance' between adenine and guanine nucleotides.
   e. **False.** AMP can be formed from 3′, 5′-cyclic AMP by phosphodiesterase action (Chapter 18), but this is not on the pathway from IMP to AMP.

4. a. **True.** Clearly, impaired excretion will cause hyperuricaemia since uric acid is normally eliminated via the kidneys.
   b. **True.** That deficiency increases PRPP concentration and this turns on de novo purine nucleotide synthesis, which will increase urate formation.
   c. **True.** PRPP turns on purine nucleotide synthesis by activating PRPP-glutamine amidotransferase.
   d. **True.** This therapy works since hypoxanthine and xanthine are more water soluble than uric acid.

5. a. **True.** Product feedback inhibition is a feature of the control of purine and pyrimidine nucleotide biosynthesis.
   b. **True.** Salvage, which conserves ATP, occurs for both purine and pyrimidine nucleotides.
   c. **True.** If all of the UTP was converted to CTP, this would impair RNA and DNA synthesis.
   d. **True.** The first three and the last two steps in UMP synthesis occur in two distinct multi-enzyme complexes
   e. **True.** CPSII utilises the amine group in glutamine whereas CPSI uses ammonia.

6. a. **False.** It inhibits dihydrofolate reductase, a key reaction in the system involved in dTMP synthesis.
   b. **False.** It inhibits dihydrofolate reductase. A metabolite of 5-FU, FdUMP, inhibits thymidylate synthetase.
   c. **False.** It inhibits this enzyme.
   d. **True.** This combination is very effective in inhibiting dTMP synthesis since FdUMP inhibits the enzyme catalysing the conversion of dUMP plus N^5, N^{10}-methylene -FH_4 to dTMP plus dihydrofolate, and methotrexate inhibits the enzyme that regenerates the tetrahydrofolate needed for the synthesis of N^5, N^{10}-methylene-FH_4.
   e. **True.** Methotrexate is a close analogue of folate.

True/false answers

1. **False.** PRPP is used in both cases.
2. **True.** There are two steps where this occurs.
3. **True.** These pathways are classic examples of this type of control. Allosteric mechanisms are involved.
4. **True.** It is vital to have tight control over the relative amounts of deoxyribonucleotides in cells if DNA replication is to occur in a controlled fashion.
5. **False.** It is high levels of uric acid that cause the symptoms seen in gout. It is relatively water insoluble and crystallises out in joints etc., causing pain.
6. **True.** Examples include 5′-fluorouracil and AZT (used in the treatment of AIDS).

Short essay answers

1. It is important to recall that there are two reactions where amino acids are made by the incorporation of ammonia. One is the glutamate dehydrogenase-

catalysed reaction in which α-ketoglutarate undergoes reductive amination. The other is the amidation of glutamate to form glutamine. In most other circumstances, it is the amide nitrogen in glutamine or the amino group in aspartate that are used where a nitrogen or an amino group is required in a biosynthetic pathway.

Glutamine

a. provides the amino group required for GMP synthesis from IMP

b. provides the amino group for carbamoyl phosphate synthesis in pyrimidine nucleotide biosynthesis

c. provides two of the ring nitrogens during de novo synthesis of the purine nucleotides

d. supplies the amide group required for the synthesis of asparagine from aspartate.

Aspartate

a. provides one of the nitrogens required during urea synthesis

b. provides the amino group that is required for the formation of AMP from IMP

c. provides one of the ring nitrogens in the de novo synthesis of the pyrimidine nucleotides

d. provides a ring nitrogen in de novo purine nucleotide synthesis.

2. The reaction in question is:

$$dUMP + N^5,N^{10}\text{-methylene-FH}_4 \rightarrow dTMP + \text{Dihydrofolate (FH}_2)$$

By the action of thymidylate synthetase, dUMP is methylated, which means that N^5,N^{10}-methylene-FH$_4$ provides both a methylene group and reducing power. The other product is FH$_2$; clearly, the continued operation of the system requires that the FH$_2$ be converted to FH$_4$ so that the latter can acquire another one-carbon unit from serine as follows:

$$FH_2 \rightarrow FH_4 \text{ (+ Serine)} \rightarrow N^5, N^{10}\text{-methylene-FH}_4$$

The formation of FH$_4$ from FH$_2$ involves dihydrofolate reductase and requires NADPH.

5'-Fluorouracil (5-FU) is useful in cancer chemotherapy because it is converted in the body to 5-fluoro-dUMP, an inhibitor of thymidylate synthetase; indeed, it is a 'suicide' inhibitor of the enzyme.

Compounds that are related to tetrahydrofolate such as methotrexate can be used in cancer chemotherapy because they inhibit dihydrofolate reductase. They are often used in combination with 5-FU to produce a more efficient inhibition of dTMP synthesis; this will inhibit the growth of rapidly growing tumours since that growth is dependent upon a high rate of DNA synthesis.

DNA structure and function

13

13.1 Genes control protein synthesis

Protein catalysts are responsible for most of the synthetic activities found in living cells but the synthesis of proteins themselves cannot be carried out entirely by other protein molecules. If it was, then how could the protein molecules responsible for synthesising new proteins themselves be synthesised? Macromolecules other than proteins must be involved. The sequences of its proteins are what makes a species a species and what makes an individual unique. Protein sequence is under the control of genes.

Nucleic acids are involved in protein synthesis

Proteins are involved in protein synthesis but information about the amino acid sequence of new proteins is provided by another class of macromolecule, by the *nucleic acids*, *DNA (deoxyribonucleic acid)* and *RNA (ribonucleic acid)*. DNA, the genetic material in most organisms, is the archive of protein sequence information, which exists in every cell that is capable of protein synthesis. This archive of genetic material is known as the *genome*.

Messenger RNA (mRNA), one form of RNA, is a working copy of the genetic material and carries the information from DNA in the nucleus to the site of protein synthesis outside the nucleus. Further RNA molecules are also involved in the cellular machinery which synthesises proteins.

The cellular machinery that synthesises proteins can make any protein, even its own protein components, if it is given the appropriate mRNA. It also requires amino acid building blocks and a supply of energy in the form of ATP and GTP.

13.2 DNA structure and role

DNA content

The size of the genome appears to increase with what we might consider to be the 'complexity' of the organism (Table 17). However, a more extensive list of organisms would show some anomalies. Some organisms have much more DNA in their genome than you might expect. A few amphibians have genomes 100 times larger than those of mammals. Similar plants can have genomes of very different size. Most eukaryotic organisms appear to have some DNA that has no identifiable function. Organisms with exceptionally large genomes are assumed to have more of this 'junk' DNA than organisms whose genomes seem to be of an appropriate size for the complexity of the organism.

Location of DNA

Most, but not all, DNA is contained in the nucleus. In higher organisms, there is some DNA in mitochondria and in some other organelles, which can synthesise a small number of the protein molecules that they contain. Human mitochondria contain circular DNA molecules of known sequence. Each molecule contains 16 569 base pairs (bp), which encode for several proteins, two ribosomal RNAs and a set of transfer RNAs (tRNAs). Proteins encoded by mitochondrial DNA include some subunits of the membrane-bound complexes of the electron transport chain (p. 85) and some subunits of the membrane-bound ATP synthase. Other subunits and the vast majority of mitochondrial membrane and matrix proteins are encoded by nuclear DNA and are imported after being synthesised outside the mitochondria.

Organisation of DNA

DNA is the component of the *chromosomes* that carries genetic information. Table 17 also shows that the length of DNA in a cell greatly exceeds any linear dimension of the cell containing it. The DNA in each nucleus in human cells is almost 1 metre long. DNA molecules must be coiled and folded. Nuclear DNA is in the form of chromosomes, which condense and become visible during cell division. Human somatic cells contain *46 chromosomes, 23 pairs*. Each chromosome contains one very long DNA molecule. Chromosomes also contain basic proteins known as *histones*, which associate with the DNA and organise its coiling and folding. Histones, although an important component of the chromosome, do not have any specific genetic role. They are highly conserved proteins. Histones from animals and plants only differ by a few amino acid residues in their sequences.

Central dogma of molecular biology

Genetic information describing the amino acid sequences of proteins is carried in coded form by base sequences in DNA. Only a small percentage of the total DNA in the human genome actually codes for protein sequences. Other base sequences mark out the parts of the DNA sequence that are used for protein synthesis. Most of the DNA in the human genome is of unknown function. In each organism, every cell with a nucleus

Table 17 DNA content of cells

	Genome size (base pairs)	Length (mm)
SV40 virus	5243	0.002
E. coli	4×10^6	1.4
Yeast	1.4×10^7	4.6
Fruitfly	1.7×10^8	56
Human	3.9×10^9	990

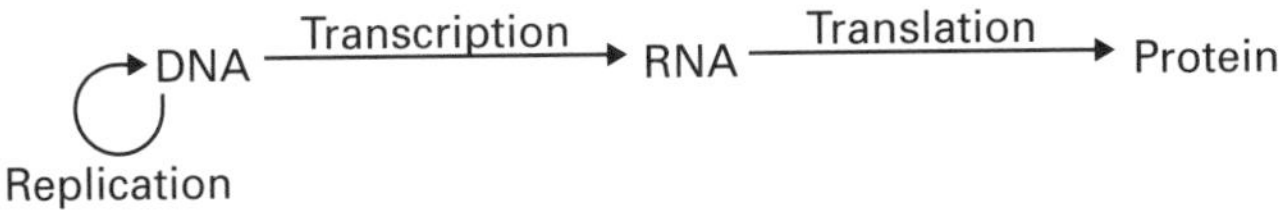

Fig. 117 The 'Central Dogma of Molecular Biology'.

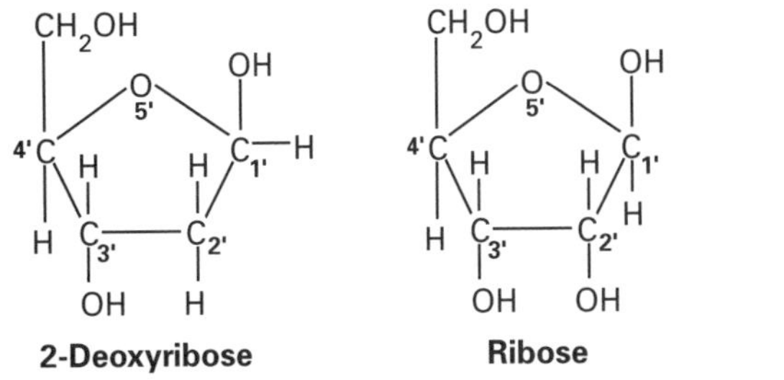

Fig. 118 Pentose sugar in DNA (deoxyribose) and RNA (ribose).

contains an identical set of DNA molecules, the genome, and, therefore, has the information to make all the protein molecules found in that organism. In practice, each cell only synthesises small subsets of all these possible proteins: proteins it needs for its specialised functions and some proteins that are made in virtually every cell. For example, proteins used by the protein synthesising machinery itself and enzymes required for basic metabolic processes, such as the production of ATP, are common to all cells.

When cells divide, each daughter cell must be provided with the complete DNA archive of sequence information. DNA molecules have a structure that allows them to replicate precisely to produce DNA molecules for each daughter cell that are identical to those found in the mother cell.

The flow of information from DNA to RNA (mRNA) to protein has been represented as the Central Dogma of Molecular Biology (Fig. 117). Of course the processes depicted, *replication, transcription* and *translation*, also require enzymes and a supply of energy and building blocks for the synthesis of new molecules.

Genetic code

The information for an organism is held in the sequences of bases in the DNA: a 'nucleic acid language'. This can be translated into amino acid sequences in proteins, which can be considered to be in 'protein language'. The process of translation from one language to the other involves the genetic code (p. 190).

Some small viruses with RNA genomes are the only exceptions to the flow of information represented by the Central Dogma (p. 206). The replication of RNA genomes either involves direct replication of RNA or the formation of a DNA version of the genome, which can then direct the formation of new RNA copies. Replication of RNA genomes is a lot more error-prone than replication of DNA; as a result, RNA viruses are very mutable and are limited in the size of the genome that they can maintain.

Structure of nucleic acids

We must study the structures of the nucleic acids if we are to understand how they perform their functions. These structures reveal how the molecules can store information and how copies of this information can be made; DNA molecules can be replicated to make identical copies for passing on to daughter cells during cell division and can also be transcribed to make RNA copies for directing protein synthesis.

Primary structure

DNA and RNA have similar covalent structures consisting of *sugar phosphate backbones* with bases attached. They are linear polymers of building blocks known as nucleotides (Chapter 12). A nucleotide comprises:

- phosphate group
- pentose sugar (Fig. 118)
  — ribose in RNA
  — 2-deoxyribose in DNA
- nitrogenous base (Fig. 119)
  — purine derivatives adenine (A) and guanine (G)
  — pyrimidine derivatives cytosine (C) and thymine (T) (DNA) or uracil (U) (RNA).

A typical nucleotide, AMP, is shown in Figure 120. A pentose sugar attached to a base but with no phosphate attached is called a *nucleoside*. Adenosine is the nucleoside composed of the base, adenine and ribose. The nucleic acid backbone chain is composed of alternating sugar and phosphate groups. Each phosphate group is esterified to the 3'-hydroxyl group on one sugar and to the 5'-hydroxyl group of the next (Fig. 121); this is known as a *phosphodiester* linkage. The chain is unbranched and may contain thousands of sugar and phosphate units in the case of RNA or millions in the case of DNA. Each sugar unit in the chain carries a nitrogenous base attached by an *N-glycosidic bond* to carbon-1, the anomeric carbon of the sugar. There is no restriction on the sequence of the bases on a single nucleic acid chain. Consequently, the base sequence can be used to encode information. Base sequences that correspond to any possible amino acid sequence for a protein can be carried on DNA.

Polarity of nucleic acids

Nucleic acid chains have direction: both RNA and DNA have ends that can be distinguished. The phosphodiester linkages result in a chain with a sugar unit with a 5'-hydroxyl not involved in a linkage at one end and a 3'-hydroxyl not involved in a linkage at the other. These ends of the chain are referred to as the 5' and 3' ends (Fig. 121). All nucleic acid chains, both DNA and RNA, are synthesised in the 5' to 3' direction, that is to say the chains are elongated by addition of new nucleotide units at the 3' ends. When we consider the association of two DNA chains to form a DNA double helix, we find they are *antiparallel*, one runs in

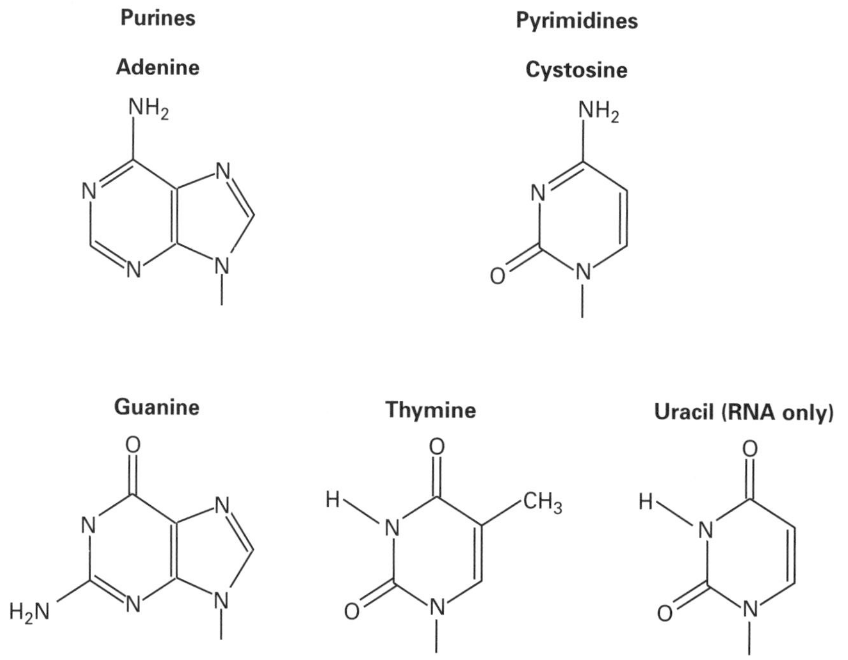

Purines

Adenine

Pyrimidines

Cystosine

Guanine

Thymine

Uracil (RNA only)

Fig. 119 Bases in DNA and RNA.

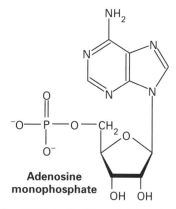

Adenosine monophosphate

Fig. 120 AMP, a typical nucleotide containing adenine, ribose and a phosphate group.

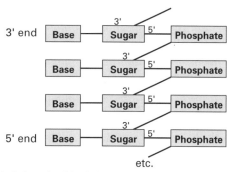

Fig. 121 Polynucleotide chain structure.

the 5' to 3' direction while the other runs in the 3' to 5' direction.

Translation of mRNA also occurs in the 5' to 3' direction. Since this is the direction for all the processes in which nucleic acids engage, nucleic acid sequences are conventionally written with the 5' end on the left and the 3' end on the right. The only exception to this

convention is when a sequence is depicted together with its complementary sequence. Since the chains are antiparallel, the lower one is shown with its 3' end on the left. Movement along a sequence is often referred to as *upstream*, towards the 5' end, or *downstream*, towards the 3' end.

Higher structural levels

In nucleic acids, as with proteins, higher levels of structure beyond the covalent primary structure must be considered when we try to relate structure to function. In the case of the nucleic acids, this involves the folding and coiling of the chains and most importantly, the specific association of one chain with another. The association of one chain with another depends on the base sequences of the chains involved. The bases on one chain must be able to make 'base pairs' with the bases on the other (see below). Two base sequences that can make base pairs with one another are said to be *complementary*.

The double helix

The most important structure which involves the association of nucleic acid chains with complementary base sequences is the *double helix* formed by DNA. It was the description of this structure by Watson and Crick in 1953 that triggered the explosion in knowledge of the biochemical basis of genetics that has occurred since then. After studying the results of X-ray crystallography studies and chemical analysis, Watson and Crick proposed that DNA existed as pairs of DNA chains having complementary base sequences. The two chains associated with each other to form a double helix with a distinct character (Fig. 122):

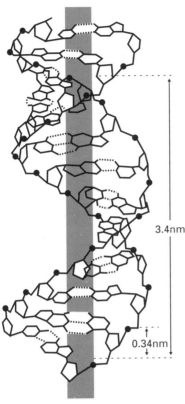

Fig. 122 The DNA double helix. The sugars are represented by pentagons and the phosphates by black circles. (From Bell, Emslie-Smith and Paterson (1976) Textbook of physiology and biochemistry, 9th edn, Edinburgh: Churchill Livingstone.)

- deoxyribose–phosphate backbones are antiparallel: one chain runs 5′ to 3′ while the other runs 3′ to 5′
- the deoxyribose–phosphate backbones wind round each other to form a helix; a complete turn of the helix occurs every 10 base pairs
- base pairs form from bases contributed one by each chain and occupy the core of the helix
- bases are planar with hydrophobic surfaces and the base pairs stack, one on top of the other like a pile of plates, to fill the core; this adds greatly to the stability of the helix
- two helical grooves, one wide and one narrow, allow access to the bases so that they can interact with proteins
- protein binding to specific base sequences is vital for the control of gene expression.

BOX 13.1
Clinical note: Many mutagens contain aromatic rings

Some mutagens (and, hence, carcinogens) have planar aromatic ring structures which can insert themselves into the stack of base pairs at the core of the DNA double helix. Examples of such carcinogens are benzanthracene found in cigarette smoke and aflatoxins produced by the action of certain moulds.

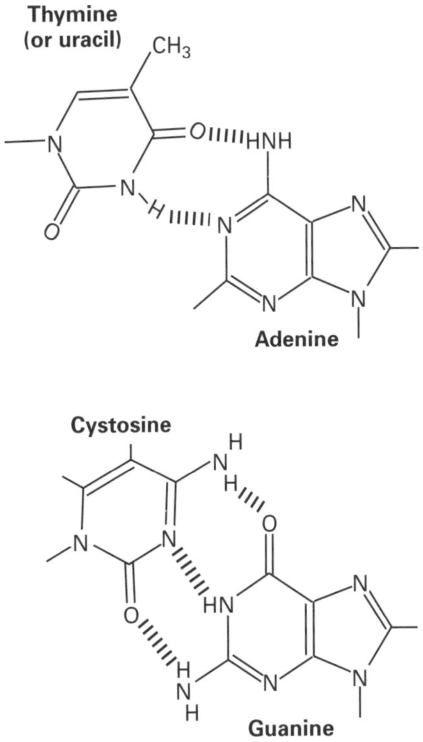

Fig. 123 Base pair formation.

Base pairing

Each base pair must form according to strict base-pairing rules. One base in each pair must be a purine, (adenine or guanine) while the other must be a pyrimidine (cytosine or thymine). Two purines together are too large to fit into the core of the helix and two pyrimidines are too small. Furthermore, hydrogen bond formation dictates that if one base is adenine, the other in the pair must be thymine, and if one base is guanine, the other must be cytosine. Thus four base pairs are possible, AT, TA, GC and CG (Fig. 123). Notice that the overall sizes and shapes of the base pairs are very similar and that the atoms on the bases which form bonds to the sugar occupy similar positions in each base pair. An AT base pair and a TA base pair are also similar and are related to each other by a twofold rotational symmetry. So also for GC and CG base pairs. The double helical structure of DNA can accommodate any sequence of base pairs. One chain in the double helix can have any sequence of bases, but this sequence of bases imposes a complementary, and hence pre-dictable, sequence on the second chain. If one chain were to be taken away or destroyed, an identical chain could be constructed to replace it by constructing a chain with a base sequence complementary to the remaining chain.

13.3 **DNA replication**

The Watson–Crick structure of DNA lends itself to direct replication. If you separate the chains and obey

Increasing density ⟶

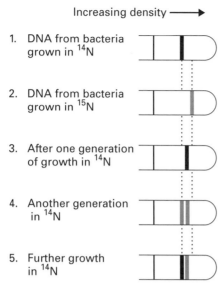

1. DNA from bacteria grown in ^{14}N

2. DNA from bacteria grown in ^{15}N

3. After one generation of growth in ^{14}N

4. Another generation in ^{14}N

5. Further growth in ^{14}N

Fig. 124 Meselson and Stahl's experiment to show semi-conservative DNA replication. DNA containing ^{14}N can be distinguished from that containing ^{15}N by ultracentrifugation in a caesium chloride density gradient, where they form bands at differing positions (tubes 1 and 2). Bacteria grown for several generations in ^{15}N and then grown for one generation in ^{14}N contain a hybrid DNA of intermediate density (tube 3). After another generation in ^{14}N, an ^{14}N band appears in addition to the hybrid band (tube 4); the latter band gets fainter during further generations (tube 5).

the base-pairing rules while constructing a new partner chain for each, the result is two double helical molecules that are exact replicas of the original. This mode of replication is described as semi-conservative. Each daughter molecule contains a complete chain from the original. Meselson and Stahl demonstrated by an elegant experiment that DNA did indeed replicate in this way (Fig. 124), but the actual replication process in cells must overcome some practical difficulties. The main difficulty is that the two chains are not separated before being copied; a continuous process of separation and copying passes along the original molecule. Only a very short section of DNA is converted to single-stranded form for copying at one time.

Replication of prokaryotic DNA starts in both directions from a single initiation site on the closed circular DNA molecule and replication proceeds until the replication sites meet on the other side of the circle.

Replication in eukaryotes, where the DNA molecules are much longer, starts at many initiation sites on each chromosome and proceeds in both directions until the replication process moving in one direction from one site meets the process moving in the other direction from the next site. The two replication processes moving apart from a single initiation site form what is termed a *replication bubble*. Each replication bubble has two regions where the DNA double helix is being unwound and replicated (Fig. 125). These regions are known as *replication forks*. To understand how DNA replication works, we have to consider events at a replication fork.

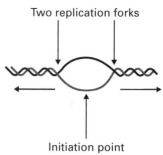

Two replication forks

Initiation point

Fig. 125 Replication bubble consisting of two replication forks proceeding in opposite directions.

Synthesis of new DNA

DNA polymerases synthesise new DNA from deoxynucleoside 5'-triphosphates. At least two forms are involved, *DNA polymerase III*, which synthesises most of the new DNA, and *DNA polymerase I*, which fills in gaps that DNA polymerase III must leave in one of the new chains at each fork. Both enzymes require a supply of deoxynucleotide units in the form of their triphosphates: dATP, dGTP, dCTP and dTTP. During the addition of each unit to the growing chain, two phosphate groups are eliminated as inorganic pyrophosphate, which is quickly hydrolysed by a pyrophosphatase. The hydrolysis of two high energy bonds in the triphosphate provides the energy for the addition of one nucleotide unit (Fig. 126).

Addition of new units only occurs at the 3' end of an existing DNA chain. Because they use deoxynucleoside 5'-triphosphates as substrates, DNA polymerases can only catalyse the addition of new nucleotides at the 3' end of an existing DNA molecule. They also require a *template*: a single-stranded DNA molecule. This controls the base sequence of the new strand, which is complementary to the template. The new strand is formed antiparallel to the template. At a replication fork, DNA polymerase III and its associated DNA unwinding proteins separate the two chains of the original double helix. The replication process is different for the two chains of the original helix, the so-called *leading* and *lagging* strands.

The leading strand

The leading strand is copied continuously as it runs

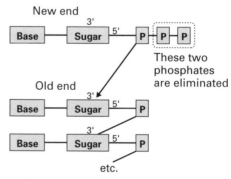

New end

These two phosphates are eliminated

Old end

etc.

Fig. 126 Addition of a nucleotide unit to a growing chain: 5' to 3' growth.

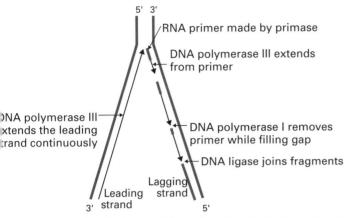

Fig. 127 Replication fork. The leading strand is directly replicated 5' to 3'. The lagging strand is replicated in Okazaki fragments from RNA primers. The RNA primers are then removed and the gaps filled with DNA.

from 3' to 5', and will be able to act as a continuous template to produce an antiparallel complementary strand (Fig. 127).

The lagging strand

Copying of the other strand, the lagging strand, cannot be continuous, since no DNA polymerase can produce a new strand in the 3' to 5' direction. New DNA for the lagging strand is synthesised in fragments, called *Okazaki fragments* after the biochemist who first described them. These fragments, which are a few hundred base units long, are then joined to form a continuous chain (Fig. 127), a process that requires the cooperation of several enzyme activities.

Formation of Okazaki fragments. Each Okazaki fragment has an *RNA primer*. Only after the leading

strand synthesis has proceeded for several hundred base units can the synthesis of the lagging strand commence to make a complementary chain for the several hundred units length of single-stranded 5' to 3' template now exposed. Synthesis of this chain must be in the direction opposite to the overall direction of movement of the replication fork. That is to say it must start in the fork and grow out from the fork. Since DNA polymerases absolutely require a 3' end of a nucleic acid chain if they are to attach new units, a primer must be provided. This primer is a short section of RNA made by a form of RNA polymerase known as *primase*. RNA polymerases do not need a 3' end to start synthesis. DNA polymerase can then add a new DNA chain to the RNA primer until it reaches the 5' end of the previous fragment.

Filling the gaps between fragments. This is done by *DNA polymerase I* which removes the RNA primer and replaces it with DNA. *DNA ligase* then joins the DNA fragments to make a continuous chain (Fig. 128) using the energy of hydrolysis of ATP or NAD$^+$ to create the phosphodiester bond.

13.4 Fidelity of DNA replication

It is evident that to copy the complete genome with very few errors requires tremendous accuracy in the copying process, 4×10^9 base pairs to be copied with hardly any error. The accuracy required is, in fact, greater than can be achieved by DNA polymerase in its synthetic reaction alone. It is thought that about 1 in 10^5 of the inserted bases are not complementary to the corresponding base in the template chain. In bacteria

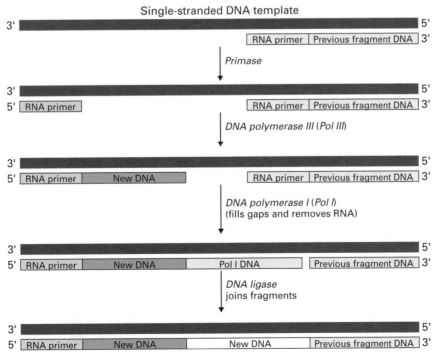

Fig. 128 Mechanism of replication of the lagging strand.

any wrongly inserted nucleotide is removed by a 3′-nuclease activity of DNA polymerase I. After inserting the wrong nucleotide, the enzyme is unable to proceed until the non-complementary nucleotide is removed. Bacterial DNA polymerase, therefore, has a 'proof-reading' function. In eukaryotes, the DNA polymerase does not have this proof-reading ability and detection and elimination of copying errors is carried out by enzymes that are also responsible for the elimination of errors from the genome.

DNA repair

As well as the errors introduced during the copying process, the DNA of the genome may from time to time sustain damage that needs to be repaired. Enzyme systems that correct errors and repair the DNA do exist. There are some diseases where the underlying bio-chemical lesion has been identified as a reduced activity of one of these enzymes. Subjects suffering from such diseases may be unable to tolerate exposure to direct sunlight, or be particularly prone to some forms of cancer.

Damage to DNA can, in principle, be repaired if one of the DNA chains remains intact in the damaged region. The damaged part of the chain can be excised or cut away and then replaced by newly synthesised DNA that is complementary to the undamaged chain. Damage to DNA can arise from a variety of causes:

- exposure of cells to intense ultraviolet light can induce photochemical reactions between bases on the DNA chains: two thymines if next to each other in a sequence can react to form a thymine dimer
- mutagenic chemicals may convert one base into another
- reactive chemical species produced by ionising radiation may react with bases and alter them
- the bond between deoxyribose and a base, particularly a purine, is not completely stable and may break leaving a sugar group without any base attached.

All these forms of damage can be detected by proteins that interact with the distorted double helix which the damage produces. *Nucleases* then excise the damaged section, DNA polymerase I fills in the gap with new DNA and DNA ligase joins the new DNA to the old.

13.5 **DNA in cells**

DNA synthesis and the cell cycle

Eukaryotic cells that are dividing do not synthesise DNA continuously but only during the S phase of the cell cycle (Fig. 129). Replication of chromosomal DNA must be complete before the start of mitosis, the process by which replicated chromosomes segregate

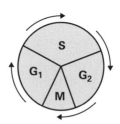

Fig. 129 The cell cycle.

equally toward opposite poles prior to cell division. DNA synthesis does not resume again until after completion of mitosis. S (for synthesis) phase in the cycle is separated from M (for mitosis) phase by gap phases (G_1 and G_2) when neither process is occurring. There is evidence that the controls responsible for the timing of the cell cycle contain 'checkpoints' that halt the cycle while DNA replication or repair is in progress.

DNA in chromosomes

Apart from the enzymes required for replication and repair, many other enzymes and proteins exist which interact with DNA. In eukaryotes, the molecule of DNA that forms a single chromosome may be several centimetres in length. It must be condensed or shortened by coiling and folding if it is to fit in the nucleus. *Histones* are proteins that bind to DNA to promote coiling of DNA and reduction of its length. The first stage of the condensation process is the formation of *nucleosomes*. These are formed by a length of DNA, about 200 base pairs long, forming a double coil around a 'bobbin' composed of histone proteins (Fig. 130). The core of the nucleosome is made up of eight histone molecules, two each of H2A, H2B, H3 and H4. A single H1 molecule per nucleosome appears to control when DNA can unwind from the core. A single nucleosome will hold DNA of about 200 base pairs in length. Chains of nucleosomes are further coiled into a solenoid structure, thus reducing the length of the DNA. DNA that is being replicated or that is being used as a template for RNA synthesis must be unwound from the nucleosome and from the higher level coiling. This is achieved by local covalent modifi-cation of the histones by acetylation, phosphorylation and other processes. Condensed DNA is protected against nuclease action while DNA that is unwound is much more easily attacked.

Mitochondria contain closed circles of DNA similar to that found in bacteria.

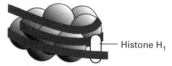

Fig. 130 Nucleosome structure with histones.

Bacterial DNA

Histones are not found in bacteria and another means of condensing the DNA is used. The DNA is in the form of a closed circle so there is no 5' or 3' end to either chain in the double helix. This circle is made to supercoil by the introduction of extra turns into the circle by enzymes known as *helicases*. Since there are no free ends to rotate, the DNA coils on itself and shortens (Fig. 131). Other enzymes known as *topoisomerases* can act as swivel points in the DNA chain and relieve the supercoiling.

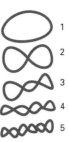

Fig. 131 Supercoiling of circular DNA.

Self-assessment: questions

Multiple choice questions

1. The following statements describe nucleic acids and proteins:
   a. Nucleic acids are involved in protein synthesis
   b. Proteins are not involved in nucleic acid synthesis
   c. Chromosomes contain DNA
   d. Chromosomes contain protein
   e. Every diploid nucleated cell in the body contains information about the amino acid sequence of every protein that can be synthesised in any cell

2. In the genomes of different species:
   a. Fruit flies have more DNA per cell than bacteria and humans have more than fruit flies but some frogs and toads have more than humans
   b. DNA is the primary genetic material in animals and RNA is the primary genetic material in plants
   c. All the DNA in a eukaryotic cell is contained in chromosomes in the nucleus
   d. Chromosomes contain large amounts of protein as well as DNA
   e. All cells in a eukaryotic organism contain the same amount of nuclear DNA per set of chromosomes

3. The following statements describe DNA and protein synthesis:
   a. The Central Dogma of Molecular Genetics concerns the flow of sequence information from DNA to RNA to protein
   b. The production of two identical DNA molecules from an original DNA molecule is known as replication; it occurs in the nucleus of eukaryotic cells
   c. The copying of base sequence information from DNA to RNA is known as transcription; it occurs outside the nucleus in eukaryotic cells
   d. The synthesis of a protein with an amino acid sequence specified by the base sequence of an RNA molecule is known as translation; it occurs outside the nucleus in eukaryotic cells
   e. DNA replication, transcription and translation are sufficient to account for the specificity of protein synthesis in all organisms except RNA viruses

4. Bases in nucleic acids:
   a. In the DNA double helix, each base pair must contain two purines or two pyrimidines
   b. The bases in DNA and RNA are joined to the sugar phosphate backbone by ester linkages to the phosphate groups
   c. DNA is usually double-stranded
   d. In double-stranded DNA, the number of adenines equals the number of thymines and the number of guanines equals the number of cytosines
   e. The two DNA chains in a double helix are antiparallel

5. Bases in DNA and RNA:
   a. Uracil is a pyrimidine base that occurs in RNA but not in DNA
   b. Thymine is a pyrimidine base that occurs in DNA but not in RNA
   c. Ribose is a pentose sugar that occurs in RNA but not in DNA
   d. Cytosine is a purine base that occurs in both RNA and DNA
   e. Adenine and guanine are purine bases that occur in both RNA and DNA

6. Nucleic acids as polynucleotides have:
   a. Two ends that can be distinguished, one has a free 5' group, whereas the other has a free 3' group
   b. A backbone consisting of alternating phosphate groups and pentose sugar units
   c. No structural restriction on the sequence of bases
   d. Nucleic acid chains that are never closed circles
   e. Nucleic acid chains that are never branched

7. DNA and RNA:
   a. Contain sugar residues joined by phosphodiester links
   b. RNA is chemically more stable than DNA
   c. Contain bases attached to 1'-carbon of the pentose sugar units
   d. Nucleotide units are joined by 3', 5'-phosphodiester bonds in DNA whereas those in RNA are joined by 2', 5' bonds
   e. When DNA is denatured by heating, the two strands in the double helix separate and the bases are no longer paired

8. Base pairs:
   a. Every base pair contains one purine base and one pyrimidine base
   b. In DNA, adenine always pairs with thymine
   c. In DNA, guanine always pairs with cytosine
   d. The specificity of base-pair formation depends on interbase hydrogen bonding
   e. The GC base pair is much larger than the AT base pair

9. The following are required for replication of DNA by DNA polymerase:
   a. A template of single-stranded DNA
   b. A DNA or RNA primer with a free 3′ end
   c. 2′-deoxy-ATP
   d. 2′-deoxy-UTP
   e. 2′-deoxy-CTP

10. In DNA replication:
    a. Addition of new nucleotide units can occur at either the 5′ or the 3′ end of the chain being extended
    b. Addition of new nucleotide units can occur continuously on the leading strand
    c. Addition of new nucleotide units cannot occur continuously on the lagging strand
    d. Each new nucleotide unit added to a growing strand should have a base that can form a complementary base pair with the corresponding base on the template strand
    e. DNA polymerase is responsible for the replication of both the leading and lagging strands

11. DNA replication:
    a. Is semi-conservative, that is to say each of the original strands from a double helix is associated with a newly synthesised strand in the daughter molecules
    b. Occurs continuously on the two DNA chains in a double helix
    c. Involves DNA polymerase, which requires a DNA template and a primer, which is usually RNA
    d. Proceeds in both directions from an initiation site, so a replication bubble is formed

    e. Of the lagging strand in DNA synthesis involves the formation of RNA primers and Okazaki fragments; the fragments are finally sealed together by the actions of DNA polymerase I and DNA ligase

12. Lagging strand replication:
    a. Occurs as a series of fragments that are then joined
    b. Produces fragments that start with an RNA primer; DNA polymerase III adds new nucleotide units to the 3′ end of this primer
    c. Results in gaps between fragments, which are filled with DNA by reverse transcriptase
    d. Produces fragments known as Okazaki fragments, which are eventually joined into a continuous strand by DNA ligase
    e. Involves DNA ligase, which is also involved in DNA repair

13. DNA in chromosomes:
    a. Is replicated continuously in dividing cells
    b. The first stage of condensation of nuclear DNA in eukaryotes involves the formation of nucleosomes
    c. Contains nucleosomes each consisting of about 200 base pairs length of double helix wound around a core composed of histone proteins
    d. In prokaryotes exists as closed circles and is condensed by supercoiling
    e. Is supercoiled. Supercoiling can be increased or decreased by enzymes

Short essay question

Describe the features of DNA that fit it for its function as the primary genetic material in most organisms.

Self-assessment: answers

Multiple choice answers

1. a. **True.** Nucleic acids are responsible for providing the sequence information for protein synthesis.
   b. **False.** proteins, particularly enzymes, are involved in nucleic acid synthesis.
   c. **True.** DNA carries the genetic information in chromosomes.
   d. **True.** Protein molecules organise the DNA in chromosomes.
   e. **True.** Every diploid nucleated cell has a complete set of chromosomes.

2. a. **True.** As a general rule, the more complex the organism, the more DNA it has in its genome, but some frogs and toads have much more DNA than would be expected.
   b. **False.** Both animals and plants have DNA as the primary genetic material.
   c. **False.** There is some DNA in mitochondria and other cellular organelles such as chloroplasts.
   d. **True.** Proteins, particularly histones, keep DNA in a condensed form.
   e. **True.** Each nucleated cell contains the whole genome.

3. a. **True.** It applies in the great majority of organisms.
   b. **True.** Nuclear DNA is replicated in the nucleus.
   c. **False.** The definition of transcription is correct but it occurs in the nucleus.
   d. **True.** The RNA is synthesised in the nucleus and then exported to direct protein synthesis.
   e. **True.** RNA viruses need further processes to replicate their genome.

4. a. **False.** Each base pair contains a purine and a pyrimidine.
   b. **False.** They are joined to carbon-1 of the sugars by glycosidic bonds.
   c. **True.** DNA is almost always found in double-stranded form.
   d. **True.** This is a consequence of specific base pairing.
   e. **True.** One runs in the 5′ to 3′ direction, the other 3′ to 5′.

5. a. **True.** Uracil does not occur in DNA.
   b. **True.** Thymine does not occur in RNA.
   c. **True.** Ribose is found in RNA and 2′-deoxyribose is found in DNA.
   d. **False.** Cytosine is a pyrimidine base.
   e. **True.** The same purines occur in DNA and RNA.

6. a. **True.** Bonds between nucleotides involve the 3′-carbon on one and the 5′-carbon on the next. Nucleotide units at the ends of chain have either a free 3′ or a free 5′ carbon.
   b. **True.** This is the same in both DNA and RNA.
   c. **True.** This allows nucleic acids to act as information carriers.
   d. **False.** Bacterial DNA usually occurs as closed circular molecules, as does mitochondrial DNA.
   e. **True.** Nucleic acids are always linear polymers.

7. a. **True.** This is the same in both DNA and RNA.
   b. **False.** RNA is much more easily hydrolysed, especially in alkali.
   c. **True.** This applies to all nucleotides and polynucleotides.
   d. **False.** Both have 3′,5′-phosphodiester bonds.
   e. **True.** This process is sometimes referred to as melting of DNA.

8. a. **True.** There is space in the core of the double helix for one purine and one pyrimidine.
   b. **True.** This base pair is abbreviated AT.
   c. **True.** This base pair is abbreviated GC.
   d. **True.** The bases in each complementary base pair have matching hydrogen bond donor and acceptor sites.
   e. **False.** GC and AT base pairs are approximately the same size.

9. a. **True.** The template directs the sequence of the new strand.
   b. **True.** DNA polymerases need primers and cannot start a chain without one.
   c. **True.** 2′-Deoxy ATP provides nucleotide residues for the new chain.
   d. **False.** Uracil does not occur in DNA. 2′-Deoxy TTP is required.
   e. **True.** 2′-Deoxy CTP provides nucleotide residues for the new chain.

10. a. **False.** Addition occurs only at the 3′ end.
    b. **True.** The leading strand grows continuously at the 3′ end.
    c. **True.** The lagging strand is replicated in fragments, not continuously.
    d. **True.** This is how the template directs the base sequence of the new strand (some mismatching can occur, which requires subsequent repair).
    e. **True.** It is a very complex enzyme.

11. a. **True.** This was shown by the experiment of Meselson and Stahl.
    b. **False.** The leading strand is replicated continuously but the lagging strand is replicated in fragments.

c. **True.** Its also requires the four deoxy nucleotide triphosphates.

d. **True.** The replication bubble consists of two replication forks.

e. **True.** This mechanism is necessary as new nucleotide units can only be added to the 3′ end of growing strands.

12. a. **True.** These are known as Okazaki fragments.
    b. **True.** DNA polymerases need a primer.
    c. **False.** The gaps are filled by DNA polymerase I.
    d. **True.** DNA ligase joins the 3′ end of one fragment to the 5′ end of the next.
    e. **True.** Damaged strands are repaired by DNA polymerase I and DNA ligase.

13. a. **False.** Nuclear DNA is replicated only during S phase of the cell cycle.
    b. **True.** DNA double helix winds around a core composed of histones.
    c. **True.** Nucleosome formations shortens the DNA molecule about sevenfold.
    d. **True.** Bacterial genomes and plasmids are circular DNA molecules.
    e. **True.** DNA gyrases and topoisomerases catalyse these processes.

Short essay answer

Points which should be mentioned include its double helical structure, which allows for straightforward replication, its ability to carry information in its sequence of bases and its chemical stability.

RNA structure and

function

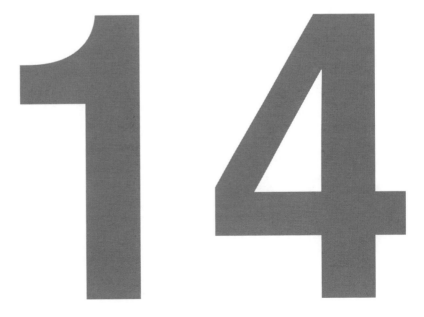

14.1 Types of RNA

Although DNA carries the information that is needed for the synthesis of proteins, it is not directly involved in protein synthesis. There are three types of RNA needed for protein synthesis:

- messenger RNA (mRNA): carries the sequence information from DNA in the nucleus to the protein synthetic machinery in the cytoplasm
- ribosomal RNA: forms about 50% of the weight of ribosomes, on which protein synthesis occurs
- transfer RNA (tRNA): acts as an adaptor matching a specific amino acid to the *codon* on the mRNA.

RNA structures

RNA has a covalent structure very similar to that of DNA. It has *ribose* in place of deoxyribose and the pyrimidine base *uracil* in place of thymine. The extra hydroxyl group on the 2' position of the sugar facilitates the cleavage of the phosphodiester bond to the hydroxyl group on the 3' hydroxyl, so RNA is more easily hydrolysed than DNA. Uracil is very similar to thymine, lacking only the methyl substituent at the 5 position on the ring. Like thymine, it can form a base pair with adenine.

RNA does not have a higher order structure on the same scale as the double helix formed by DNA. Nevertheless, structures containing some base-pairing do exist and are important. Table 18 summarises the properties and functions of the various RNAs.

Transfer RNAs

There are 30 to 40 distinct tRNA molecules, each responsible for bringing a single amino acid to the growing polypeptide chain. Each of these tRNA molecules contains a sequence of approximately 80 nucleotide units and has the same basic shape. Base pairing by parts of these sequences leads to folded forms in a 'clover leaf' structure, containing three major stem loops (Fig. 132). Base pairing occurs between different parts of the same chain, which folds back on itself; the remaining unpaired bases are exposed in loops where the chain turns. There are three bases at the end of one loop that are not base paired and form the *anti-codon*, which binds to the mRNA. Amino acids are attached to the 3' end of the tRNA which carries their specific anti-codon by amino acyl tRNA synthetases (p. 191).

Ribosomal RNA

The molecules of ribosomal RNA also contain sequences that bring about folding to form a structure

Table 18 Principal forms of eukaryotic RNA

Form of RNA	Size (bases)	Role
mRNA	varies with size of protein to be synthesised	Carries protein sequence information from nucleus to ribosomes. Some mRNA species are very short-lived, others more stable. mRNA is processed in the nucleus from initial transcripts
Ribosomal RNA		
16S	1542	Together with about 20 proteins, makes up the structure of the small ribosomal subunit
23S	about 3000	23S and 5S rRNA with about 30 proteins, make up the structure of the small ribosomal subunit
5S	about 120	Small ribosomal subunit
tRNA	about 80	There are between 30 and 40 different species to act as adaptors, matching amino acids to codons
Small nuclear RNAs (snRNAs)	up to 200	Associated with proteins to form complexes involved in splicing during mRNA processing
Small cytoplasmic RNA (scRNA)	about 300	Associates with proteins to form a signal recognition particle that is involved in intracellular transport of newly synthesised proteins
RNA primers	about 5	Primers for Okazaki fragments during replication of the lagging strand in DNA replication (Chapter 13); these primers are then replaced by DNA

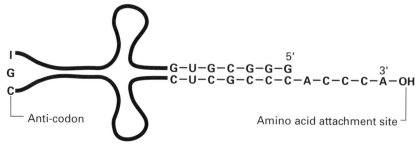

Fig. 132 Secondary structure of tRNA.

containing many stem loops. Ribosomal RNA adopts a specific three-dimensional configuration that is required for its function. The role of ribosomes is discussed in Chapter 15.

Messenger RNA

mRNA has a base sequence that directs the synthesis of a protein with a particular amino acid sequence so it cannot adopt a specific three-dimensional shape by base-pairing. Nevertheless, stem loops may form in sections of the mRNA sequence that are not used for coding.

Other RNAs

Other forms of RNA exist, especially in eukaryotic cells. RNA molecules having specific catalytic action participate in the processing and maturation of eukaryotic RNA before it leaves the nucleus. Further RNA molecules direct newly synthesised proteins to their destinations in the cell. These forms of RNA have specific three-dimensional structures that depend on base pairing.

14.2 Transcription: synthesis of RNA

RNA is synthesised by *RNA polymerase* from the precursor nucleoside triphosphates ATP, GTP, UTP and CTP. RNA polymerase, like DNA polymerase, requires a template to direct the sequence of the RNA product. The template in this case is DNA and the enzyme synthesises an RNA molecule that has a sequence which is complementary to one chain of the DNA molecule. Each adenine in the DNA sequence is copied as uracil, each thymine as adenine, each guanine as cytosine and each cytosine as guanine. As in DNA synthesis, pyrophosphate is eliminated during the polymerisation, and the subsequent hydrolysis of this drives the reaction in the direction of synthesis. The growing RNA chain has each new nucleotide unit added at its 3' end. As in DNA synthesis, the template and the new chain are antiparallel, so the DNA chain is copied in its 3' to 5' direction. For any one region of the double helix only one chain acts as a template. In other regions the other chain is used, i.e. all the coding sequences are not on just one of the two chains. In eukaryotes, different molecular species of RNA polymerase catalyse the synthesis of mRNA, ribosomal RNA and tRNA (Table 19). The process of RNA synthesis can be considered in three phases:

- initiation
- elongation
- termination.

Initiation

Initiation has been much studied because it is during this phase that the starting points on the DNA sequence

Table 19 RNA polymerases in eukaryotic cells

Form	RNA species for which transcript is produced
I	23S and 16S ribosomal RNA
II	mRNA
III	tRNAs and 5S ribosomal RNA

are identified. These starting points are known as *promoters*. It is the efficiency of initiation at each promoter that determines how much of each particular mRNA is made and hence how much of the corresponding protein. Some promoters are subject to control and can be switched on and off. Control of promoter action is the most important mechanism by which the cell controls the proteins that it synthesises and the amount of each.

Formation of a transcription complex

RNA polymerase binds at promoter sequences. RNA polymerase is responsible for all RNA synthesis in prokaryotes and is simpler than the eukaryotic enzymes. It contains five subunits, two alpha subunits, two similar beta subunits (β and β'), and the sigma subunit. The sigma subunit is involved in promoter recognition and in the formation of a *transcription complex* before the synthesis of each RNA molecule. It is not required for elongation. Promoters are recognised by their sequences. By convention, the base in DNA that is complementary to the first base in the RNA molecule is designated +1. The bases of the template are then numbered in sequence, +2, +3 and so on. Bases further down the chain in this direction are said to be *downstream*. The base on the upstream side of +1 is designated –1.

The recognition sequences for the promoter are situated around –10 and –35. Promoter sequences are similar but not identical; they are said to resemble a consensus sequence. Around –10, the sequence often include the bases TATA. If DNA is to act as a template for RNA synthesis, the DNA chains must be temporarily unwound and separated. This involves breaking the base pairs and it may be significant that the section of chain where separation is initiated consists predominantly of AT base pairs. Adenine forms only two hydrogen bonds with thymine, whereas a guanine–cytosine base pair is stabilised by three hydrogen bonds. The TATA sequence is, therefore, more easily separated than a sequence made up of GC base pairs. A schematic drawing to represent initiation and elongation during transcription is shown as Figure 133.

Elongation

Once the initiation complex is formed and nucleotide units are bound to start transcription, the sigma unit is no longer required and dissociates. Core enzyme of RNA polymerase then catalyses elongation of the RNA chain as it moves along the DNA.

1. Initiation: *RNA polymerase* binds at promoter

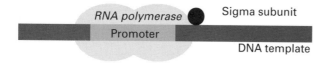

2. DNA chain separation

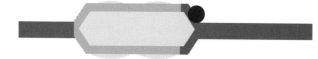

3. Transcription starts

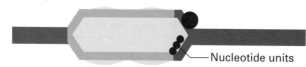

4. Elongation

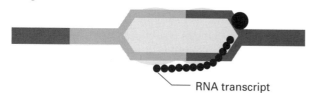

Fig. 133 Transcription: initiation and elongation.

Termination

RNA polymerase continues elongating the RNA transcript until it encounters a termination sequence. This sequence is recognised by a termination protein called the *rho factor*, which binds to DNA and separates the enzyme from its template.

14.3 Control of transcription

Protein synthesis is largely controlled by transcription. Specific DNA-binding proteins control initiation at many promoters and cells have the ability to switch the synthesis of specific proteins on and off. In each cell proteins can be classified as:

- constitutive, synthesised whatever the circumstances
- repressible, normally synthesised but synthesis can be turned off
- inducible, not normally synthesised but synthesis can be turned on.

Repression is often seen in anabolic pathways where a surplus of the end-product of the pathway represses synthesis of all the enzymes in the path. Repressible proteins in bacteria include the enzymes responsible for the synthesis of some amino acids or other cellular building blocks. If these amino acids or building blocks are abundant in the growth medium then bacteria can save energy and material by repressing the synthesis of these enzymes.

Inducible proteins often carry out functions that the cell does not always need, such as the catabolism of some rarely encountered nutrient. *E. coli* can grow on glucose and a variety of other sugars including lactose. The enzymes for glucose catabolism are constitutive but those for lactose catabolism are inducible: they are only synthesised if lactose is present and if glucose is absent. The mechanism by which this control is exerted on the synthesis of lactose-catabolising proteins in *E. coli* is well understood (see below).

Control of transcription in prokaryotes

Control of protein synthesis in bacteria has been much studied and some important control mechanisms have been described.

Control of the lac operon in E. coli

Lactose is a disaccharide containing a galactose unit joined to a glucose by a glycosidic bond joining carbon-1, the anomeric carbon of galactose, to carbon-4, of glucose. It is a β-galactoside and must be hydrolysed before it can be catabolised. *Beta-galactosidase* is one of the enzymes required for lactose utilisation in *E. coli*. A *lactose transporter protein* is also required for entry of lactose into the bacterium. These two proteins and a third protein, a *transacetylase*, whose function is not clear, are only synthesised when *E. coli* is grown in the presence of lactose or some synthetic analogues of lactose. Synthesis of these proteins is inhibited if glucose is present. *E. coli* can use glucose for energy and as a carbon source so lactose utilisation is not required if glucose is present. If *E. coli* cells growing in a glucose-containing medium are transferred to a medium containing lactose but no glucose, growth ceases and only resumes after a 'lag' phase lasting about 20 min. The proteins required for lactose catabolism are synthesised from amino acids during this interval. They are not produced by the activation of previously synthesised inactive precursors.

Bacterial genes for proteins with related functions often map side by side on the bacterial genome and form a group of genes that are controlled as a unit. Such a group of genes is called an *operon*. The structural genes of the operon are transcribed to give a single mRNA molecule that carries within its length sequences corresponding to the sequences of the polypeptide chains. The three proteins required for lactose catabolism are coded for by the three structural genes of the *lac* operon, *lac z*, *lac y* and *lac a*, which code for β-galactosidase, the galactoside transporter protein and the transacetylase, respectively. A map of the genes of the *lac* operon is given in Figure 134.

Downstream from the promoter of the *lac* operon there is a base sequence, the *operator*, which controls initiation at the promoter. This base sequence is rec-

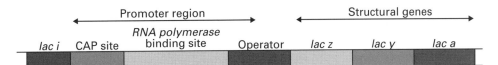

Fig. 134 Map of the *lac* operon of *E. coli* (not to scale).

ognised by an allosteric control protein, the lac *repressor protein*. When this protein coded for by the *lac i* gene binds to the operator, initiation of RNA synthesis at the promoter is completely blocked. The second ligand of the repressor protein is *allolactose*, made from lactose by β-galactosidase, which is always present in the bacterium but at a very low level of activity if it has not been induced. When the repressor binds allolactose it is no longer able to bind to the operator and initiation at the promoter can occur (Fig. 135). Lactose thus induces the proteins required for its own catabolism.

Role of glucose

Glucose can decrease transcription of the lac operon. The *lac* promoter does not bind RNA polymerase with high affinity so that even with lactose present very little transcription occurs. The efficiency of the promoter is greatly increased if another protein binds to its control sequence, which is beside and upstream of the promoter. This protein is the *catabolite gene activator protein* or *CAP* protein and the control sequence to which it binds is known as the *CAP site*. When the CAP protein binds to its site it can make contacts with RNA polymerase that greatly favour the initiation of transcription. The CAP protein is also an allosteric protein and can only bind to its site if it has first bound a molecule of the signal molecule *cyclic AMP*. Cells that are catabolising glucose contain very low concentrations of cyclic AMP so induction of the lactose-catabolising proteins does not occur if glucose is available. This control by glucose of operons involved in the synthesis of enzymes required for the catabolism of lactose and other sugars is known as *catabolite repression* (Fig. 136).

Control of the trp *operon in* E. coli

E. coli can synthesise the tryptophan it needs for protein synthesis if this amino acid is not available in the growth medium. The enzymes required are coded for by genes carried on the *trp* operon, which is controlled as a single unit. *E. coli* either synthesises all the enzymes coded for by the genes on the *trp* operon or none of them. Control is again exerted by an allosteric repressor protein that binds to an operator sequence between the promoter and the structural genes. In this case, the repressor protein on its own cannot bind to the operator to block transcription. Only when it has bound its other ligand, (tryptophan, of course) can it bind to the operator. Tryptophan acts as a co-repressor (Fig. 137). The presence of tryptophan in the growth medium, therefore, switches off the synthesis of the enzymes required for tryptophan synthesis.

Control of termination

Termination of transcription can also control protein synthesis. In some bacteriophages the production of different proteins at differents stages of the phage infection cycle is controlled by proteins that act as anti-termination factors. In the presence of these factors, RNA polymerase no longer responds to the termination signal and reads through it to transcribe a further section of the phage genome.

Control of transcription in eukaryotes

As might be expected, the processes controlling transcription in eukaryotes are much more complex than those found in bacteria. Proteins have to be synthesised that are appropriate to each cell type and its state of differentiation and growth. Protein synthesis must also respond to nutritional state and to stimulation by hormones, particularly steroids and those from the thyroid.

Operons do not occur in eukaryotes. Each gene has its own promoter and control sequences. Identification of these control sequences is a very active area of research at the present time. They have been found not only upstream and downstream of the genes being controlled but within the genes themselves. Some control sequences are remote, being thousands of bases away from the genes they control. Eukaryotic genes are subject to control by several *DNA-binding proteins*, each specific for its particular control sequence. Some of these proteins recognise sequences that identify genes coding for proteins required in a particular cell type; others are allosteric and will only bind to their control sequences if they have also bound a specific steroid or thyroid hormone. The action of each promoter appears to depend on an exact combination of control proteins, which have bound to their specific sequences. These control proteins not only bind to control sequences on the DNA but often bind to each other. Only such a combinatorial mechanism could possibly account for the specific expression of the large number of genes found in the eukaryotic genome.

Many of the proteins that control transcription have been isolated and have had their structures determined. The structures often show shared structural motifs for interacting with specific DNA sequences (e.g. *zinc fingers*) or for interacting with each other, (e.g. *leucine zippers*) (Fig. 138). For transcription to occur at any potential promoter, the correct combination of DNA-binding proteins must be built up, with each protein binding to its specific DNA sequence and able

No inducer present

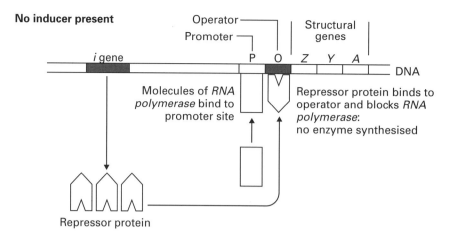

Inducer present

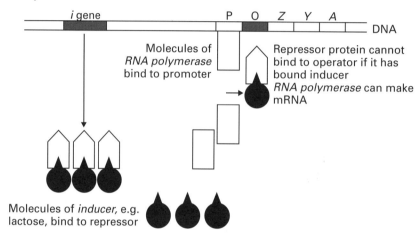

Induction process

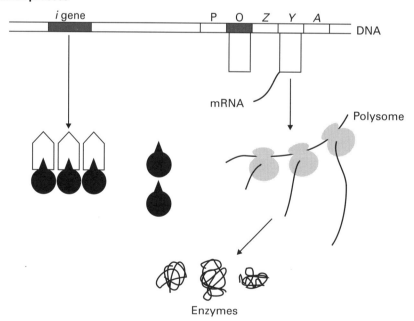

Fig. 135 Repressor function in the *lac* operon: an example of an inducible operon.

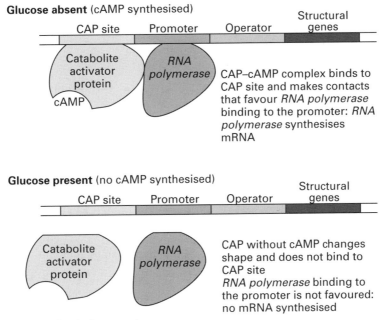

Glucose absent (cAMP synthesised)

CAP–cAMP complex binds to CAP site and makes contacts that favour *RNA polymerase* binding to the promoter: *RNA polymerase* synthesises mRNA

Glucose present (no cAMP synthesised)

CAP without cAMP changes shape and does not bind to CAP site
RNA polymerase binding to the promoter is not favoured: no mRNA synthesised

Fig. 136 Catabolic repression.

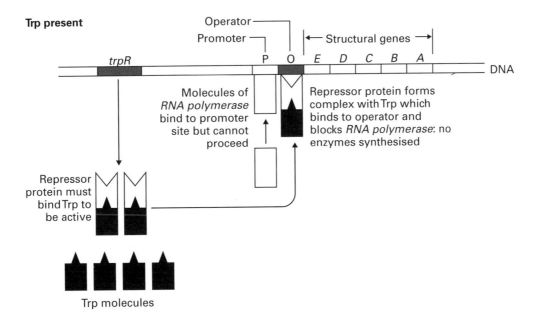

Trp present

Molecules of *RNA polymerase* bind to promoter site but cannot proceed

Repressor protein forms complex with Trp which binds to operator and blocks *RNA polymerase*: no enzymes synthesised

Repressor protein must bind Trp to be active

Trp molecules

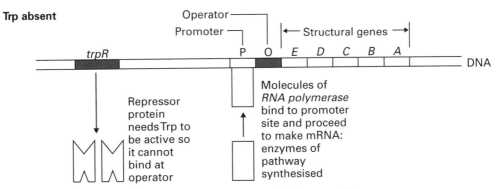

Trp absent

Repressor protein needs Trp to be active so it cannot bind at operator

Molecules of *RNA polymerase* bind to promoter site and proceed to make mRNA: enzymes of pathway synthesised

Fig. 137 Co-repressor function in the *trp* operon; an example of a repressible operon.

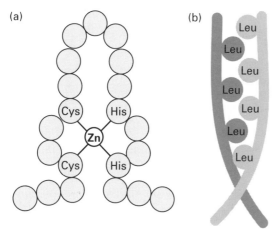

Fig. 138 Structural motifs in DNA-binding proteins: (a) zinc finger; (b) leucine zipper.

to interact with the other DNA-bound proteins in the complex.

Zinc fingers have a zinc ion bound by two cysteine and two histidine side chains; this stabilises a finger-shaped structure that can make contact with the bases within the major groove of DNA. Other amino acid side chains vary to give interaction with specific base sequences.

Leucine zippers. Protein subunits with a leucine zipper have leucine residues at every seventh position in an alpha helix. Such subunits can be brought together by these to form homo- or heterodimers. Other parts of the subunits bind to specific sequences within DNA.

14.4 RNA processing

After being produced by RNA polymerase, most RNA molecules are extensively modified before reaching their functional state.

Transfer RNA

tRNA contains several modified bases as well as the usual ones. tRNA sequences are transcribed in long sequences that are then cleaved to give precursor tRNA molecules. These have some bases methylated and others rearranged so that they are attached to the ribose by carbon–carbon bonds. Every functional tRNA molecule has the sequence CCA at its 3′ end. In

eukaryotic cells, this sequence is added enzymatically to a precursor molecule after it has left the nucleus.

Ribosomal RNA

Ribosomal RNA is also transcribed as a long precursor sequence that is then cleaved to give the three RNA molecules that are components of the ribosomal subunits. Ribosomal RNA is transcribed from DNA sequences in the nucleolus of the eukaryotic cell, which contains multiple copies of the ribosomal RNA genes. These multiple copies are necessary to allow the high rate of transcription that is needed to form all the ribosomal RNA needed for ribosome formation.

Messenger RNA

mRNA in eukaryotes is subject to several different modifications before becoming functional.

RNA capping and tailing

The ends of mRNA molecules are modified, probably to protect them from rapid degradation by exonuclease action. The 5′ end has a methylated guanine-containing nucleotide unit (cap) attached by a 5′ to 5′ phosphodiester bond, i.e. it has the reverse of the usual orientation. The 3′ end of the RNA transcript has a few hundred adenine-containing nucleotide units added enzymatically, a process known as *tailing*. Possession of this *poly A* tail by most eukaryotic mRNA molecules is exploited for their purification. Their tails will hybridise with a nucleic acid containing only thymine (polyT), so they will stick to an affinity chromatography column on which polyT has been immobilised.

RNA splicing

Eukaryotic structural genes are not stored as continuous base sequences in DNA. Sequences called *exons* which do code for protein sequence are separated by intervening sequences or *introns*. Both exons and introns are transcribed into a primary RNA transcript from which the introns, which are often hundreds of nucleotide units long, must be precisely *spliced* out of the RNA before it can be used as messenger. Sites where splicing is to occur are marked by specific base sequences. These are recognised by catalytic RNA–protein complexes known as *spliceosomes*. The intron is removed and the exons that were formerly at each end

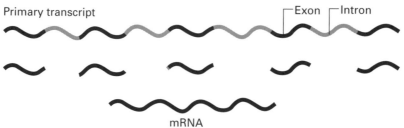

Fig. 139 Splicing of RNA.

of the intron are joined to form a continuous chain (Fig. 139). Some mRNA molecules are formed from many exons joined in this way. The gene for human haemoglobin beta chains contains three exons separated by two introns.

Splicing of the original transcript may not be carried out in the same way in different cell types. By using alternative splice sites, different cell-specific mRNAs, and hence proteins, can be synthesised from identical original transcripts.

BOX 14.1
Clinical note: Some genetic defects are caused by splicing errors

Splicing must be carried out with great precision. It can be affected by alterations in base sequence, i.e. by mutations. Some *thalassaemias* (inherited disorders of haemoglobin synthesis) are caused by mutations that alter the base sequence at splice sites.

Self-assessment: questions

Multiple choice questions

1. The following are properties of RNA:
   a. RNA occurs in the cytosol of eukaryotic cells but not in the nucleus
   b. RNA does not form structures in which base pairing is important
   c. Uracil, which is found in RNA, is similar to thymine but has an additional methyl group
   d. mRNA molecules occur in a large range of sizes but tRNA molecules are all very similar in size
   e. Ribosomes are made of ribosomal RNA and ribosomal proteins. Eukaryotic ribosomes are made up of two subunits, the smaller, 40S containing 40 nucleotide units and the larger 60S containing 60 nucleotide subunits

2. The following are needed for RNA synthesis:
   a. ATP
   b. UTP
   c. GTP
   d. A DNA primer
   e. A DNA template

3. RNA synthesis:
   a. Occurs in the 5' to 3' direction
   b. Eliminates pyrophosphate during the addition of every nucleotide unit in RNA synthesis
   c. Uses a template that is read in the 3' to 5' direction
   d. For structural genes which map close together on the bacterial genome may produce a single molecule of mRNA, a polycistronic messenger that codes for several polypeptide chains
   e. Is initiated at special DNA sequences known as start codons

4. In RNA synthesis:
   a. Promoter sequences are rich in AT base pairs at the point where the DNA chains are unwound
   b. Initiation of transcription is an important control point for the control of protein synthesis
   c. Prokaryotes have a single RNA polymerase while eukaryotes have separate enzymes for the synthesis of different classes of RNA
   d. Termination is by stop codons
   e. Only one strand of the DNA double helix is used as a template, the other strand does not code for protein synthesis but functions during DNA replication

5. In protein synthesis in bacteria:
   a. Proteins can be classified as constitutive, inducible or repressible
   b. Proteins required for lactose catabolism are examples of inducible proteins
   c. Proteins required for tryptophan synthesis are examples of repressible proteins
   d. Induction of the proteins required for lactose catabolism does not occur when glucose is available
   e. Induction of the proteins required for lactose catabolism does not occur in a bacterial cell containing a higher than normal concentration of cyclic AMP

6. The following statements describe promoters and operators:
   a. Transcription starts at a sequence on DNA that can bind RNA polymerase and that is known as an operator
   b. Operators are usually upstream of the promoters that they control
   c. Repressors are proteins that bind to specific DNA sequences and block transcription
   d. Some bacterial repressors have binding sites for a metabolite or building block molecule. This molecule, known as a co-repressor, must be bound to the repressor before the repressor can bind to its operator and block transcription
   e. Some bacterial repressors have binding sites for a molecule that can be used by the bacteria as an energy or carbon source. This molecule, known as an inducer, binds to the repressor and stops it binding to its operator and blocking transcription

7. Transcription in eukaryotes involves:
   a. Structural genes which are arranged in operons with a single promoter for several genes
   b. Control sequences to which regulatory proteins bind which are clustered around the promoter
   c. Regulation by zinc fingers and leucine zippers, which are structural motifs found in proteins in eukaryotes
   d. Histone proteins, which are responsible for the specific control of protein synthesis
   e. DNA-binding proteins that often have binding sites for steroid or thyroid hormones

8. In RNA processing in eukaryotes:
   a. The first transcript of ribosomal RNA is subject to specific cleavage before becoming functional
   b. tRNA contains several modified bases as well as adenine, cytosine, guanine and uracil
   c. mRNA has a methylated guanine nucleotide added to its 5′ end
   d. mRNA has a long tail of poly A added to its 3′ end
   e. RNA splicing is the joining of intron sequences with the elimination of exons

Short essay question

Write an essay about the central role of transcription in controlling the activities of prokaryotic and eukaryotic cells.

Self-assessment: answers

Multiple choice answers

1. a. **False.** RNA is synthesised in the nucleus and moves out after processing.
   b. **False.** Base pairing occurs in some RNA structures, e.g. tRNA, ribosomes.
   c. **False.** It is thymine that has the additional methyl group.
   d. **True.** tRNA molecules all contain about 80 nucleotide units. mRNA varies in size depending on the length of the polypeptide for which it codes.
   e. **False.** 40S and 60S refer to the sedimentation constants of the subunits.

2. a. **True.** This is used to add adenine-containing nucleotide units.
   b. **True.** This is used to add uracil-containing nucleotide units.
   c. **True.** This is used to add guanine-containing nucleotide units.
   d. **False.** No primer is needed for RNA synthesis.
   e. **True.** This directs the base sequence of the new RNA molecule.

3. a. **True.** All nucleic acid chain synthesis occurs in this direction.
   b. **True.** The nucleoside triphosphate eliminates two phosphate groups as pyrophosphate during the addition of each nucleotide unit to the chain.
   c. **True.** Template and newly synthesised strand are antiparallel in all nucleic acid synthesis.
   d. **True.** This does not occur in eukaryotes.
   e. **False.** The special sequences are known as promoters.

4. a. **True.** Chain separation must occur at promoters. AT base pairs are more easily broken than are GCs.
   b. **True.** Control of transcription allows the cell to control the synthesis of each specific protein.
   c. **True.** Eukaryotes have separate RNA polymerases for mRNA, tRNA and ribosomal RNA.
   d. **False.** Stop codons are signals in mRNA for the termination of translation.
   e. **True.** If one strand of DNA codes for a useful polypeptide, it is most improbable that the complementary strand will also do so.

5. a. **True.** Constitutive (made all the time), inducible (made only when needed) and repressible (normally made but synthesis is switched off if not needed).

   b. **True.** The *lac* operon was the first inducible operon to be studied.
   c. **True.** Enzymes for the synthesis of tryptophan and several other amino acids are repressible.
   d. **True.** This phenomenon is known as catabolite repression.
   e. **False.** Induction of the Lac proteins requires a higher than normal concentration as cyclic AMP.

6. a. **False.** The sequence where transcription starts is known as a promoter.
   b. **False.** Operators are usually downstream of the promoters they control.
   c. **True.** They bind to sequences known as operators.
   d. **True.** As in the control of the *trp* operon.
   e. **True.** As in the control of the *lac* operon.

7. a. **False.** This organisation of genes is only found in prokaryotes.
   b. **False.** Control sequences in eukaryotes are often remote from the promoter.
   c. **True.** These motifs allow these proteins to bind to DNA and to each other.
   d. **False.** Histones are the same in every cell of an organism and vary only slightly from species to species.
   e. **True.** This is how such hormones are able to control the synthesis of proteins.

8. a. **True.** Both ribosomal RNA and tRNA are cleaved from longer precursors.
   b. **True.** These bases are modified after transcription.
   c. **True.** Addition of this nucleotide unit is known as 'capping'.
   d. **True.** Addition of this poly A sequence is known as 'tailing'.
   e. **False.** It is the introns that are eliminated. The exon sequences are joined together to form the mature mRNA.

Short essay answer

Several points should be mentioned. Controlling transcription is the most important way in which cells control the proteins that they make. It obviously saves material and energy if cells only make mRNA for the proteins that they actually need. Transcription ensures appropriate amplification of the genetic information before it is used. One or two structural genes can be transcribed to give thousands of mRNA molecules, which can in turn be translated to give millions of protein molecules.

The synthesis of proteins

15

Many activities of the cell, particularly growth, cell division, adaptation and repair, involve the synthesis of new protein molecules. Even in the adult human when growth has ceased, turnover of tissue protein involves the synthesis of hundreds of grams of protein every day (Chapter 9).

Different cells synthesise different proteins. The mechanism of protein synthesis must account for the large number of proteins that are found in a typical cell and for the specificity of these proteins. It also has to explain how different proteins are synthesised in different cells of the same organism. Muscle cells make some proteins found only in muscle, and liver cells make proteins found only in liver, yet other proteins such as some enzymes catalysing glycolysis are common to many different cell types. In protein synthesis, the amino acids that make up the polypeptide chains must be joined in the required order by peptide bonds. The information concerning the order of the amino acids is supplied by mRNA, which is translated at the ribosomes (Chapter 14). mRNA is translated in the same direction as it is synthesised, in the 5′ to 3′ direction. Translation starts near but not at the 5′ end. Prokaryotic mRNA, which may code for more than one polypeptide chain, may contain further starting points along its length. The identification of the precise starting points for translation is an important feature of the initiation of polypeptide synthesis.

15.1 The genetic code

The correspondence between the base sequence in RNA and the amino acid sequence of the protein is known as the genetic code. The sequence of bases on the DNA and mRNA is divided into groups of three bases, each of which is treated as an instruction to insert a specific amino acid in the growing chain (or sometimes to terminate the chain). The group of three bases is known as a *codon* and the matching set of three bases on the tRNA that brings the amino acids into line for protein synthesis is called the *anticodon*. Since there are four bases there are $4 \times 4 \times 4$ or 64 possible codons. Of these, 61 out of the 64 specify an amino acid while the remaining three are *chain termination signals*. The genetic code is set out in Table 20. The same code applies in prokaryotes and eukaryotes, that is to say the code is universal. Only a very few minor exceptions to the universality of the code have been identified. The nucleic acid sequence and the amino acid sequence it codes are said to be colinear; that is, the base triplets are in the same order as the amino acids in the corresponding protein chain.

Some amino acids are represented by just one codon, others by two or four and some even by six: the code is said to be *degenerate*. While it is possible to translate a nucleic acid base sequence into an amino acid

Table 20 The genetic code

First position	Second position				Third position
	U	C	A	G	
U	Phe	Ser	Tyr	Cys	U
	Phe	Ser	Tyr	Cys	C
	Leu	Ser	Stop	Stop	A
	Leu	Ser	Stop	Trp	G
C	Leu	Pro	His	Arg	U
	Leu	Pro	His	Arg	C
	Leu	Pro	Gln	Arg	A
	Leu	Pro	Gln	Arg	G
A	Ile	Thr	Asn	Ser	U
	Ile	Thr	Asn	Ser	C
	Ile	Thr	Lys	Arg	A
	Met	Thr	Lys	Arg	G
G	Val	Ala	Asp	Gly	U
	Val	Ala	Asp	Gly	C
	Val	Ala	Glu	Gly	A
	Val	Ala	Glu	Gly	G

sequence, the reverse process is not possible. Given the amino acid sequence of a polypeptide, the base sequence of the mRNA involved in its synthesis cannot be predicted. As many amino acids are represented by more than one codon, there is no way of telling which one of these codons was used in any instance.

Do not attempt to memorise the genetic code table but notice that:

- Where multiple codons represent one amino acid these codons are often similar. For example UUU and UUC both represent phenylalanine and UAU and UAC both represent tyrosine. In this and in other cases where there are just two codons representing an amino acid, the codons are identical in the first two positions and the third positions contain either the purines A and G or the pyrimidines C and U.
- In the cases of amino acids that are represented by four codons, these codons always have the same first and second bases, the identity of the third base being immaterial. Thus GGX always represents glycine whether X is A or G or C or U.
- Chemically similar amino acids are often represented by similar codons, as in the case of phenylalanine and tyrosine (above) or in the case of aspartate (GAU or GAC) and glutamate (GAA or GAG).

The effect of mutations

The code is unpunctuated, that is to say there is no feature in the structure of mRNA that shows where one codon ends and the next one begins. Translation, once started, proceeds three bases at a time along the messenger in the 5′ to 3′ direction. Any change that affects the sequence will alter the protein product.

Frame shift mutations

If an extra base were to be inserted in the sequence, the whole message would be corrupted and the sequence of the protein that was synthesised would be completely changed subsequent to the site of the insertion. The same would happen if one base were to be deleted. Such changes are known as frameshift mutations.

Point mutations

The replacement of one base by another is much less damaging. If the replacement occurs in the third position of a codon, either the original amino acid or one similar to it will be used. Changes in the first or second positions will almost always result in a change of amino acid but since only one codon has been altered, only one amino acid will be changed in the sequence. This may not alter the activity of the protein or it may result in poor or no activity, e.g. a single base change resulting in valine instead of glutamate in haemoglobin causes sickle cell disease (p. 63). If the change creates a stop codon, incomplete proteins will form.

Range of potential sequences

The code is also *non-overlapping*. The meaning of each codon depends only on its own base sequence and not on any other sequence in the mRNA. This makes it possible to synthesise a polypeptide containing any sequence of the 20 amino acids. The nature of the code imposes no restriction on the protein sequences that can be produced.

15.2 Synthesis of protein chains

tRNA molecules act as adaptors

Selection of the amino acid specified by each codon is achieved by having tRNA molecules (p. 178) that attach and activate the amino acids and bring them to the required position in the growing polypeptide chain. The anticodon on the tRNA is complementary (under somewhat less strict base-pairing rules than apply during DNA replication and transcription) to codons on the messenger. Between them, the tRNA molecules can form base pairs with all the 61 codons which specify amino acids. Some of the tRNA molecules can pair with more than one codon, but when they do this, all the codons they pair with must specify the same amino acid. The codon and anticodon are antiparallel when they associate by base pairing: the third position of the codon is the base at the 3' end of the codon, while the third position of the anticodon is at its 5' end.

Wobble

Base pairing is strict between the first and second bases

Table 21 'Wobble' pairing

Third position in codon	
Anticodon Base	Codon bases matched
C	G
A	U
G	C or U
U	G or A
Inosine	U, C or A

of the codon and the first and second bases of the anticodon. Base pairing is less strict in the third position, a phenomenon named *Wobble* by Crick (Table 21). For example, an inosine base in the third position of the anticodon can base pair with A, U and C in the third position of the codon. Wobble allows all 61 codons specifying amino acids to be recognised by less than 40 species of tRNA molecule.

Attachment of amino acids to tRNA

The tRNA molecules are charged with their specific amino acids by a set of enzymes, the *aminoacyl-tRNA synthetases*. Each amino acid has one of these enzymes which specifically attaches it to its tRNA. These enzymes, which require ATP as well as the amino acid and the tRNA molecule, attach the amino acid to its tRNA by an ester linkage between the carboxyl group of the amino acid and a hydroxyl group on the ribose of the adenosine at the 3' end of the tRNA molecule. The reaction proceeds in two stages. ATP is used to adenylate the amino acid on its carboxyl group and pyrophosphate (PP_i) is eliminated. During the second stage the amino acid is transferred to the tRNA molecule. The reaction is irreversible since the pyrophosphate is hydrolysed to two molecules of inorganic phosphate by pyrophosphatase.

$$\text{Amino acid} + \text{ATP} \rightarrow \text{Aminoacyl-AMP} + PP_i$$
$$\text{Aminoacyl-AMP} + \text{tRNA} \rightarrow \text{Aminoacyl-tRNA} + \text{AMP}$$
$$PP_i + H_2O \rightarrow 2P_i$$

Each of these aminoacyl-tRNA synthetases shows very high specificity and will only join its amino acid to its corresponding tRNA. Some of these enzymes must distinguish between very similar amino acids, pairs such as valine and leucine or glycine and alanine differ only by a single methylene group. Some of the synthetases have associated hydrolase activities, which proof-read and correct the mistake if the 'wrong' amino acid is joined to a tRNA. The proof-reading is by a double sieve mechanism. Leucine should never be mistaken for valine since it is larger and will not fit an active centre that was specific for valine, but valine can be mistaken for leucine since it fits an active centre created to fit the larger leucine. The hydrolase associated with leucyl-tRNA synthetase is specific for valyl-tRNA$_{leu}$, which can fit its active centre and be hydrolysed. When the synthetase makes the correct leucyl-tRNA$_{leu}$ it is too large to fit the active centre of the hydrolase and will not be cleaved.

Role of ribosomes

The constituents required for protein synthesis are brought together by ribosomes, ribonucleoprotein structures found in the cytoplasm. These subcellular particles, which can be seen in the electron microscope, are particularly numerous in tissues such as liver and pancreas where protein synthesis is most active. They can be isolated from disrupted bacteria or from homogenised cells by high speed centrifugation. Ribosomes prepared in this way are often found in the form of *polysomes*, several ribosomes associated with a single mRNA molecule. These ribosomes are simultaneously translating the single messenger but with the resulting polypeptide chains at different stages of completion. Each individual ribosome can engage in the synthesis of only one polypeptide chain at a time. Ribosomes are not specific for the polypeptide sequences that they synthesise. The sequences they produce depend on the mRNA message.

Biochemists separate ribosomes from other cellular materials using ultracentrifugation, so ribosomes and their subunits are identified by their sedimentation constants, measures of the rates at which they sediment in the ultracentrifuge (Table 22). The sedimentation constant of a particle depends on its size, shape and density. Sedimentation constants are quoted in Svedberg (S) units. Prokaryotic ribosomes are smaller than those from eukaryotes.

Ribosomes are composed of three RNA molecules and about 50 proteins, forming two subunits with distinct functions. The small and large ribosomal subunits only come together during protein synthesis. They join the assembly responsible for translation one after the other, first the small subunit, then the large.

Phases of chain synthesis

Synthesis of a polypeptide chain can be considered in three phases, *initiation*, *elongation* and *termination*.

Chain initiation

Initiation of a new chain is a critical stage in protein synthesis because it is at this stage that the 'reading frame' is set for translation. Bases on mRNA are recognised in groups of three, but there is no structural

Table 22 Prokaryotic and eukaryotic ribosomal subunits

| | Sedimentation constant (Svedberg units(S)) | |
	Prokaryotic	Eukaryotic
Ribosome	70	80
Large subunit	50	60
Small subunit	30	40

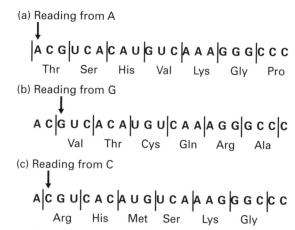

Fig. 140 Reading frame for translation: moving the start position alters the triplet sequence and gives three different polypeptide sequences.

feature on the RNA to act as punctuation to indicate which of the three possible reading frames is to be used. Use of either of the two incorrect reading frames would produce a polypeptide that was completely unrelated in sequence to the required polypeptide (Fig. 140). Mechanisms for initiation and setting of the correct reading frame differ slightly between prokaryotes and eukaryotes.

Initiation in prokaryotes

In prokaryotes, the small ribosomal subunit binds to a ribosome-binding sequence by base pairing with a complementary sequence in the ribosomal RNA of the small subunit. The ribosome-binding sequence, also known as a *Shine–Dalgarno sequence*, is located within the untranslated region upstream from each translated region of the mRNA. These sequences are rich in A and G but are not identical. Different mRNAs bind the ribosomal subunit with different affinities, this being yet another way in which the amount of protein produced can be controlled. Once bound to mRNA, the ribosomal subunit moves downstream until it encounters a start codon: AUG (Fig. 141).

AUG codes for the amino acid methionine, which is found at the N-terminus of prokaryotic proteins when they are first synthesised although it may be cleaved off later. A special form of tRNA$_{Met}$ is used for initiation. This is first charged with methionine, which is thus activated in its carboxyl group. The amino group of the amino acid is then modified by the addition of a *methanoyl (formyl)* group.

Initiation in eukaryotes

In eukaryotes, each mRNA molecule codes for a single polypeptide chain and there is no sequence corresponding to the Shine–Dalgarno ribosome-binding sequence. Recognition appears to depend on the presence of the cap, the modified G nucleotide found at the 5' end of every eukaryotic mRNA. Once bound, the small ribosomal subunit moves along the mRNA until an AUG start codon is encountered. A

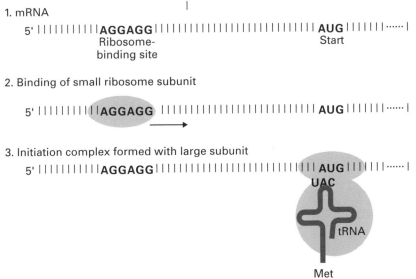

1. mRNA

5' | | | | | | | | | | |**AGGAGG**| | | | | | | | | | | | | | | | | | | | | | | | | | | |**AUG**| | | | | | |·······|
Ribosome-
binding site   Start

2. Binding of small ribosome subunit

5' | | | | | | | | | | | |**AGGAGG**| | | | | | | | | | | | | | | | | | | | | | | | | | |**AUG**| | | | | | |·······|

⟶

3. Initiation complex formed with large subunit

5' | | | | | | | | | | | |**AGGAGG**| | | | | | | | | | | | | | | | | | | | | | | | | | | | | | | |**AUG**| | | | | | |·······|
UAC

tRNA

Met

Fig. 141 Initiation of translation in prokaryotes.

species of tRNA that carries methionine is required for initiation. The N-terminal methionine is not formylated in eukaryotes. Another tRNA is used for inserting methionine residues where they are needed in other positions in the polypeptide sequence.

Initiation complex formation
Having located the start codon, AUG, the small ribosomal subunit binds the large subunit and formyl-methionyl-tRNA$_{Met}$, (or methionyl-tRNA$_{Met}$ in eukaryotes,) and creates an initiation complex. Assembly of the initiation complex also involves three protein initiation factors. The reading frame for translation is set and the elongation phase of translation can begin.

Chain elongation

The ribosome has two sites where it can bind tRNA, a *P* or *peptidyl* site and an *A* or *amino* acyl site. In the initiation complex, methionyl-tRNA$_{Met}$ occupies the P site. Later it will be occupied by a tRNA carrying the growing polypeptide chain. There are three stages during each round of the elongation process (Fig. 142).

In the first stage a tRNA molecule charged with its amino acid binds to the A site. Which tRNA and thus

which amino acid binds at the A site depends on the next three bases on the mRNA. The binding of each charged tRNA molecule to the ribosome is an energy-requiring process and involves a catalytic protein or elongation factor. One molecule of GTP is hydrolysed to GDP and phosphate for every aminoacyl-tRNA that is bound.

In the second stage, with a tRNA molecule bound at both sites, a new peptide bond can be formed. The amino acid, or peptide, bound by its carboxyl group to the tRNA in the P site is transferred to the amino group of the amino acid bound to the tRNA in the A site. Synthesis of this new peptide bond is driven by the (ATP) energy used earlier to activate the amino acid by joining it to its tRNA.

In the third stage the growing peptide chain attached to tRNA in the A site is translocated. The tRNA in the P site, now without any attached amino acid or peptide, is ejected and moves away to pick up another molecule of its amino acid. The tRNA in the A site, which carries the growing polypeptide chain, moves into the P site as the ribosome moves along the mRNA molecule. The A site is now vacant so another round of elongation can begin. Translocation is another energy-requiring process and, like tRNA binding, it involves a catalytic protein, another elongation factor and the hydrolysis of GTP to GDP and phosphate.

Energy requirements of peptide bond synthesis
Each round of elongation requires the equivalent of four molecules of ATP to be hydrolysed to ADP and phosphate. Two of these four are used to drive the activation of the amino acid by joining it to its tRNA. One molecule of ATP is used directly and one indirectly to convert the AMP formed into ADP. The two GDP molecules produced by the use of one GTP to drive tRNA binding and another to drive translocation are each reconverted to GTP by phosphate transfer from ATP.

BOX 15.1
Clinical note: Many antibiotics inhibit protein syntheses in bacteria

Several antibiotics in clinical use are inhibitors of protein synthesis, particularly in bacteria. Chloramphenicol inhibits peptide bond formation in prokaryotes. Tetracycline inhibits binding of aminoacyl tRNAs to ribosomes in both eukaryotes and prokaryotes but cannot cross eukaryotic membranes. Erythromycin blocks translocation of the peptidyl tRNA during elongation.

1. Initiation complex

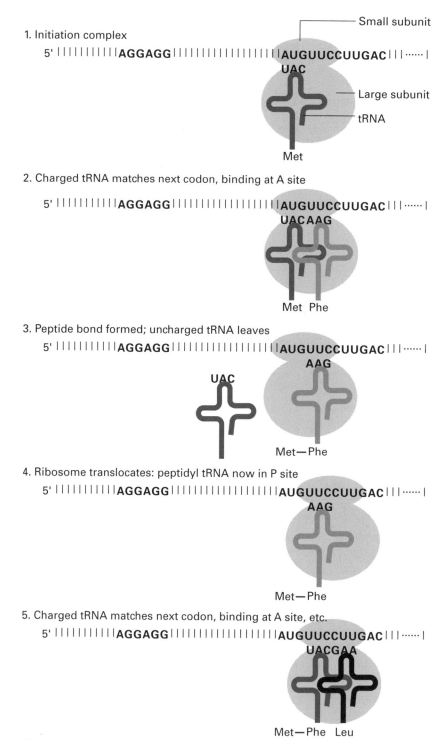

Fig. 142 The elongation phase of protein synthesis.

Chain termination

Elongation steps continue until the ribosome encounters a codon for which there is no corresponding tRNA. There are three such codons, *UAA, UAG* and *UGA*. These codons trigger release factors, enzymes that cleave the completed polypeptide from the tRNA which carried the C-terminal amino acid. The final tRNA can then dissociate and the ribosomal subunits separate, ready to start the translation of another molecule of mRNA.

As one ribosome moves along an mRNA molecule, enough of the 5′ end of the mRNA will become available for another ribosome to attach and start translation of the same messenger. As a result, several ribosomes may be simultaneously translating one mRNA molecule, each with a polypeptide at a different stage of completion. Ribosomes isolated from reticulocytes, red cell precursor cells in which mRNA coding for haemoglobin polypeptide chains is being translated, are found in clusters of four or five, held together by mRNA. In prokaryotes, an mRNA molecule does not even have to be completely transcribed before its translation can begin.

15.3 Post-translational modification and transport of proteins

Once synthesised, polypeptide chains are often substantially modified before becoming functional proteins. Typically, amino acid side chains may be modified and specific peptide bonds cleaved. This post-translational modification is often associated with the transport of the newly synthesised protein to its destination inside or outside the cell.

Signal sequences

Polypeptide chains that are to be transported to different destinations within the cell often contain sequences known as signal sequences that act as address labels during the transport process. The signal sequence that marks a protein for transport to the Golgi apparatus via the endoplasmic reticulum is typical. This sequence is at the N-terminal end of the polypeptide chain and is, therefore, synthesised before the remainder of the chain. It is often cleaved off after the protein reaches its destination. Its sequence varies somewhat but is generally about 20 residues long and contains a highly hydrophobic stretch of about 12 residues and also one positively charged residue.

Once the signal sequence has been synthesised, it is taken up by the transport system, which carries it across the *endoplasmic reticulum* membrane and the synthesis of the rest of the chain is coupled to its movement through the membrane (Fig. 143). This prevents the polypeptide chain from folding before it passes through. Folding occurs after the chain has crossed the membrane.

The newly synthesised signal sequence, attached to its ribosome, is recognised by a *signal recognition particle* (SRP), a ribonucleoprotein particle, which binds to it. This binding arrests further translation temporarily. The complex binds to an SRP receptor on the endoplasmic reticulum and the signal peptide is taken

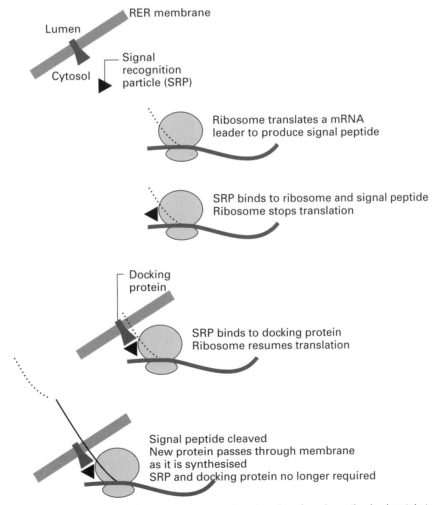

Fig. 143 The use of a signal sequence to ensure translocation of newly synthesised protein to the endoplasmic reticulum before sufficient protein is formed to start folding. RER, rough endoplasmic reticulum.

(a) Inside the cell

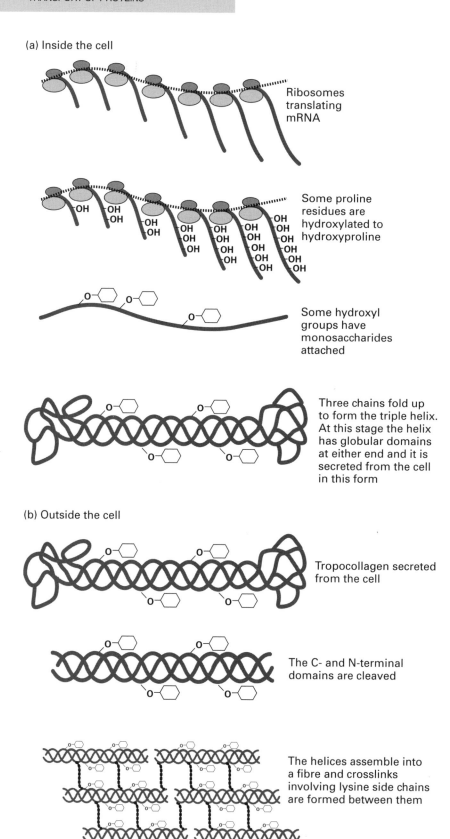

Ribosomes
translating
mRNA

Some proline
residues are
hydroxylated to
hydroxyproline

Some hydroxyl
groups have
monosaccharides
attached

Three chains fold up
to form the triple helix.
At this stage the helix
has globular domains
at either end and it is
secreted from the cell
in this form

(b) Outside the cell

Tropocollagen secreted
from the cell

The C- and N-terminal
domains are cleaved

The helices assemble into
a fibre and crosslinks
involving lysine side chains
are formed between them

Fig. 144 Post-translational transport and modification of collagen.

up by the translocation machinery and fed through a pore in the membrane. At this point the SRP is no longer required. It can dissociate from the complex and the ribosome can resume translation. Elongation of the polypeptide and its passage through the ER membrane can now occur concurrently.

Different signal sequences mark proteins for entry to mitochondria. Most mitochondrial proteins are synthesised in the cytosol and carry N-terminal sequences that are recognised by transport mechanisms in the mitochondrial membrane. Folding is delayed by *chaperonins* since folded proteins are not readily transported across intracellular membranes. Chaperonins are cytosolic proteins one function of which is to bind unfolded peptide chains and deliver them to the transport mechanism. Once in the mitochondrial matrix the chains fold to their functional forms.

Collagen biosynthesis

The transport and processing steps that occur between synthesis of a polypeptide chain and the formation of a functional protein can be illustrated by considering collagen biosynthesis. Collagen is an extracellular structural protein that has some of its amino acid side chains modified after translation, both by hydroxylation and by the addition of carbohydrate groups. Each collagen triple helix consists of three chains, which are synthesised as precursors and then modified and secreted to form mature collagen fibres. As illustrated in Figure 144, the steps in this process include:

- recognition of a leader sequence in preprocollagen so that the chain is taken up into the endoplasmic reticulum
- cleavage of the leader sequence by an enzyme known as signal peptidase
- attachment of carbohydrate groups to amino acid side chains
- hydroxylation of some proline and lysine side chains by a process involving ascorbic acid and molecular oxygen
- passage of precursors through the Golgi apparatus, with modification of carbohydrate groups and formation of triple helices. Formation of a triple helix involves aggregation of C-terminal extensions and the winding of three chains from their C-terminals towards their N-terminals, forming procollagen
- secretion from cells as procollagen, packaged in membrane-bounded vesicles formed from the Golgi apparatus
- removal of C- and N-terminal extensions on the triple helices by extracellular proteases
- aggregation of triple helical molecules (tropocollagen) to form fibres
- Crosslinking between triple helices.

Self-assessment: questions

Multiple choice questions

Consult a copy of the genetic code (p. 190) while answering questions 1–4.

1. In amino acid representation by codons:
   a. No amino acids are represented by only one codon in the genetic code
   b. Some amino acids are represented by two codons in the genetic code
   c. Some amino acids are represented by four codons in the genetic code
   d. Some amino acids are represented by more than four codons in the genetic code
   e. Amino acids that have chemically similar side chains often have similar codons

2. When an amino acid is represented by four different codons, these codons are identical:
   a. In the first position only
   b. In the first and second positions
   c. In the first and third positions
   d. In the second and third positions
   e. In the third position only

3. When an amino acid is represented by either of two different codons:
   a. These codons are identical in the first and second positions and can have either purine or either pyrimidine in the third position
   b. These codons are identical in the first and third positions and can have either purine or either pyrimidine in the middle position
   c. These codons are identical in the second and third positions and can have either purine or either pyrimidine in the third position
   d. Only the first base is identical in the two codons
   e. Only the third base is identical in the two codons

4. A mutation that changes:
   a. The first base of a codon will always change the amino acid to which the codon corresponds
   b. The second base of a codon will always change the amino acid to which the codon corresponds
   c. The third base of a codon will always change the amino acid to which the codon corresponds
   d. The first base of a codon will never change the amino acid to which the codon corresponds
   e. The third base of a codon will never change the amino acid to which the codon corresponds

5. The following are needed for protein synthesis:
   a. GTP
   b. Nucleosomes
   c. Amino acids
   d. tRNA
   e. mRNA

6. The following statements describe the genetic code:
   a. A codon is a group of three bases in mRNA that directs the insertion of a specified amino acid during protein synthesis
   b. The genetic code is unambiguous, that is to say for a given codon there is only one possible translation
   c. The genetic code is degenerate, that is to say there is often more than one codon corresponding to each amino acid
   d. The genetic code is almost but not quite universal
   e. mRNA is translated in the 3′ to 5′ direction and polypeptide chain synthesis starts at the N-terminal end

7. Codons:
   a. May contain bases other than A, C, G and U
   b. There is no structural feature in mRNA that shows where one codon ends and the next begins
   c. Exist in 64 possible combinations
   d. Correspond to amino acids in 61 cases
   e. Include 2 of the 64 codons to correspond to stop signals and one to show where the new polypeptide chain begins

8. Codon recognition by anticodons:
   a. Occurs at three consecutive bases carried on a loop of a tRNA molecule
   b. Involves complementary base pairs forming between bases in the anticodon and bases in the codon
   c. Involves the base at the 5′ end of the codon pairing with the base at the 3′ end of the anticodon
   d. Has base pairing rules that are not so strict for the 3′ base of the anticodon as for the other two bases in the anticodon
   e. Involves 'Wobble', the ability of one anticodon to recognise more than one codon

9. The following statements describe tRNA molecules:
   a. There are 61 different species of tRNA molecule, one for each codon that corresponds to an amino acid
   b. There are 20 different species of tRNA molecule, one for each amino acid that can occur in proteins
   c. Some tRNA molecules can carry more than one amino acid

d. Some amino acids can be carried by more than one tRNA molecule

e. Special tRNA molecules are needed to recognise stop codons

10. The following statements describe amino acid activation:
    a. Amino acids are joined to their cognate tRNA molecules by specific enzymes known as aminoacyl-tRNA synthetases
    b. Aminoacyl-tRNA synthetases hydrolyse ATP to ADP and inorganic phosphate at the same time as they join amino acids to their tRNA molecules
    c. Amino acids are joined to tRNA by an ester bond between the α-carboxyl group on the amino acid and a hydroxyl group on the ribose at the 3′ end of the tRNA
    d. Some aminoacyl-tRNA synthetases can hydrolyse the product if they join the wrong amino acid to a tRNA molecule
    e. Aminoacyl-tRNA synthetases are responsible for the specificity of matching an amino acid to its tRNA

11. Formation of an initiation complex for polypeptide synthesis in prokaryotes directly requires:
    a. mRNA
    b. Formyl methionyl-tRNA$_{Met}$
    c. 30S ribosomal subunit
    d. 50S ribosomal subunit
    e. ATP

12. In the elongation phase of protein synthesis:
    a. For each amino acid added, two molecules of GTP are converted to GDP and inorganic phosphate
    b. For each amino acid added, the tRNA molecule to which the growing peptide chain is attached must be translocated from the A (amino acyl) site on the ribosome to the P (peptidyl site)
    c. For each amino acid added, a loaded tRNA molecule is bound to the A site
    d. Each new polypeptide bond is formed between the C-terminal end of the growing chain and the α-amino group of the amino acid bound to tRNA in the P site
    e. Amino acids are activated by being attached to tRNA, so no ATP hydrolysis is directly needed for peptide bond formation

13. Termination of polypeptide synthesis:
    a. Occurs whenever a ribosome encounters a stop codon in the translation reading frame
    b. Occurs at the stop codons UAA, UAG and UGA
    c. Occurs when special tRNA molecules that carry no amino acid recognise stop codons
    d. Involves the cleavage of the bond joining the final amino acid in the chain to its tRNA
    e. Is followed by separation of the ribosomal subunits, which dissociate from the mRNA

14. In post-translational modification of newly synthesised polypeptides:
    a. Many proteins are chemically modified before becoming functional proteins
    b. Chemical modification is often associated with transport to destinations inside and outside the cell
    c. Cleavage of specific peptide bonds is often required to form functional proteins
    d. Amino acid side chains may be chemically modified by enzyme action
    e. For proteins that function outside the cell, modification is complete before they are secreted from the cell in which they were synthesised

15. In post-translational modification and transport:
    a. Proteins are made in the compartment of the cell in which they are to function
    b. Insulin is synthesised as part of a larger precursor protein that folds to form a structure containing insulin, which is then cut out by limited proteolysis
    c. Proteins are transported through the nuclear membrane if they carry a signal sequence that is recognised by an SRP (signal recognition particle)
    d. When a newly synthesised signal sequence is recognised by an SRP, the ribosome to which it is attached stops protein synthesis
    e. Proline hydroxylation in the formation of collagen is carried out while the proline is attached to its tRNA molecule

Short essay question

Explain why mutations caused by the insertion of an extra base, or the deletion of a base from a gene, are often much more serious than mutations produced by the change of a single base.

Self-assessment: answers

Multiple choice answers

1. a. **False.** Methionine and tryptophan are each represented by only one codon.
    b. **True.** For example, histidine, aspartate and glutamate.
    c. **True.** For example, alanine, valine, proline and glycine.
    d. **True.** Serine, leucine and arginine are each represented by six codons.
    e. **True.** For example, all the amino acids with hydrophobic side chains have U as the second base in their codons.

2. a. **False.** The codons are identical in the first and second positions.
    b. **True.** Look at the genetic code table.
    c. **False.** The third position can be any of the four bases.
    d. **False.** The codons are identical in the first and second positions.
    e. **False.** The third position can be any of the four bases.

3. a. **True.** For example, histidine, aspartate, glutamate or lysine.
    b. **False.** It is the bases in the first two positions that are identical.
    c. **False.** It is the bases in the first two positions that are identical.
    d. **False.** The second base is identical too.
    e. **False.** Only the third base differs between the codons.

4. a. **False.** Leucine represented by UUA, UUG, CUA and CUG is one exception (see also arginine).
    b. **True.** There is no exception.
    c. **False.** Eight amino acids are specified by the first two bases and can have any base in the third position.
    d. **False.** Change in the first base often changes the amino acid but there are exceptions, e.g. leucine is coded for by UUA and CUA.
    e. **False.** Sometimes the third base is important.

5. a. **True.** GTP is needed for aminoacyl-tRNA binding and translocation.
    b. **False.** Ribosomes are needed. Nucleosomes are found in chromosomes.
    c. **True.** As building blocks.
    d. **True.** For amino acid activation.
    e. **True.** To provide sequence information.

6. a. **True.** By definition.
    b. **True.** Each codon represents a single amino acid.
    c. **True.** There are 61 codons to represent 20 amino acids.
    d. **True.** There are very few exceptions.
    e. **False.** mRNA is translated in the 5' to 3' direction.

7. a. **False.** It is anticodons that contain other bases.
    b. **True.** The genetic code is said to be 'unpunctuated'.
    c. **True.** Four possible bases in each of the three positions ($4 \times 4 \times 4$).
    d. **True.** The other three are stop codons.
    e. **False.** There are three stop codons. The start codon also codes for methionine.

8. a. **True.** By definition
    b. **True.** Recognition is achieved by complementary base pairing.
    c. **True.** As for all base pairing, the sequences are antiparallel.
    d. **False.** The base-pairing rules are relaxed between the 5' base on the anticodon and the 3' base on the codon.
    e. **True.** The term was coined by Crick.

9. a. **False.** Some tRNA molecules can recognise more than one codon.
    b. **False.** Some amino acids need more than one tRNA molecule to recognise all their codons.
    c. **False.** Fidelity of protein synthesis depends on each tRNA being loaded with a single amino acid.
    d. **True.** When they are represented by more codons than one tRNA molecule can recognise.
    e. **False.** Stop codons are recognised by proteins associated with ribosomes.

10. a. **True.** These enzymes are responsible for ensuring that the tRNA molecules are correctly loaded.
    b. **False.** AMP and pyrophosphate are produced from ATP.
    c. **True.** This activates the carboxyl group for peptide bond formation.
    d. **True.** Some have associated hydrolases that can cleave any amino acid wrongly attached to the tRNA.
    e. **True.** There is no direct recognition between an tRNA and its amino acid; the aminoacyl synthetases bring them together.

11. a. **True.** Initiation complex formation starts with the small ribosomal subunit binding to mRNA.
    b. **True.** Formyl methionyl-tRNA$_{Met}$ matches the start codon.
    c. **True.** The 30S (small) ribosomal subunit binds to the Shine–Dalgarno sequence, upstream from the start codon.
    d. **True.** The 50S (large) ribosomal subunit completes the initiation complex.
    e. **False.** ATP is not directly required.

12. a. **True.** One for the binding of each aminoacyl-tRNA to its codon and one for the translocation step.
    b. **True.** To make room for the binding of the next aminoacyl-tRNA.
    c. **True.** This is the site where each aminoacyl-tRNA is matched to the next codon.
    d. **False.** The latest amino acid in the chain is bound to its tRNA in the A site when the new peptide bond is formed.
    e. **True.** ATP is only involved in aminoacyl-tRNA synthetase action, not directly in peptide bond formation.

13. a. **True.** No tRNA matches a stop codon.
    b. **True.** U followed by two purines. UGG, which also matches this pattern, codes for tryptophan.
    c. **False.** Proteins known as release factors are involved, not tRNA molecules.
    d. **True.** The peptide is transferred to a water molecule, not a further amino acid as in elongation.
    e. **True.** So that they can participate in the synthesis of further polypeptides.

14. a. **True.** Especially proteins that are to be secreted from the cell.
    b. **True.** Signal sequences are often removed once they have completed their function.

c. **True.** Collagen, insulin and trypsin are examples.
    d. **True.** For example, formation of hydroxyproline and hydroxylysine residues from proline and lysine in collagen formation.
    e. **False.** For example, zymogens must be activated after they are secreted.

15. a. **False.** Most proteins are transported to the site where they are to function.
    b. **True.** Insulin needs the extra sequence to fold correctly.
    c. **False.** An SRP mediates transport through the endoplasmic reticulum.
    d. **True.** It stops temporarily while the complex docks on the endoplasmic reticulum membrane.
    e. **False.** It occurs with proline incorporated in a precursor protein.

Short essay answer

Changing a single base may not even change the amino acid if the change occurs in the third position of a codon. If it does change the amino acid, there is a high probability that the change will introduce an amino acid that is chemically similar, for instance one non-polar amino acid side chain will be replaced by another non-polar side chain. Unless the amino acid is at a very critical point in the sequence, function of the protein might well be preserved.

Inserting or deleting a single base will alter the reading frame and produce a frameshift mutation. There will be a loss of function of the protein unless the mutation is very close to the C-terminal. Downstream from a frameshift mutation, every codon and every amino acid is altered. Also, insertion and deletion mutations often bring stop codons into the altered reading frame. One way to recognise the true reading frame in a newly determined DNA sequence is the relative absence of stop codons.

Molecular aspects of viruses

16

16.1 Virus composition and structure

Viruses are subcellular *parasites* that must infect the cells of other organisms to propagate themselves. They are much smaller and simpler than cells in their structures and they have a very limited genome; as a result, they rely on their host cell to provide most of the synthetic machinery needed for viral replication. They can be considered as genetic elements that invade a host cell and take over its cellular machinery to replicate themselves before moving on to infect further cells.

Use of viruses as model systems

Viruses are much studied because they are of such medical and agricultural importance. They are also studied because, with their small size and relative simplicity, they can be used as model systems for the study of processes seen in more complex life forms. Many virus genomes are strictly limited in size by the structure of the virus, so when the complete base sequence of a viral genome is determined, a function can be identified for most parts of the sequence. This is in contrast to the genomes of eukaryotes, where much of the sequence may well have no function.

Examples of processes where viruses provide useful model systems follow.

Assembly of macromolecular structures. Viruses have very small genomes so they must build their structures with a very limited number of proteins. Study of mutant viruses allows the pathways of virus construction to be explored.

Programmed gene expression. Viruses must express their genes in a time-dependent manner if the infection process is to be successful. Control systems governing the expression of viral genes are model systems for development in higher organisms. Viral control systems capable of switching between different possible life cycles have also been discovered and studied.

Evolutionary strategy and host – parasite relationship. Successful parasites tend to inflict minimal damage on their hosts so that a flourishing population of hosts remains for the parasite to infect. New strains of a virus that start by being particularly damaging to their hosts evolve to become less virulent. Evolution can be particularly rapid in viruses because of their vast numbers and short generation times. The evolution of viruses is easily studied within the human lifespan. Viruses have evolved that can infect a very wide range of living cells: animals, plants and bacteria.

Biochemical studies. Bacterial viruses, also known as *bacteriophage* or *phage*, are widely used in biochemical studies both as objects of study and as tools for gene sequencing, gene transfer, gene expression and gene cloning. Table 23, which shows a short list of much-studied viruses and bacteriophages, illustrates the wide range of hosts used, the varied nature of their genetic material and the range of sizes for viral genomes.

Viral genome

Viruses always contain a genome composed of nucleic acid. The nature and amount of nucleic acid can vary depending on the virus. Virus genomes can contain either DNA or RNA and in each case it may be single stranded or double stranded. Plant viruses are all RNA viruses. Usually the nucleic acid forms a single molecule, but in a few cases it is segmented: the genome of the influenza molecule exists as eight RNA molecules. The number of genes in a virus can vary from less than ten to several hundred. For reasons that will be described below, DNA viruses tend to have larger genomes than RNA viruses.

Table 23 Examples of viruses

Type	Example	Genome size (genes)	Host/effects
DNA viruses			*E. coli*
Single-stranded (a few bacteriophage)	Phage M13		
Double-stranded (very common)	Phage λ		*E. coli*: lysogeny or cell lysis
	Herpes	70	Human: cold sores, genital lesions
	Simian virus 40 (SV40)	5	Monkeys: tumours in rodents
	Smallpox virus		Human: smallpox
RNA viruses			
Single-stranded (very common)	Polio	8	Human: infantile paralysis, poliomyelitis
	Tobacco mosaic virus (TMV)	6	Tobacco plant: lesions on leaves
	Human immunodeficiency virus (HIV)	7	Human: acquired immunodeficiency syndrome (AIDS)
	Influenza	12	Human and other animals: respiratory disease
	Rous sarcoma	4	Birds: tumours in chickens
Double-stranded (a few animal viruses)	Reovirus	22	Human: infant enteritis

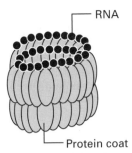

Fig. 145 Tobacco mosiac virus. Only a short section of the long cylinder is shown.

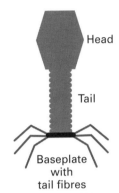

Fig. 146 Structure of bacteriophage T4.

Viral proteins

The nucleic acid forming the viral genome is covered by a protein coat or *capsid*. In cylindrical viruses like tobacco mosaic virus, the coat is built from many copies of a single protein component arranged in a regular helix around the genome (Fig. 145). In this virus, a single-stranded RNA chain of 6390 nucleotides is packaged by 2130 identical molecules of a protein that contains 168 amino acid residues. Spherical (or more strictly icosahedral, shaped like a solid having 20 faces) viruses build their capsids with as few as three protein components. Some spherical bacteriophages, such as bacteriophage T4, have further protein components forming a tail, which is used to inject the viral genes into the host bacterium during the infection process (Fig. 146). This phage was used in classic experiments to demonstrate that only the DNA was required to enter a cell for infection to occur. The protein components all remained outside the cell.

Some spherical viruses have a membranous envelope surrounding the capsid. This membrane is derived from the host cell in which the virus was assembled but also contains virus-specific membrane proteins. A few viruses must carry one or two molecules of an enzyme needed for virus replication.

Use of host functions

Viruses depend on the metabolic pathways of their host cells to provide building blocks, amino acids and nucleotides for building the next generation of viruses. Host cell metabolism also provides ATP for energy since viruses have no way to synthesise it. Viruses provide mRNA, but the host cells provide ribosomes, tRNA and amino acid-activating enzymes for the synthesis of viral proteins. This high dependence on host processes has made viruses difficult targets to attack by chemotherapy. Most drugs that could block viral replication would also block some vital function of the host cell.

16.2 Viral multiplication

Virus multiplication occurs in three stages: *infection*, *replication* and *release*.

Infection

For a virus to infect its host it must somehow get its nucleic acid into the cell. Different viruses achieve this in different ways but it generally involves binding of part of the virus to a receptor on the host. This receptor is often a protein with a normal useful function in the host. This is one reason why each virus is only able to infect a limited range of host cells.

Bacteriophage T4, which infects *E. coli*, has a hollow tail structure with a baseplate carrying fibres at its end (Fig. 146). The baseplate and fibres recognise and bind to a structure on the bacterial surface. The viral DNA is then injected into the bacteria leaving all the bacterial protein outside.

Viruses with envelopes may achieve entry by endocytosis, the virus binding to a membrane receptor on the surface of the host. Human immunodeficiency virus (HIV) binds to the CD4 receptor on T lymphocytes. Cells with no CD4 receptors cannot be infected. The viral envelope and the cell membrane fuse, releasing the viral capsid, which contains the viral nucleic acid, into the cell.

Replication

A virus must replicate its nucleic acid and also bring about the synthesis of its protein components if it is to multiply and produce more virus particles. DNA animal viruses enter the nuclei of their host cells, which contain all the synthetic machinery and materials used by the host for replication of its own DNA. Some viruses stimulate division of host cells that were not currently dividing, thus increasing their ability to replicate DNA.

Replication of RNA viruses
RNA viruses entering a host cell will find no enzymes there already that can replicate RNA, so RNA viruses must possess enzymes to do this. Different RNA viruses employ different strategies; these are additional processes (Fig. 147) that modify those outlined in the Central Dogma of Molecular Biology (p. 165). The various strategies for replicating viral RNA can be used to group the viruses into classes (Fig. 148):

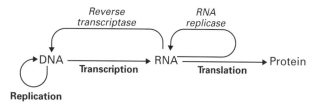

Fig. 147 Information flow in organisms. Either reverse transcriptase or RNA replicase is required for replication of the genome of RNA viruses.

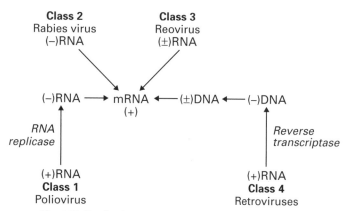

Fig. 148 Replication strategies of viruses with RNA genomes.

Class 1. The single-stranded genome consists of positive-strand RNA, which can be used directly as a messenger in the host cell. To replicate its genome, the virus must use the positive strand as a template to make a negative strand. This is achieved with *RNA replicase*, an RNA polymerase that uses an RNA template to specify the base sequence of its product. Once a negative strand is made, it can be used to make more viral RNA. RNA replicase may be part of the viral particle or may be synthesised by the ribosomes of the host using viral RNA as messenger.

Class 2. The single-stranded genome consists of negative-strand RNA, which can be copied to make new viral genomes but must be used as a template for positive-strand synthesis before synthesis of virus-coded proteins can begin.

Class 3. The genome is double-stranded.

Class 4. The single-stranded genome is positive and is replicated by a DNA polymerase, *reverse transcriptase*, that can use RNA as a template (so violating the 'central dogma' that information flows from DNA to RNA). The DNA made is incorporated into a chromosome of the host cell and can be transcribed to RNA for use as messenger and to construct new viral particles. Viruses such as HIV that use reverse transcriptase are known as *retroviruses*.

The enzymes that RNA viruses use to replicate their RNA are less accurate than DNA polymerase III since they have no proof-reading ability. RNA viruses are, therefore, much more vulnerable to mutation than DNA viruses and are not able to sustain such large genomes. RNA replication would introduce so many

---

BOX 16.1
Clinical note: Therapy for retrovirus infection

Since reverse transcriptase is not required by the host cell, it would appear to be a potential target for chemotherapy against HIV and other retroviruses. Inhibitors of reverse transcriptase such as AZT (azidothymidine), a nucleoside analogue, have indeed been used to treat HIV infection. However, its use imposes a strong selection pressure on the virus, which responds by mutation of its reverse transcriptase to produce an enzyme much less susceptible to inhibition by AZT (Box 12.2, p. 157). Long-lasting control of virus multiplication cannot, therefore, be achieved by treatment with this single inhibitor. *Multiple drug* treatment regimens currently offer better prospects for successful therapy.

---

errors into a large genome that viable viruses would rarely be produced.

Release

Virus particles are assembled from new viral nucleic acid and virus-coded proteins synthesised within the host cell. They must emerge before they are capable of further infection. Phage λ codes for an enzyme that lyses the host bacterium and releases the next generation of phage particles, killing the host cell in the process. Synthesis of this enzyme must obviously be carefully timed by the phage since its premature action would destroy the host cell before the new phages could assemble.

Viruses that acquire an envelope leave the host cell by exocytosis taking part of the plasma membrane with them. This membrane contains virus-coded membrane proteins that the new virus particles use during infection of their next hosts.

16.3 Viruses can coexist with their hosts

Not all viruses multiply themselves immediately after they infect a suitable host cell. More successful strategies are available. One such strategy is that used by phage λ.

By using its so-called *lytic pathway*, phage λ can infect *E. coli*, multiply and produce over 100 copies of itself that emerge about half an hour after infection. A few cycles of infection in this manner would soon exhaust the supply of potential hosts. But phage λ has another pathway, its *lysogenic pathway* (Fig. 149). In this pathway, after the phage has first infected the host cell, the phage DNA, which was injected in a linear form, circularises and then integrates with the circular DNA

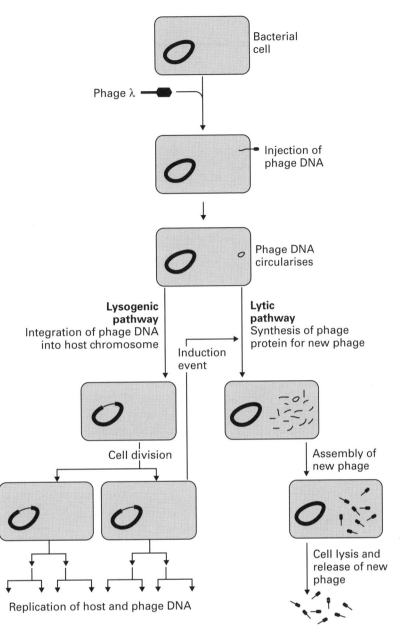

Fig. 149 The lytic and lysogenic.

molecule of its host. Once integrated, it produces a repressor protein that suppresses the synthesis of all phage proteins except the repressor itself. Each time the host cell divides thereafter, another copy of phage DNA is made, still integrated in the bacterial DNA. If conditions for bacterial growth become less than ideal, the stress response by the bacteria may trigger excision of the phage DNA and expression of all the phage genes, in other words the phage reverts to its lytic pathway.

Self-assessment: questions

Multiple choice questions

1. In viruses and their hosts:
   a. Viruses can use animal cells and bacterial cells as hosts but not plant cells
   b. Each virus can usually only infect a limited range of cell types
   c. Viruses that have bacterial hosts are known as bacteriophages
   d. New strains of viruses usually evolve to become more damaging to their hosts
   e. Some bacteriophage have hollow tails through which they inject their DNA into their bacterial hosts

2. Viral genomes:
   a. May be RNA or DNA
   b. Can be double-stranded DNA or single-stranded DNA
   c. In some viruses are double-stranded RNA and in some are single-stranded
   d. In RNA viruses tend to be larger than in DNA viruses
   e. Always consist of a single nucleic acid molecule

3. In viral structure:
   a. Some viruses have a membranous envelope and others have not
   b. Viruses with envelopes make them from host membrane proteins and viral phospholipid
   c. All viruses have a protein coat known as a capsid
   d. Some viruses are cylindrical in shape with a nucleic acid core covered by protein
   e. Viruses always contain nucleic acid but never contain enzymes

4. Viruses:
   a. Must enter a host cell to replicate
   b. Rely on the metabolic activity of their host cells for ATP
   c. Obtain the building block molecules for their own replication from the cell they have infected

   d. Depend so much on host enzymes that enzyme inhibitors can never be used to control virus replication
   e. Use host cell ribosomes but use viral mRNA and viral tRNA for the synthesis of viral protein

5. RNA viruses:
   a. Need processes not described in the Central Dogma of Molecular Biology
   b. May use viral RNA as mRNA to direct the synthesis of viral proteins
   c. Are generally less liable to mutate than DNA viruses
   d. Cannot use host cell enzymes to replicate their nucleic acid
   e. May use an RNA polymerase that can use an RNA template to replicate their nucleic acid

6. Retroviruses:
   a. Are RNA viruses
   b. Use reverse transcriptase to make DNA transcripts of viral RNA
   c. Contain reverse transcriptase, which is a DNA polymerase that uses an RNA template
   d. Include the human immunodeficiency virus, HIV
   e. Contains reverse transcriptase, which copies base sequences more accurately than DNA polymerase III

7. Bacteriophage λ:
   a. Uses *E. coli* as its host
   b. Injects a linear DNA molecule into its host
   c. Can incorporate its DNA into the DNA of its host
   d. In its lytic pathway only expresses one gene to make a repressor protein
   e. Is interesting to study but bacteriophages are of no practical importance since they only infect bacteria

Short essay question

Why study viruses?

Self-assessment: answers

Multiple choice answers

1. a. **False.** Some viruses can use plant cells as hosts. All plant viruses are RNA viruses.
   b. **True.** Each virus is adapted to infect its host cell and replicate there.
   c. **True.** Often abbreviated to phage.
   d. **False.** Both virus and host evolve to make viral infection less damaging.
   e. **True.** This is one way in which phage DNA can enter the host cell.

2. a. **True.** Viruses with each kind of nucleic acid are found.
   b. **True.** The great majority of DNA viruses are double-stranded.
   c. **True.** The great majority of RNA viruses are single-stranded.
   d. **False.** RNA replication is less accurate than that of DNA so RNA viruses cannot maintain very large genomes.
   e. **False.** Some viral genomes contain more than one nucleic acid molecule, e.g. influenza virus has a genome consisting of eight RNA molecules.

3. a. **True.** Not all viruses have an envelope.
   b. **False.** The phospholipid is from the host and the proteins from the virus.
   c. **True.** Viral nucleic acid is always packaged in protein.
   d. **True.** For example, tobacco mosaic virus, a much-studied plant virus.
   e. **False.** Many virus particles contain one or two enzyme molecules, e.g. reverse transcriptase in HIV.

4. a. **True.** Viruses rely on host cells for many of their replication processes.
   b. **True.** Viruses need energy for synthesis of their nucleic acids and proteins
   c. **True.** For example, amino acids for synthesis of viral protein.
   d. **False.** Viruses present a few targets for control by drugs, e.g. inhibitors of reverse transcriptase and viral protease in HIV.
   e. **False.** Viral mRNA is used but the host cell provides the tRNA.

5. a. **True.** The Central Dogma makes no provision for replication of RNA.
   b. **True.** Those with positive-strand RNA.
   c. **False.** They are more likely to mutate; RNA replication is less accurate than that of DNA.
   d. **True.** Host cells do not have enzymes to replicate RNA.
   e. **True.** The RNA polymerase is known as RNA replicase.

6. a. **True.** They reverse transcribe their RNA to form DNA sequences.
   b. **True.** This is the common property of all retroviruses.
   c. **True.** It catalyses the reverse of transcription, forming DNA using an RNA template.
   d. **True.** Not the first one discovered but the most important at present.
   e. **False.** Reverse transcription is more error prone than DNA replication. HIV is very mutable.

7. a. **True.** Phage λ is one of the most-studied phages; *E. coli* is the most-studied bacterium.
   b. **True.** The DNA is linear when injected but forms a circle once inside.
   c. **True.** In the lysogenic pathway.
   d. **False.** It is in its lysogenic pathway that phage λ only expresses one gene.
   e. **False.** Phage are important vectors in genetic engineering.

Short essay answer

The follow list indicates some reasons:

- medical importance: many diseases are caused by viruses
- agricultural importance: many animal and plant diseases are caused by viruses
- genetic engineering: viruses widely used as vectors.

In addition, viruses provide excellent model systems for studying the following: gene organisation, control of gene expression, virus capsids as models for the assembly of macromolecular structures, virus entry to and exit from host cells as models for endocytosis and exocytosis.

It has been suggested that benign viruses could be used as vehicles to introduce genes to cells selectively and so alleviate inherited disease. For example, in cystic fibrosis where the inactivity of a chloride channel leads to lung damage, it may be feasible to introduce the missing gene into the cells where its absence is causing disease.

Biochemical functions of the liver

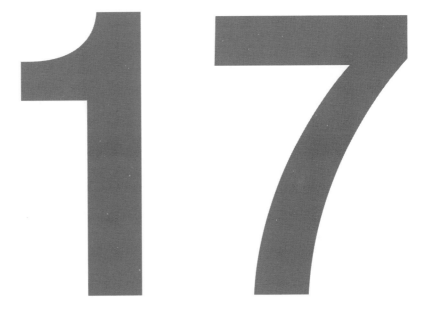

17.1 Carbohydrate, lipid and amino acid metabolism

Almost every major metabolic pathway is present in the liver and, clearly, it is has a vital role to play in fuel balance, facilitated by its anatomical location and the fact that it receives fuels and metabolites directly from the gut via the portal vein.

Carbohydrate metabolism

Table 24 contains core information related to carbohydrate metabolism in the liver. The liver has the ability to store glucose in the form of glycogen in the fed state and break down glycogen and make glucose from non-carbohydrate precursors in the fasted state and during exercise (Chapters 11). Fructose and galactose, produced by the digestion of dietary sucrose and lactose, respectively, are both converted to glucose in the liver.

Ethanol metabolism

The liver is an important site for ethanol metabolism. By the action of NAD^+-dependent *alcohol dehydrogenase*, ethanol is converted to acetaldehyde. The oxidation of acetaldehyde yields acetyl-CoA. If a large amount of ethanol is being metabolised, the resultant increase in NADH reduces TCA cycle activity and diverts acetyl-CoA to fatty acid and triacylglycerol synthesis. This can contribute to the development of fatty liver (vide infra).

Another route for ethanol metabolism involves a cytochrome P-450 ethanol-oxidising system (MEOS) located in the smooth endoplasmic reticulum. The product is again acetaldehyde.

Lipid metabolism

Table 25 contains core information related to lipid metabolism in the liver. Some fat is synthesised in the liver in the fed state; the activity of this pathway depends upon the nutritional status of the subject. People on high-fat diets typical in Western societies have low activity of the key enzymes of fatty acid synthesis. Most of the glucose that they take up in the liver is converted to glycogen. However, fatty acids derived from chylomicron remnants are converted to triacylglycerols by a pathway that uses glycerol 3-phosphate derived from glucose metabolism. Any triacylglycerol synthesised in the liver is exported as VLDL. Fatty acids are oxidised to provide ATP in the fasted state and they are also the precursors of ketone bodies. The liver is the major organ involved in cholesterol biosynthesis. Bile acid biosynthesis is unique to the liver and the formation of bile in that organ is critical for lipid digestion. Large amounts of vitamin A are stored in the lipocytes of the liver. The liver is the site for the synthesis of 25-hydroxy-vitamin D, the precursor of calcitriol (p. 226), formed in the kidney.

Fatty liver

The accumulation of triacylglycerols in the liver is indicative of abnormal function and leads to liver damage. A cause of fatty liver can be failure of normal lipoprotein synthesis caused by a variety of factors. One such is where there is a deficiency of choline, hence choline is called a lipotropic factor.

Amino acid metabolism

When a person's diet contains protein in excess of requirements for protein synthesis much of the amino acids produced by protein digestion is catabolised in the liver, where it can be converted to glycogen and triacylglycerol or completely oxidised to generate ATP (Table 26). The liver is the only organ in the body with a functional urea cycle. Under fasted conditions, the conversion of amino acid carbons to glucose by the gluconeogenic pathway achieves great significance. Most of the plasma proteins are synthesised in the liver (Chapter 20).

Table 24 Carbohydrate metabolism in the liver

Activity	Pathways	Control
Maintenance of blood glucose	Glycogenolysis and gluconeogenesis	High glucagon/insulin ratio
Fuel storage	Glycogenesis, fatty acid synthesis	High insulin/glucagon ratio
Ribose phosphate and NADPH generation	Pentose phosphate cycle	
Utilisation of other carbohydrates	Fructose and galactose metabolism	

Table 25 Lipid metabolism in the liver

Activity	Pathways
Production of fatty acids	Fatty acid synthesis from glucose, amino acids
Utilisation of fatty acids	Beta-oxidation
Production of ketone bodies	Mitochondrial synthesis from fatty acids and ketogenic amino acids
Cholesterol biosynthesis Production of bile acids Phospholipid synthesis Lipoprotein synthesis	Biosynthesis from cholesterol
Provision of 25-Hydroxy-vitamin D Storage of vitamin A	Synthesis from vitamin D

Table 26 Amino acid metabolism in the liver

Activity	Pathways
Energy metabolism	Individual pathways then the TCA cycle and oxidative phosphorylation
Urea synthesis	The liver is the sole site in the body
Glucose/glycogen production	Gluconeogenesis from glucogenic amino acids, e.g. alanine

17.2 Metabolism of xenobiotics

The turn-over of many biologically active endogenous compounds (e.g. hormones) and almost all drugs occurs in the liver; the enzymes involved are localised in the smooth endoplasmic reticulum. The enzyme systems are inducible and their activity often determines the duration of action of the drugs they metabolise. Drug metabolism usually achieves two goals:

- inactivation of the compound
- increased water solubility of the compound.

Increased water solubility facilitates elimination by the kidneys or in bile. Drug metabolism occurs in two phases.

Phase 1. Initial metabolism often involves members of a gene family called *cytochromes P-450*, which are mixed-function oxidases. These enzymes, which have broad specificity, catalyse oxidations and demethylations of naturally occurring compounds and xenobiotics which are lipophilic.

Phase 2. These reactions involve polar molecules being added to the products of phase 1 to produce water-soluble end-products that are finally excreted via the kidney or via bile, for example:

- benzoic acid with glycine
- steroids and phenols with glucuronic acid
- indoles and steroids with sulphuric acid
- aromatic acids with glutamine.

Hormone inactivation

The liver is responsible for much of the inactivation of hormones, a process essential to the fine control of hormone levels in blood. Examples include:

- metabolism and inactivation of adrenaline and noradrenaline by monoamine oxidase and catechol *O*-methyl transferase (COMT) and conjugation of their products with glucuronic acid
- deiodination of thyroxine and triiodothyronine
- insulin reduction to separate A and B chains by insulin–glutathione transhydrogenase; these separate chains can then be hydrolysed

---

BOX 17.1
Clinical note: Drug interactions

Some of the cytochromes P-450 are induced by drugs and this can complicate therapy with a second drug that is also a substrate of the induced enzyme. Similarly, in multiple drug therapy or liver disease, there may be competition for the drug-metabolising enzymes. This tends to be most important with drugs with a narrow therapeutic index, e.g. warfarin, digoxin or cyclosporin.

- metabolism and inactivation of steroid hormones such as cortisol, testosterone, progesterone and oestradiol by double bond reduction and conjugation of hydroxyl groups with glucuronic or sulphuric acids to form very water-soluble products
- further hydroxylation of steroids.

17.3 Bile pigment metabolism

Bile pigments are hydrophobic metabolites of the haem rings in haem proteins. They are taken into the liver and converted to water-soluble metabolites that are secreted into bile. Problems with uptake, conjugation or secretion of bile pigments lead to *jaundice*.

Bile pigments are produced from haem in the spleen

Bile pigments are formed from haem proteins, with most being derived from senescent erythrocytes by conversion of the haem of haemoglobin to *biliverdin* and subsequent reduction to *bilirubin* in cells of the reticuloendothelial system, predominantly in the spleen. Other proteins, such as the electron transport chain cytochromes and cytochromes P-450, are also sources of bilirubin; they have a short half-life whereas haemoglobin has a long half-life because of the long life of erythrocytes. Tissues forming bile pigments contain a highly active enzyme system, *haem oxygenase*, which is associated with the smooth endoplasmic reticulum (Fig. 150). In the presence of oxygen and NADPH, a membrane-bound cytochrome P-450 oxidises one of the carbons that bridges the pyrrole rings and releases it as carbon monoxide. This effectively opens the porphyrin ring to yield the linear, tetrapyrrole chain of biliverdin. The globin (or other apoprotein portion) is hydrolysed to free amino acids, which will be reconverted in part to newly synthesized protein. The iron that is released when the haem is cleaved will be almost quantitatively retained for recycling into new haemoproteins. Biliverdin rarely accumulates or escapes from cells because it is acted upon as soon as it is formed by a very active, soluble reductase enzyme that also requires NADPH. The product is bilirubin, the principal bile pigment found in the body.

Bilirubin is transported to the liver

Bilirubin made in the reticuloendothelial system diffuses into the bloodstream where it forms a soluble complex with albumin in the plasma. Upon reaching the hepatic cells, the albumin–bilirubin complex dissociates, and free bilirubin is taken up using *bilitranslocase* (Fig. 150). It then becomes bound to a specific carrier protein (ligandin) in the cytosol.

(a) Synthesis of bilirubin in spleen

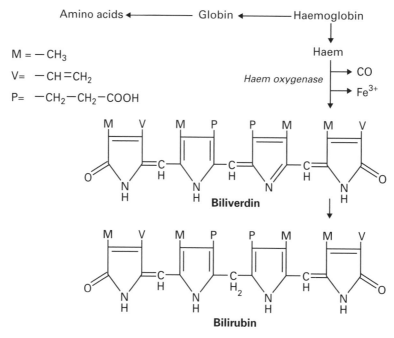

(b) Bilirubin metabolism in liver

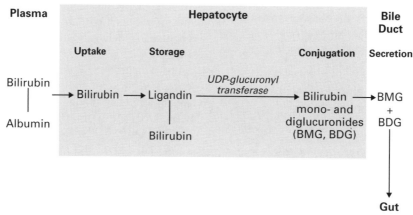

Fig. 150 Bilirubin synthesis in the spleen (a) and its metabolism in the liver (b).

Bilirubin conjugation with glucuronic acid precedes secretion into bile

A major function of the liver is to convert the bilirubin to a water-soluble form by attaching sugar derivatives onto two of the pyrrole rings, a process called *conjugation*. The sugar derivative, glucuronic acid, is added in its activated form, UDP-glucuronic acid; this is derived in the liver by the action of a soluble dehydrogenase upon UDP-glucose. A specific enzyme in the endoplasmic reticulum, *UDP-glucuronyl transferase*, catalyses the addition of glucuronic acid to propionyl side-chains in ester linkages. The resulting conjugated form of the bile pigment, bilirubin diglucuronide (BDG), has the hydrophilic sugar residues to offset the hydrophobic property of the rest of the molecule.

Bilirubin is secreted into bile

The conjugated and unconjugated bilirubin molecules may then be passed from the hepatic cells into the bile canaliculi, utilising the ATP-dependent canalicular multidrug resistance-like protein (CMRP). They then percolate down the biliary tree to the gallbladder before being released into the intestinal tract. In the intestine, BDG is metabolised to urobilinogen, some of which is reabsorbed and is in turn excreted in urine, i.e. we have an enterohepatic circulation of bile pigment metabolites. Urobilinogen that is not reabsorbed is excreted in faeces.

Excess levels of bile pigments cause jaundice

When bile pigments accumulate in the blood and other body fluids either because of excessive formation or because of inadequate removal in the bile, they may produce an intense yellow coloration of the skin. This condition, termed icterus or jaundice, may result from:

- massive breakdown of erythrocytes (haemolysis) leading to overproduction of bilirubin from haemoglobin catabolism
- a defect in the mechanisms by which the liver disposes of the normal flux of bilirubin.

Neonatal jaundice has to be treated

This is really a normal event since the glucuronyl transferase and ligandin system is still immature during the first few days of life. However, premature babies can achieve very high levels of unconjugated bilirubin; if it gets into the CNS, leading to kernicterus, there is the possibility of a motor disorder. Treatment is usually by phototherapy, where the bilirubin is converted to a water-soluble (easily excreted) derivative in the skin. You can see this treatment in any neonatal unit of a hospital.

Other forms of jaundice

These can be due to:

- defects in bilirubin uptake (Gilbert's disease)
- absence of glucuronyl transferase activity (Crigler–Najjar disease)
- defective hepatic excretion (Dubin–Johnson syndrome)
- hepatitis/cirrhosis (viral hepatitis or alcoholic cirrhosis)
- biliary obstruction (obstructive jaundice caused by stones, cancer etc.).

17.4 Liver function tests

It is important to realise that as much as 80% of the liver cells can be damaged or removed with no evidence of abnormality of liver function, i.e. the liver has great reserve activity. In this way, significant liver damage is not usually associated with an abnormal glucose tolerance test, even though we know that much of the glucose is usually metabolised in the liver during such a test.

Liver function tests (LFTs) include:

- the measurement of serum albumin and prothrombin time (PT) of plasma as indices of synthetic ability of the liver
- the measurement of alkaline phosphatase as a test for cholestasis
- the measurement of aminotransferases (AST and ALT) as a test for inflammation and necrosis
- measurement of serum bilirubin.

Elevated PT is a very sensitive test for the synthetic capability of the liver and is dependent upon the fact that factor VII, involved in the extrinsic pathway and measured by PT (Chapter 20), is a blood coagulation factor that has a relatively short half-life. Since factor VII is a vitamin K-dependent blood coagulation factor, the vitamin K status of any subject being evaluated has to be considered in interpreting data.

Serum alkaline phosphatase is derived from liver, bone, intestine, placenta and kidney. It is possible to measure the liver isozyme and an increase in its level in serum is associated with obstructive and cholestatic liver disease.

When the liver is damaged, as in viral hepatitis, enzymes present in high concentrations in hepatocytes appear in serum in increased amounts. Of the aminotransferases, alanine aminotransferase (ALT) is more liver specific (it is involved in the gluconeogenic pathway from alanine to glucose).

Self-assessment: questions

Multiple choice questions

1. Metabolic pathways found in the liver include:
   a. Glycolysis
   b. Fatty acid oxidation
   c. Glycogenesis
   d. Pentose phosphate pathway
   e. Purine and pyrimidine nucleotide biosynthesis

2. Bile pigment metabolism in the liver includes:
   a. Conjugation of bilirubin to produce the mono- and diglucuronide derivatives
   b. Conversion of biliverdin to bilirubin
   c. Production of urobilinogen
   d. Secretion of bilirubin glucuronides into the bile canaliculi
   e. Uptake of bilirubin from the bilirubin–albumin complex found in plasma

3. Lipid metabolism in the liver includes:
   a. Phospholipid synthesis
   b. Cholesterol synthesis
   c. Bile salt synthesis
   d. Ketone body utilisation
   e. Triacylglycerol synthesis

4. The following statements describe liver function:
   a. A deficiency of choline can cause fatty liver
   b. LDL is the lipoprotein made in the liver to transport triglycerides to adipose tissue
   c. Drug inactivation in the liver is based on the principle that the liver converts the drug to a more lipophilic metabolite
   d. Factor VII, one of the coagulation factors made in the liver, has a very short half-life
   e. High levels of alkaline phosphatate and bilirubin diglucuronide in blood suggest obstructed bile flow

True/false questions

Are the following statements true or false?

1. The liver has a large reserve capacity in terms of its ability to handle glucose loads.
2. In normal subjects in the fed state, gluconeogenesis in the liver is stimulated.
3. The liver is the site for synthesis of 25-hydroxy-cholecalciferol.
4. The liver is the site of action of vitamin K metabolism in the body.
5. The source of glucuronic acid for bilirubin diglucuronide synthesis is UDP-glucuronate.
6. Neonatal jaundice is caused by the high efficiency of bilirubin conjugation in the newborn.
7. Drug-metabolising enzymes in the liver are chiefly located in the mitochondria.
8. Bile acids and bile pigments are both metabolites of the haem ring in haemoglobin and cytochromes.
9. A dietary deficiency of choline can lead to the development of 'fatty liver'.

Short essay questions

1. Explain in a few sentences the reason why the measurement of prothrombin time, a blood coagulation test, provides critical information about protein synthesis in the liver.
2. Suggest four possible reasons for jaundice developing in a patient, based on your knowledge of bile pigment formation and metabolism.

Self-assessment: answers

Multiple choice answers

1. a. **True.** Glycolysis is the first pathway when one is converting glucose to fatty acids in the liver. It also provides glycerol 3-phosphate for triacylglycerol synthesis.
   b. **True.** Fatty acids are important fuels for the liver especially in the fasted state.
   c. **True.** This pathway is stimulated in the fed state to replenish the liver's glycogen stores.
   d. **True.** There is a need for NADPH in the liver for many reactions including those of drug metabolism.
   e. **True.** Given the high activity of protein synthesis in the liver, there is a big demand for purine and pyrimidine nucleotide biosynthesis in order to make DNA and RNA.

2. a. **True.** These are water-soluble derivatives that are secreted into bile.
   b. **False.** Bilirubin is made from biliverdin chiefly in the spleen.
   c. **False.** This bile pigment is made in the colon.
   d. **True.** Conjugated bilirubin is secreted into bile using an ATP-dependent transporter.
   e. **True.** Bilirubin is extracted from albumin before entering the hepatocyte (albumin does not accompany it).

3. a. **True.** At a high rate.
   b. **True.** The liver is the major site for cholesterol synthesis in the body.
   c. **True.** Bile salts are made from cholesterol in the liver.
   d. **False.** The liver is the site for ketone body synthesis; they are utilised elsewhere.
   e. **True.** Fatty acids made in the liver or taken up in the fed state are converted to triacylglycerols and then incorporated into VLDL.

4. a. **True.** Choline is a lipotropic agent no doubt related to its role in phospholipid and therefore lipoprotein synthesis.
   b. **False.** It is VLDL that is made to transport triacylglycerols.
   c. **False.** Usually the derivatives are more hydrophilic, allowing them to be more readily transported for excretion.
   d. **True.** It is that short half-life that results in the prothrombin time being abnormal in patients with liver malfunction.
   e. **True.** The bile is the usual excretory route for both. Bile obstruction leads to large increases in both in blood, diagnostic of the condition.

True/false answers

1. **True.** This means that glucose tolerance is not a sensitive test of liver malfunction.
2. **False.** Why make more glucose when one has fed?
3. **True.** Cholecalciferol can be made in skin and 25-hydroxylation in the liver gives the precursor of the hormone (calcitriol), which is made in the kidney.
4. **True.** Several vitamin K-dependent proteins involved in blood coagulation, including prothrombin, are made in the liver.
5. **True.** UDP is the 'carrier' for biosynthetic reactions that incorporate carbohydrates and some carbohydrate derivatives into molecules.
6. **False.** Quite the opposite is true; newborn babies often have elevated unconjugated bilirubin levels in their plasma.
7. **False.** Most are located in the smooth endoplasmic reticulum.
8. **False.** Bile acids are formed from cholesterol in the liver; bile pigments are made in the spleen from haem.
9. **True.** Choline is required for the synthesis of phosphatidylcholine, a phospholipid involved in lipid transport.

Short essay answers

1. Prothrombin time (PT) is used by haematologists as a way of quantifying the activity of the extrinsic pathway of blood coagulation (Chapter 20). The range of normal values is small, which means that even a 2 or 3 second prolongation of the PT can be significant and must be pursued. Factor VII is involved in this pathway and is a vitamin K-dependent factor synthesised in the liver. It is distinguished from most other plasma proteins by having a very short half-life. If a patient has hepatocellular disease, liver protein synthesis will be impaired and this is quickly reflected in a prolonged PT. It is important to recognise that since factor VII is a vitamin K-dependent factor, a prolonged PT can also be caused by vitamin K deficiency. In such cases, the injection of vitamin K will return the PT value to the normal range.

2. Jaundice is the condition when excess concentrations of bilirubin are present in blood. The bilirubin can be either free (unconjugated) or in the form of bilirubin diglucuronide (conjugated). Possible reasons for hyperbilirubinaemia include:
   a. haemolytic anaemia, where there is a high rate of lysis of red blood cells: this can overload the ability of the body to deal with bilirubin, the end-product of haem metabolism

b. impaired uptake of bilirubin from blood (where it is transported bound to albumin) into liver: an unconjugated hyperbilirubinaemia would result

c. impaired activity of the UDP-glucuronyl transferase system in the liver bilirubin diglucuronide formation: the end result would again be unconjugated hyperbilirubinaemia

d. obstruction to the flow of bile from the liver to the gallbladder and gut: bilirubin diglucuronide will accumulate in blood (along with some unconjugated bilirubin) resulting in conjugated hyperbilirubinaemia and, in this case, excessive levels of bile pigment in urine, making it dark.

The biochemistry of
the endocrine system

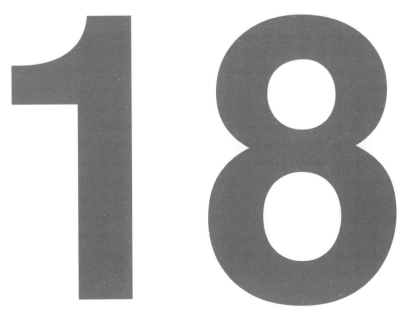

18.1 General aspects

One of the axioms of physiology is the relative constancy of the internal environment of the body, i.e. **homeostasis**. The endocrine and nervous systems regulate almost all metabolic and homeostatic activities in humans and these two regulatory systems interact. Most endocrine secretions are influenced directly or indirectly by the brain. Various feedback loops exist to provide a stable internal milieu (ionic or fuel homeostasis) or a coordinated series of actions (growth and reproduction).

The homeostatic role of the endocrine system is usually divided into five major areas (summarised in Table 27).

Chemical nature of hormones

Rather than memorising a particular hormone's detailed chemical structure, it is important to appreciate the nature of its chemical structure since, to a large degree, that is what determines how it is made, how it is transported and how it acts. There are three general chemical classes:

Table 27 The scope of endocrine regulation

System	Hormones involved
Ionic homeostasis	
Control of Na^+/K^+ ratios in blood	Aldosterone
Control of $[Ca^{2+}]$ in blood	Parathyroid hormone, calcitonin, calcitriol
Control of water balance	Antidiuretic hormone
Fuel homeostasis	
Control of blood glucose concentration	Insulin in the fed state Glucagon, adrenaline, cortisol, growth hormone in the fasting state and during exercise
Basal metabolic rate	Thyroid hormones
Regulation of growth	
Growth of cartilage	Growth hormone, mediated by insulin-like growth factor (IGF-1; somatomedin C)
Growth and development	Growth hormone, thyroid hormones
Regulation of reproduction, sexual differentiation and lactation	
Control of gonadal function	Luteinising hormone (LH), Follicle-stimulating hormone (FSH), testosterone, oestradiol
Control of lactation	Prolactin, oxytocin
Pregnancy	Human chorionic gonadotrophin (hCG), human chorionic somatomammotrophin (hCS), progesterone, oestradiol
Gastrointestinal activity	
Pepsin and acid production	Gastrin
Bicarbonate release from pancreas	Secretin
Release of bile from gallbladder	Cholecystokinin
Enzyme release from pancreas	Cholecystokinin

- **Peptides.** These include large complex polypeptides that contain disulphide bonds and may be glycosylated, as well as linear peptides with as few as three amino acid residues.
- **Amino acid derivatives.** These are either made from single amino acids or from the coupling of two amino acids. Examples are the catecholamines, adrenaline and noradrenaline and the thyroid hormones thyroxine (T_4) and triiodothyronine (T_3).
- **Steroids.** Steroid hormones such as cortisol, progesterone, aldosterone, androgens and oestrogens contain an intact steroid nucleus whereas in calcitriol the steroid nucleus has been disrupted.

The biosynthesis of hormones

Peptide hormones are coded for by particular genes and synthesised by the standard protein biosynthetic machinery (Chapter 15). There are usually multiple copies of the genes for shorter peptides, and single hormone molecules are derived by post-translational proteolysis. Some hormones may be synthesised as separate subunits, which then associate, e.g. the glycoprotein hormones of the adenohypophysis.

Since peptide hormones are to be secreted from the cells of origin, the mechanism of production is similar to that for other secreted proteins (p. 195). The classic example of this is insulin, which is synthesised in the pancreatic beta cell as preproinsulin containing a signal peptide sequence that is removed generating proinsulin. The action of intracellular peptidases on proinsulin yields insulin plus a connecting peptide (C-peptide).

Preproinsulin $\rightarrow$ Proinsulin $\rightarrow$ Insulin + C-peptide

Other hormones where there are large prohormones include growth hormone, parathyroid hormone, ACTH and glucagon.

Amino acid derivatives are synthesised by unique pathways, each having several enzymatic steps. There are two groups of this type of hormone:

- The key feature of the biosynthetic pathway for the *thyroid hormones* (Fig. 151) is that the protein thyroglobulin is synthesised in the follicular epithelial cells of the thyroid gland (Fig. 152). This protein contains a large number of tyrosine residues that can be iodinated. Iodide derived from the diet is taken up by the thyroid as an active process. There is uptake into kidney, gastric and salivary glands, too, but the difference is that only in the thyroid is the iodine used to iodinate a protein. A *thyroperoxidase* catalyses the oxidation of iodide to iodine as well as the iodination of tyrosyl residues leading to the formation of mono-iodotyrosine (MIT) and di-iodotyrosine (DIT) within thyroglobulin. Two DIT molecles couple to form T_4 and a small amount of T_3 is also generated. Thyroglobulin is an exportable glycoprotein. It is stored in the colloid from where it can be internalised by micropinocytosis. When

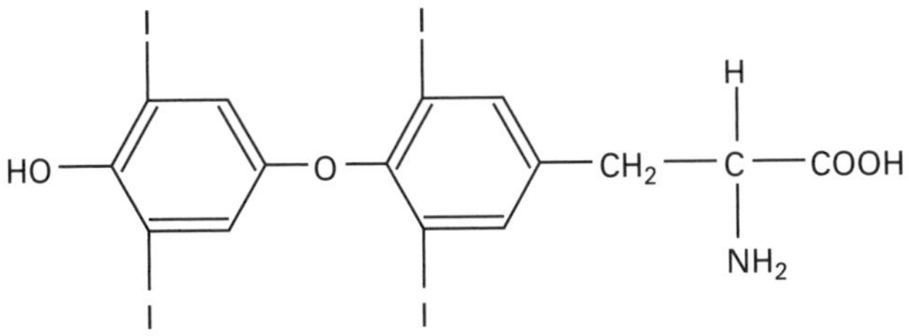

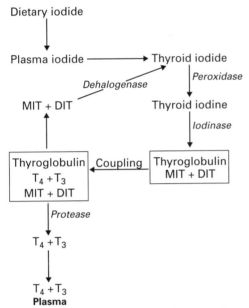

Fig. 151 The structure of the thyroid hormones.

Thyroxine (T$_4$)

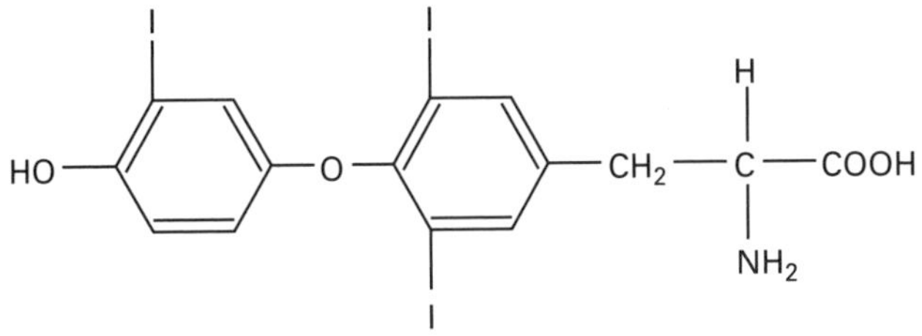

Triiodothyronine (T$_3$)

Fig. 152 Thyroid hormone biosynthesis. MIT, monoiodotyrosine; DIT, diiodotyrosine.

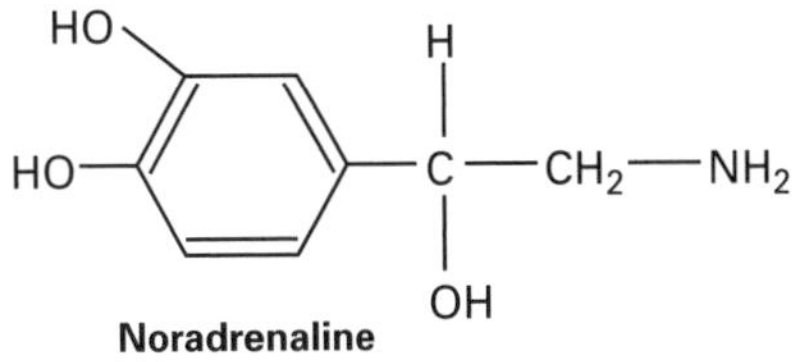

Noradrenaline

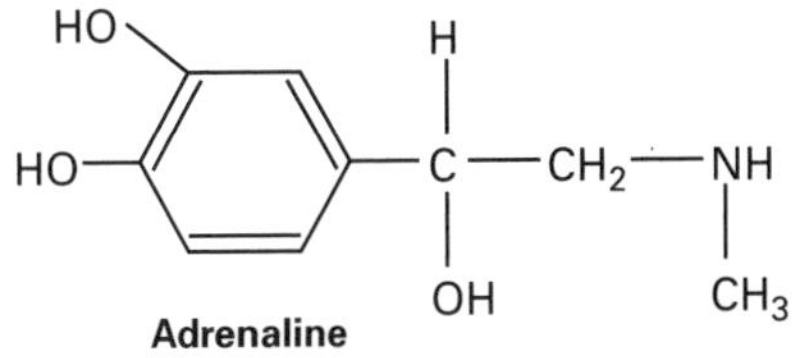

Adrenaline

Fig. 153 The structures of adrenaline and noradrenaline.

Tyrosine $\xrightarrow{\textit{Tyrosine hydroxylase}}$ Dihydroxyphenylalanine (I– DOPA)

$\downarrow -CO_2$

Noradrenaline $\xleftarrow{\textit{Dopamine } \beta\text{– hydroxylase}}$ Dopamine

$\downarrow \textit{PNMT}$

Adrenaline

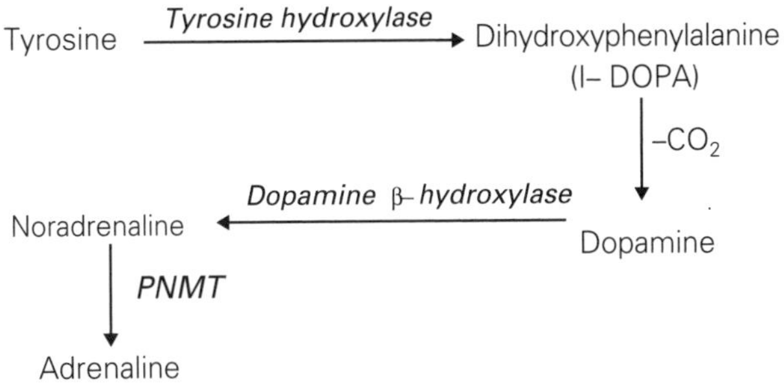

Fig. 154 Catecholamine biosynthesis. PNMT, phenylethanolamine *N*-methyl transferase.

thyroid hormones are required, the internalised thyroglobulin interacts with lysosomes to form secondary lysosomes and the thyroglobulin is digested to its constituent amino acids (including T$_4$, T$_3$, MIT and DIT) by the action of lysosomal proteases. T$_4$ and much less T$_3$ are then secreted into blood. Much more iodine is present in MIT and DIT than in T$_4$ and T$_3$ and that iodine is salvaged by the action of a thyroidal dehalogenase.

- *Adrenaline and noradrenaline* (Fig. 153) are synthesised in the chromaffin cells of tissues such as the adrenal medulla as well as in the brain and in sympathetic nerve endings (Fig. 154). Phenylethanolamine *N*-methyl transferase (PNMT) is induced by high concentrations of glucocorticoid, a situation brought about by the anatomical relationship of the adrenal medulla and adrenal

cortex. Adrenaline is stored complexed to ATP in granules within the chromaffin cells. The rate-limiting step is catalysed by *tyrosine hydroxylase*, a mixed-function oxidase that requires tetrahydrobiopterin as coenzyme.

Steroid hormones are also synthesised by unique pathways, each having several enzymatic steps. There are many types of steroid hormones but they are all derived from cholesterol, a sterol with 27 carbons. The steroid hormone products depend upon the tissue but overall the pathway can be described as:

$$C27 \rightarrow C21 \rightarrow C19 \rightarrow C18$$

In the critical first step, cholesterol undergoes side-chain cleavage, losing six carbons to give *pregnenolone*, the precursor of all the steroid hormones.

The structures of the steroid hormones are shown in Figure 155.

- The C21 steroids are *progesterone*, plus the corticosteroids, *aldosterone and cortisol*
- The C19 steroids are androgens such as *testosterone* and *dehydroepiandrosterone* (DHEA)
- The C18 steroids are the oestrogens; *oestradiol* is the most important.

Oxygens are added in the conversion of pregnenolone to the steroid hormones; the oxygens are derived from molecular oxygen in reactions catalysed by a family of haem-containing enzymes called cytochromes P-450 which require NADPH as cofactor.

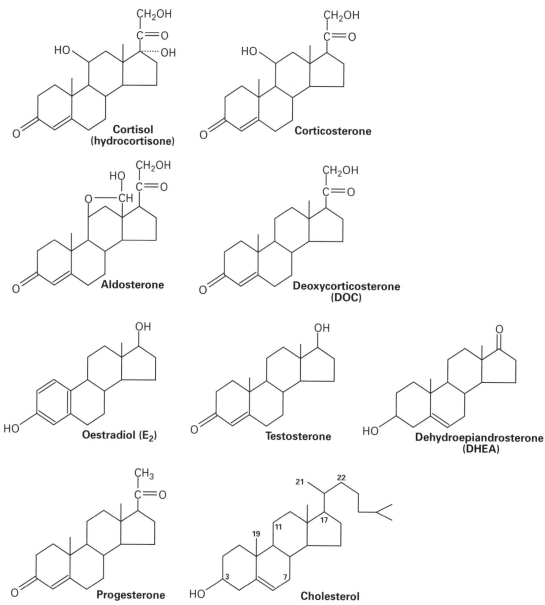

Fig. 155 The structures of steroid hormones and cholesterol.

Steroid hormone biosynthesis is complex and the following are key points:

- aldosterone and cortisol are made in the adrenal cortex, a gland which exhibits 'functional zonation'. Aldosterone, the hormone controlling sodium and potassium balance in the body, is made in the outermost *zona glomerulosa*. Cortisol, the major glucocorticoid (p. 140), is made in the inner *zona fasciculata*
- progesterone is made in the corpus luteum and also in the placenta during pregnancy
- androgens such as testosterone are made in the male and female gonads
- testosterone is the precursor of oestradiol; the conversion involves an enzyme called *aromatase*; aromatase is also found outside of the gonads, e.g. in adipose tissue.

Physicochemical properties of hormones

Another classification focuses on the water or lipid solubility of the hormone in question. Hormones in the water-soluble class – peptide hormones and catecholamines – have a number of key differences from the lipophilic hormones – thyroid hormones and steroid hormones (Table 28).

Water-soluble hormones are transported in the plasma in the free state, have short half-lives (this affects treatment regimens) and since they do not pass readily through lipid bilayers, they act by binding to specific receptor molecules on the plasma membranes of target cells.

Lipophilic hormones are transported mostly bound to plasma proteins but it is the free fraction that is biologically active and controlled. The total concentration of a lipophilic hormone will change if the concentration

Table 28 Contrasting properties of hydrophilic and lipophilic hormones

	Hydrophilic hormones[a]	Lipophilic hormones[b]
Transport in blood	Free	Transport protein involved
Half-life	Short	Long
Receptor site	Plasma membrane	Nucleus
Extra-glandular activation	Rare	Common
Mechanism of action	Second messenger	Transcription factor

[a]Proteins and peptides as well as catecholamines such as adrenaline and noradrenaline.
[b]Lipophilic hormones have limited water solubility and include all steroid hormones and the thyroid hormones T_4 and T_3.

Table 29 Hormones of the hypothalamus

Hormone	Chemistry	Target
Thyrotrophin-releasing hormone (TRH, TRF)	Tripeptide pyroGlu–His–Pro–NH$_2$	Thyrotrophs
Gonadotrophin-releasing hormone (GnRH, LHRH)	Decapeptide	Gonadotrophs (LH and FSH)
Growth hormone-releasing hormone (GHRH, GRF)	Peptide (44 amino acid residues)	Somatotrophs
Growth hormone-inhibiting hormone (somatostatin)	Tetradecapeptide	Somatotrophs
Corticotrophin-releasing hormone (CRH, CRF)	Peptide (41 amino acid residues)	Corticotrophs

Table 30 Hormones of the pituitary

Hormones	Produced by	Site of action
Adenohypophysis		
Glycoprotein hormones		
Thyroid-stimulating hormone (TSH)	Thyrotroph	Follicular epithelial cells of the thyroid
Luteinising hormone (LH)	Gonadotroph	Ovarian follicle, corpus luteum, Leydig cells
Follicle-stimulating hormone (FSH)	Gonadotroph	Ovarian follicle, Sertoli cells
Large polypeptides		
Growth hormone (GH, STH)	Somatotroph	Liver (IGF-1), adipocytes, general
Prolactin (PRL)	Mammotroph	Mammary gland (possibly other sites)
Small peptides		
Adrenocorticotrophic hormone (ACTH, corticotrophin)	Corticotroph	Adrenal cortex, adipocytes
β-Endorphin (β-EP) β-Lipotrophin (β-LPH) α-Melanocyte-stimulating hormone (α-MSH)	Corticotroph and neuro-intermediary lobe	Brain Melanocytes
Neurohypophysis		
Small peptides		
Antidiuretic hormone (ADH, vasopressin)	Supraoptic and paraventricular nuclei (SON and PVN)	Kidney
Oxytocin (OT)	PVN and SON	Mammary gland, uterus

of its transport protein is altered; an understanding of this is important when clinicians interpret hormone assay data on their patients. They have longer half-lives and can cross lipid bilayers to target receptors normally present in the nuclei of target cells. Some lipophilic hormones, thyroxine and testosterone are examples, undergo extra-glandular bioactivation. Thyroxine is converted to the much more active triiodothyronine in thyroid hormone target tissues. Testosterone, which is secreted from the gonads and elsewhere in the body, is converted to oestradiol, a female sex hormone, or to 5α-dihydrotestosterone, the androgen involved in the development of the secondary male sexual characteristics.

18.2 Hormones of the hypothalamus and pituitary

The overall importance of the adenohypophyseal and neurohypophyseal hormones is well illustrated by the consequences of hypophysectomy:

- atrophy of the gonads, adrenal cortex and thyroid accompanied by decreased secretion of sex hormones, cortisol and thyroid hormones
- interruption of the ovarian (menstrual) cycle and decreased ability to respond to stress
- inhibition of growth and development in young animals and increased sensitivity to insulin
- temporary diabetes insipidus.

The hormones secreted from the pituitary are listed in Table 30. Those arising from the anterior pituitary are controlled by releasing and inhibitory hormones that are made in the hypothalamus (Table 29); they travel to the pituitary via the pituitary portal veins. Antidiuretic hormone and oxytocin are made in the hypothalamus and travel down nerve tracts that terminate in the posterior pituitary from which these hormones are released into blood.

Hormones of the anterior pituitary include:
- large polypeptide hormones; growth hormone and prolactin
- glycoprotein hormones, thyroid stimulating hormone (TSH), luteinising hormone (LH) and follicle stimulating hormone (FSH). The alpha subunits of these hormones are homologous! It is the beta subunits that specify for function
- small peptides including adrenocorticotropic hormone (ACTH), α-melanocyte stimulating hormone (α-MSH) and β-endorphin. These three peptides are made from a large precursor called pro-opiomelanocortin (POMC).

Hormones of the posterior pituitary are:

- antidiuretic hormone and oxytocin, both formed from large precursors.

18.3 The hypothalamic–pituitary–adrenal cortical axis

Cortisol (hydrocortisone) is the principal glucocorticoid secreted by the human adrenal cortex. It is vital in our response to stress and has effects on almost all tissues in the body. The production of cortisol is controlled by corticotrophin-releasing hormone (CRH) secreted by the hypothalamus, which in turn stimulates release of ACTH (corticotrophin) from the anterior pituitary (Fig. 156).

Aldosterone is a mineralocorticoid which increases sodium retention and potassium excretion by effects on the distal convoluted tubule and collecting ducts. Other tissues affected by aldosterone include sweat, salivary and intestinal glands. Its production is controlled by the renin–angiotensin system; renin made in the juxta-glomerular cells of the kidney is released in response to sodium or volume depletion. In blood it catalyses the formation of angiotensin I from angiotensinogen, a precursor protein made in the liver. In the lungs, *angiotension-converting enzyme (ACE)* permits conversion of angiotensin I to angiotensin II, with the latter stimulating aldosterone production and secretion by increasing P-450$_{scc}$ activity. High potassium also stimulates aldosterone secretion by a direct effect on zona glomerulosa cells.

Pathology

As with many endocrine glands, there can be under-secretion or oversecretion of adrenal cortical hormones.

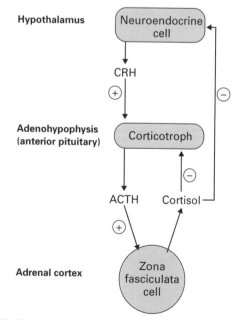

Fig. 156 The hypothalamic–pituitary–adrenal axis.

Since aldosterone and cortisol secretion are both controlled by other hormones (angiotensin II and ACTH, respectively), adrenal hypofunction and hyperfunction can be either primary or secondary. Diagnosis often relies on suppression and stimulation tests, which depend upon negative feedback control mechanisms.

18.4 The hypothalamic–pituitary–gonadal axis

Complex interactions existing between the components of this system are critical for sexual differentiation, puberty, the ovarian cycle and spermatogenesis. Gonadotropin-releasing hormone (GnRH) from the hypothalamus controls the secretion of two hormones from the anterior pituitary: LH; luteotropin and follicle stimulating hormone FSH; these, in turn, are responsible for the control of the gonads (Fig. 157). The female gonad (ovary) produces the steroid hormones *oestradiol* and *progesterone*. The male gonad (testis) makes *testosterone* which has a vital role in male sexual differentiation and the development of the male phenotype. Negative feedback control is an essential feature of this endocrine axis. Hormones produced during pregnancy in the placenta include *progesterone, oestrogens* and human chorionic gonadotrophin (hCG). The oestrogens are produced from androgens much of which arises from the fetal adrenal.

Testosterone. In *males* the Leydig cells (interstitial cells) produce testosterone from cholesterol under the control of LH. Within the male gonad, testosterone is also a prohormone serving as a precursor for the formation of oestrogen in the Sertoli cells as well as DHT, the androgen that controls the development of secondary male sex characteristics. Testosterone also has an anabolic effect leading to increased size of kidney, heart, and skeletal muscle mass as well as having behavioural effects, i.e. it is largely responsible for the development of the male phenotype. Testosterone is the precursor of 5α-dihydrotestosterone (DHT), which is essential for differentiation of the urogenital sinus and tubercle to prostate and external genitalia. This is an example of testosterone acting as a prohormone. The formation of DHT requires the presence of a steroid *5α-reductase* in target tissues. An XY fetus lacking 5α-reductase will be born without a phallus and appear to be female.

In *females* testosterone serves as the precursor of oestradiol. The latter crucial hormone is made in granulosa cells of the pre-ovulatory ovary from testosterone made in thecal cells. LH stimulates androgen production by thecal cells and FSH stimulates oestrogen production by activating granulosa cell aromatase.

Oestrogens and progesterone. They are both synthesised in the ovary and their levels fluctuate during ovarian cycles. A rise in oestradiol secretion near the mid-point of the ovarian cycle leads to in-

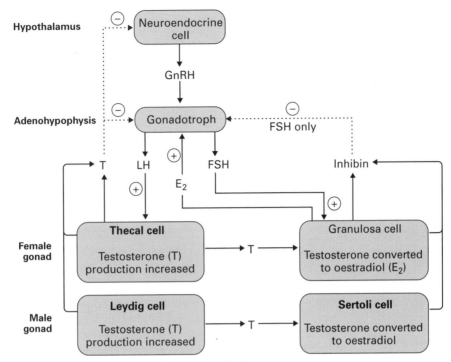

Fig. 157 The hypothalamic–pituitary–gonadal axis.

creased LH secretion and soon thereafter to ovulation.

Progesterone is synthesised from cholesterol and is produced in large amounts by the corpus luteum. Increased oestradiol and progesterone are required for essential proliferative changes in the uterus in the luteal phase of the ovarian cycle.

18.5 The hypothalamic–pituitary–thyroid axis

The thyroid hormones, thyroxine (T_4) and triiodo-thyronine (T_3), are iodinated amino acids that have significant effects on almost all tissues in the body. Their production is controlled by thyroid stimulating hormone (TSH, thyrotrophin) originating in the anterior pituitary. TSH, in turn, is regulated by thyrotrophin releasing hormone (TRH) secreted from the hypothalamus (Fig. 158).

Important points about the thyroid hormones are:

- T_4 is the major hormone secreted by the thyroid and it serves as the precursor of T_3
- T_3 is much more active than T_4
- T_4 and T_3 are bound to a very large degree by plasma proteins; thyroxine-binding globulin (TBG) made in the liver is the principal plasma protein involved.

Pathology

Thyroid hypofunction and hyperfunction can be either primary or secondary.

Graves' disease is a common form of hyper-thyroidism where patients have in their blood thyroid-

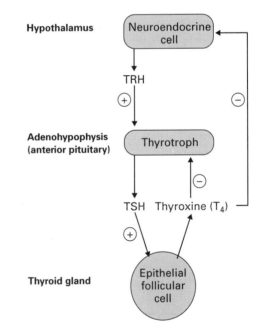

Fig. 158 The hypothalamic–pituitary–thyroidal axis.

stimulating antibodies (TSI), which bind to TSH receptors and cause thyroid hyperactivity. Serum T_4 and T_3 are elevated and, therefore TSH levels in these patients will be much below normal (negative feedback control again).

Primary hypothyroidism can involve congenital defects in thyroid hormone biosynthesis or destruction of the thyroid by thyroid autoantibodies. If hypothyroidism exists in a subject during growth and development, he or she may show mental retardation as well as stunted growth (cretinism). It is now established practice to test newborn children to ensure that they are not hypothyroid. Chronic iodine deficiency leads to *goitre* (an enlarged thyroid gland) and areas of the world where endemic goitre is common have low iodide in the environment. It is most common in mountainous regions, e.g. Alps, Himalayas and Andes.

18.6 The endocrine control of calcium and phosphate

Calcium through its presence in bones and teeth is the major mineral in the body but it has many other critical roles. Therefore, it is not at all surprising that calcium levels in the plasma and in the cytoplasm of cells are finely controlled. The control is mainly through the action of parathyroid hormone (PTH) and calcitriol, a hormone derived from vitamin D. Calcium and phosphate are intimately linked in bone but their metabolic roles in cells are quite different.

Functions of calcium ions

Intracellular:

- muscle contraction; cell motility; secretion phenomena; nerve function; growth and differentiation; second messenger involved in the action of many hormones

Extracellular:

- cell adhesion; aggregation of platelets; membrane integrity; blood coagulation.

Functions of phosphate ions

Intracellular:

- buffering; energy metabolism (sugar phosphates, ATP); component of membranes (phospholipids); component of nucleic acids; modification of many enzymes through cycles of phosphorylation–dephosphorylation; in signal molecules (2,3-BPG, cyclic AMP, inositol triphosphate)

Extracellular:

- buffering (especially important in urine).

Hormonal control of calcium and phosphate absorption/excretion

In any normal individual, there are only very minute fluctuations in plasma calcium ion levels despite variable intake of calcium in the diet and the potential to excrete calcium in urine. This implies close regulation. This is done by the parathyroid glands located behind the thyroid in the neck region. These glands (usually four in number in humans) synthesise and secrete *parathyroid hormone*, which, in effect, protects against hypocalcaemia by direct actions on bone and kidney and indirect actions on the gastrointestinal tract. Vitamin D (cholecalciferol) is a fat-soluble vitamin that has been known for a long time to be essential for efficient calcium absorption. Lack of vitamin D is classically associated with the development of rickets and osteomalacia in growing

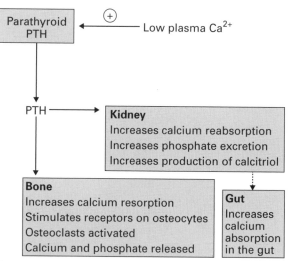

Fig. 159 Actions of parathyroid hormone.

children, leading to impaired bone formation and the classic picture of bow legs. It became clear that vitamin D per se could not be directly involved in promoting increased calcium absorption in the gut and that it was the precursor of *calcitriol* which was the hormone involved in the control of calcium absorption. Evidence was obtained that another hormone was involved in the control of plasma calcium. *Calcitonin* is produced experimentally in the thyroid/parathyroid complex specifically in response to hypercalcaemia. The key points are:

Parathyroid hormone (Fig. 159)

- Polypeptide made in the chief cells of the parathyroid gland.
- Secretion is triggered by low plasma calcium ion levels; high plasma calcium ion levels have the opposite effect.
- Action on kidney increases calcium reabsorption and phosphate excretion. It also increases calcitriol production.
- PTH increases bone resorption. PTH is usually described as acting on bone resorption by increasing osteoclastic activity. Osteoclasts produce acid hydrolases and acids that aid in resorption. However, osteoclasts do not possess PTH receptors so the activation of osteoclasts is indirect via effects on osteoblasts (which do have PTH receptors), which then release factors that stimulate osteoclasts (i.e. it is a paracrine system). The dissolution of bone mineral leads to the release of calcium and phosphate into blood.

Calcitriol (Fig. 160)

- 25-Hydroxycholecalciferol is converted to calcitriol in the kidney proximal tubule by the action of a 1-hydroxylase stimulated by PTH.
- When calcium levels are normal, the 25-hydroxycholecalciferol is converted to inactive 24,25-dihydroxycholecalciferol.
- Calcitriol acts on the gut to increase the synthesis of

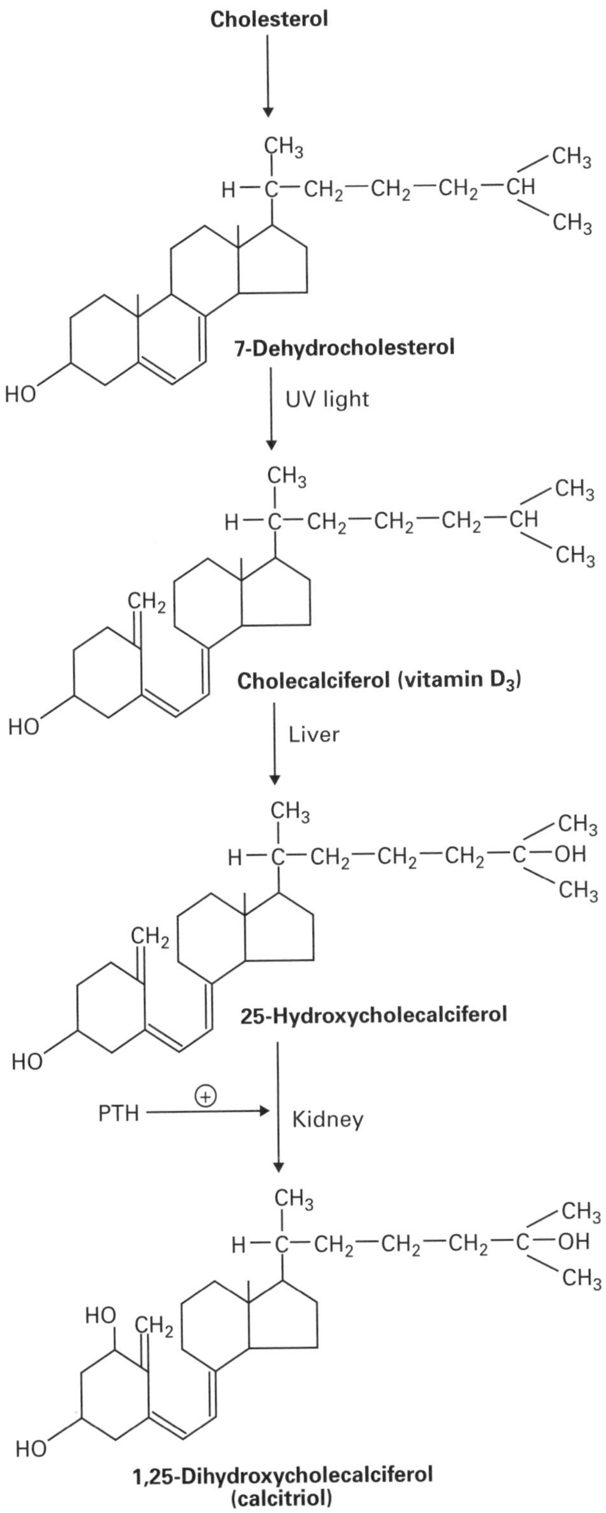

Cholesterol

Fig. 160 The synthesis of cholecalciferol (vitamin D_3) in the skin and its role as the prohormone of calcitriol.

a calcium-binding protein and also to increase phosphate absorption. The calcitriol receptor in the gut is a nuclear protein analogous to those for steroid hormones.

- **Pathology.** Low intake or low production of vitamin D leads to osteomalacia. Impaired bone formation can also occur if there is a lack of 1-hydroxylase in the kidney such that calcitriol synthesis is impaired.

Calcitonin

- Calcitonin is a peptide made in the parafollicular cells of the thyroid gland (T_4 is made in the epithelial follicular cells).
- Presumably secreted in response to high plasma levels of calcium ions. However, it is thought to be of little physiological importance in humans, except (possibly) in pregnancy, where it could have a role in promoting loading of calcium into the bones of the mother.
- Calcitonin is very active when administered to humans and has therapeutic uses.
- Calcitonin promotes the laying down of calcium into bone and it inhibits calcium reabsorption in the kidney.

18.7 Hormones of the adrenal medulla

The adrenal medulla and cortex are embryologically, anatomically and functionally separate. The medulla receives some of its blood supply from the cortex. It receives a rich nerve supply of preganglionic sympathetic fibres. The adrenal medulla has the ability to synthesise catecholamines such as adrenaline and noradrenaline starting from the amino acid tyrosine (Figs 153 and 154). As a part of the sympathetic nervous system it plays an important role in our response to stress, exercise and hypoglycaemia. These hormones have multiple effects including stimulation of muscle and liver glycogenolysis.

18.8 The endocrine pancreas

The islets of Langerhans make up the endocrine pancreas, which contains four cell types:

- alpha cells secrete *glucagon*
- beta-cells secrete *insulin*
- delta-cells secrete *somatostatin*
- PP cells secrete *pancreatic polypeptide (PP)*.

Insulin and glucagon are the key hormones controlling fuel balance in the body. Their multiple actions are discussed in Chapters 8 and 11.

18.9 Other hormonal systems

Erythropoieitin

The remarkable constancy of the circulating red cell mass in adults suggests that the process of erythropoiesis is rigidly controlled. Exposure to low oxygen tensions increases erythropoiesis whereas hyperoxia reverses this. The glycoprotein hormone erythropoietin stimulates erythropoiesis and its production in the kidney is sensitive to changes in pO_2. Erythropoietin binds to a cell surface receptor in erythroid progenitor cells in bone marrow.

Atrial natriuretic factor

Atrial natriuretic factor (ANF) is a small peptide that is synthesised in cardiocytes in the right atrium. It has actions at several sites including the kidney, where it increases sodium excretion and inhibits renin secretion. The latter effect will lead to decreased activity of the renin–angiotensin system, lower aldosterone secretion and, again, increased sodium excretion. It also inhibits ADH secretion from the posterior pituitary. The sum of these actions is to counteract any increase in the sodium and water content of the body. It also acts on peripheral resistance arteries by a mechanism involving a receptor with innate guanylate cyclase activity. The resulting increase in cyclic GMP leads to phosphorylation of key proteins.

18.10 Mechanisms of hormone action

All hormones influence processes in the body by interacting with protein receptors located in target tissues. Since each hormone has a unique chemical structure it should be obvious that a receptor must recognise that unique structure: binding elicits a signal that is trans-

duced in the target cell. The two major sub-groups of hormones – water soluble and lipid soluble – generate signals that are quite distinct from one another and have receptors that are in the cell plasma membrane or within the cell, respectively.

Transduction of signals from water-soluble hormones

There are three types of signal transduction systems known:

- cyclic AMP
- inositol phosphates and diacylglycerol (DAG)
- tyrosine kinase family of receptors.

Cyclic 3′,5′-AMP

The discovery of a *second messenger* in the transduction of signals from adrenaline and glucagon was a major advance in understanding the transmission of signals within cells. The compound was an adenine nucleotide called adenosine 3′,5′-monophosphate (Fig. 161), otherwise known as cyclic AMP. It is produced by the action of the enzyme *adenylate cyclase* on ATP. Cyclic AMP activates a protein kinase (protein kinase A (PKA)) by binding to and removing inhibitory subunits of the enzyme, thus liberating the active catalytic subunits. PKA then phosphorylates hydroxyls on serine or threonine in certain proteins leading to dramatic changes in their activities. For example, the binding of adrenaline to β-adrenoceptors on skeletal muscle leads to an increase in cyclic AMP, activation of PKA and

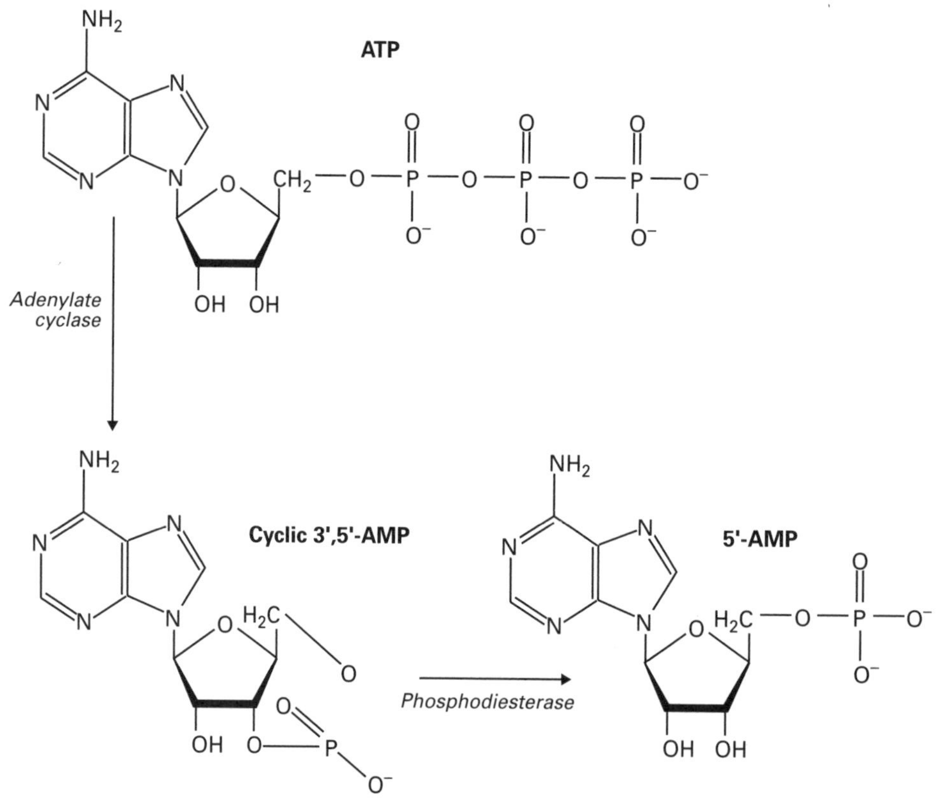

Fig. 161 Cyclic AMP production and metabolism.

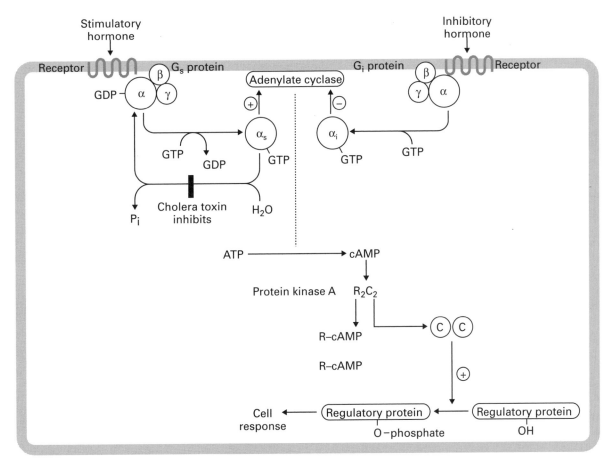

Fig. 162 The cyclic AMP (cAMP) signal transduction pathway.

phosphorylation and activation of phosphorylase kinase; this then converts inactive phosphorylase *b* to active phosphorylase *a* with a resultant increase in glycogenolysis in muscle (p. 95). A similar series of events are associated with the activation of liver phosphorylase by the action of glucagon. Cyclic AMP levels are returned to basal levels by the action of a phosphodiesterase (PDE), which converts the cyclic AMP to AMP (Fig. 161).

The transmission of the signal from the hormone outside the cell to the adenylate cyclase inside the cell involves G-proteins. Following binding of certain hormones to their receptors, GTP binds to the alpha subunit of the G-protein (G_s) causing it to dissociate. The $G_{s\alpha}$-GTP binds to adenylate cyclase, leading to its activation. The signal transduction pathway is shown in Figure 162. Also shown is the switch-off pathway involving a GTPase activity, also present in the $G_{s\alpha}$ subunit.

Other hormones bind to receptors that are linked to a related G-protein, G_i, which suppresses adenylate cyclase activity and thus reduces cyclic AMP levels in target tissues. The mechanism is similar to that seen with G_s in that when the hormone binds to receptor GTP displaces GDP from G_i and $G_{i\alpha}$-GTP dissociates from the $\beta\gamma$ subunits and binds to adenylate cyclase, leading to its inhibition (Fig. 162). The $G_{i\alpha}$, like the $G_{s\alpha}$ subunit, has GTPase activity which is involved in switching off this system. One example of such a

BOX 18.1
Clinical note: Cholera toxin

Further insight into the details of the pathway involving G_s comes from studies with cholera toxin, the agent in cholera patients that causes massive loss of sodium and water and diarrhoea. Cholera toxin in cells of the gastrointestinal tract uses NAD^+ to bring about the ADP-ribosylation of the $G_{s\alpha}$ subunit, leading to inhibition of its GTPase. As a result, G_s is permanently activated and large amounts of cyclic AMP are formed and maintained, leading to the gut changes.

hormone is somatostatin interacting with α_2-adrenoceptors. For inhibitory hormones to have an effect, G_s must already be activated by a stimulatory hormone.

Clearly, cyclic AMP is a very significant second messenger and its action will depend upon the specific characteristics of the cell in which it is produced. Although most of the initial studies on its effects have related to phosphorylation/dephosphorylation of key enzymes in metabolic pathways, it is also involved in the control of gene expression. That mechanism involves a transcription factor – cyclic AMP response element binding protein (CREB) – which becomes active upon phosphorylation by PKA and which can bind to a DNA promoter sequence (CRE). Altered gene expression

BOX 18.2
Clinical note: Pertussis toxin

Further insight into the G_i pathway has come from the study of the action of pertussis toxin, the active agent produced by Bordetella pertussis involved in whooping cough. Pertussis toxin can ADP-ribosylate the $G_{i\alpha}$ subunit but only when in its GDP-bound inactive state. GTP cannot exchange for GDP and the net effect is to increase cyclic AMP levels. When this occurs in the respiratory tract, there is excessive secretion of fluid from cells of the airways.

results, leading to the transcription of genes containing such CRE sequences.

It is the balance between adenylate cyclase forming cyclic AMP and phosphodiesterase activity breaking it down that will determine metabolic activity in a target cell (Fig. 161). Drugs present in tea and coffee, theophylline and caffeine, are inhibitors of cyclic AMP phosphodiesterase and they have significant effects upon body functions such as cardiac output and renal diuresis.

Inositol phosphates and diacylglycerol
Several hormones act by changing the intracellular calcium ion concentration, leading to the activation of protein kinase C (PKC). One way in which this occurs is by activation of phosphoinositide-specific phospholipase C (PI-PLC) following binding of such a hormone to its receptor with, in some cases, another G-protein, G_q, functioning in the pathway. The substrate for PI-PLC action is phosphatidyl inositol bisphosphate (PIP$_2$), a phospholipid present in the inner layer of the phospholipid bilayer that makes up the plasma membrane. The products are diacylglycerol (DAG) and inositol 1,4,5-trisphosphate (IP$_3$) (Fig. 163), which act as second messengers (Fig. 164). IP$_3$ causes the release of calcium that is sequestered in the endoplasmic reticulum. This leads to activation of several systems including those involving calmodulin (e.g. phosphorylase kinase). DAG is an activator of PKC, which brings about the phosphorylation of serine and threonine residues in other key proteins (that are not substrates for PKA). Examples of hormones that act through this signal transduction mechanism are angiotensin II, controlling aldosterone secretion in the adrenal cortex; TRH, controlling TSH secretion from the anterior pituitary; and adrenaline, acting through α_1-adrenoceptors to control glycogenolysis in the liver (in muscle adrenaline acts through cyclic AMP–PKA systems). Several products of IP$_3$ metabolism have biological activity.

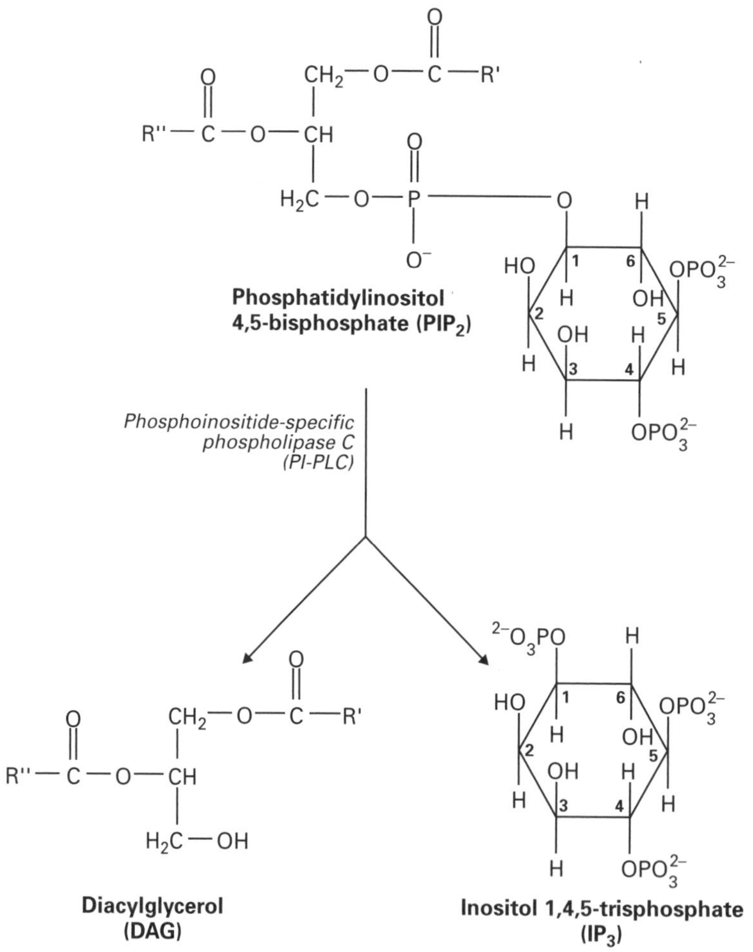

Fig. 163 Generation of two second messengers from PIP$_2$.

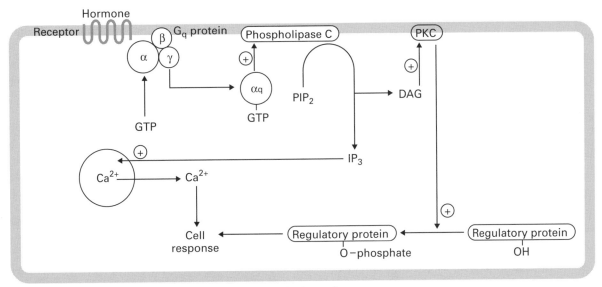

Fig. 164 The inositol phosphate, diacylglycerol signal transduction pathway.

BOX 18.3
Clinical note: Lithium inhibition of IP$_3$ metabolism

Some of the IP$_3$ metabolising enzymes are inhibited by lithium; this may explain how it acts in the treatment of dementia.

The tyrosine kinase family of receptors

A third type of signal transduction system is involved with the action of insulin and various growth factors on target cells. The insulin receptor structure is shown in Figure 165. The activation of tyrosine kinase activity in the receptor that follows binding of insulin is followed by phosphorylation of many systems in complex signalling pathways that involve the inositol phosphate metabolites. The end result in the case of insulin action on glycogen metabolism in liver and muscle is dephosphorylation of both glycogen synthetase and phosphorylase kinase (p. 95), resulting in activation and inhibition, respectively. In cardiac muscle the important action is activation of PFK-1 and, therefore, increased ATP production.

Other growth factors include:

- insulin-like growth factor I (IGF-1): the mediator of growth hormone action on cartilage
- epidermal growth factor (EGF): stimulates growth of epidermal and epithelial cells
- platelet-derived growth factor (PDGF): stimulates growth of mesenchymal and glial cells
- transforming growth factor alpha (TGFα): related to EGF.

There is great interest in growth factors given the fact that several oncogene products are growth factors.

Transduction of signals from lipid-soluble hormones

Thyroid and steroid hormones are lipid soluble and are able to enter many if not all cells in the body and influence their function. Their intracellular receptors are members of a super family of nuclear receptors. The C-terminal regions, which show the greatest heterology, are the hormone-binding domain of these receptors. The DNA-binding domain of the receptor consists of two zinc fingers and is highly conserved; for example, the sequence of the glucocorticoid receptor in this region differs only in three residues from that of the mineralocorticoid receptor (Table 31). The N-terminal domain of these receptors is rather variable.

Having entered a target cell, these hormones bind to

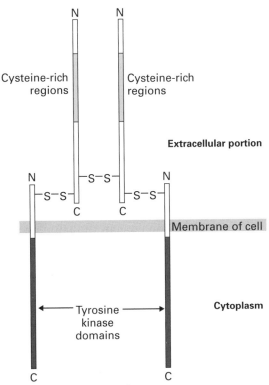

Fig. 165 Topology of the insulin receptor.

Table 31 The nuclear receptor superfamily

Receptor for	Homology compared with the glucocorticoid receptor	
	DNA-binding domain	Ligand-binding domain
Mineralocorticoids (MR)	94	57
Progesterone (PR)	90	55
Androgens (AR)	77	50
Oestrogens (ER)	52	30
Thyroid hormones (T_3R)	47	17
Calcitriol (VDR)	42	<15
Retinoic acid (RAR)	45	15

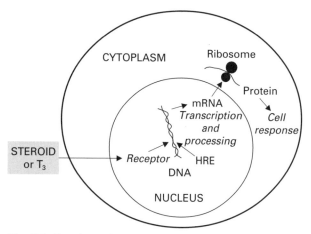

Fig. 166 Signal transduction steroid and thyroid hormones.

cytosolic- or nuclear-located receptors which are associated with chaperone proteins (Fig. 166). In the absence of hormone, the chaperones maintain the receptors in an inactive state. Binding of hormone dissociates this complex and the hormone–receptor complex binds to specific DNA sequences termed hormone-response elements (HRE), which are about 15 base pairs long with a partial palindromic sequence. The outcome is transcription of specific genes and synthesis of specific proteins that bring about the physiological effect of the hormone in question.

It is of interest that cortisol (a glucocorticoid) and aldosterone both bind efficiently to the mineralocorticoid receptor (MR) in kidney. Given the fact that the circulating cortisol concentration far exceeds that of aldosterone, the question must be asked will the receptor not always be fully occupied by cortisol and, therefore, never be responsive to aldosterone. The answer is that in aldosterone target tissues such as the kidney, the receptor is protected by an enzyme, *11β-hydroxysteroid dehydrogenase type II*, which metabolises any cortisol to its inactive metabolite, cortisone.

Other messenger systems

Surprisingly, it has been shown that the gas nitric oxide (NO) is an intercellular messenger; it is of particular importance in the blood vessels where it influences their dilation. NO is released by endothelial cells under the influence of changes in intracellular calcium levels. Nitroglycerine, a substance used to alleviate the pain caused by insufficient blood flow to heart muscle (angina), acts as a vasodilator with the mediator being NO. NO is produced by the action of the enzyme *NO synthase* using arginine as substrate, the product being citrulline. Guanylate cyclase is activated by NO and, as a result, cyclic GMP levels increase. Cyclic GMP stimulates a cyclic GMP-dependent protein kinase that brings about relaxation of smooth muscle.

Self-assessment: questions

Multiple choice questions

1. The following statements describe the endocrine system:
   a. Insulin, TSH, cortisol and thyroxine are all very water soluble
   b. Hormones involved in the control of calcium metabolism in the body are all made and secreted from the parathyroid glands
   c. The two major hormones involved in controlling fuel balance in the body are made and secreted from the islets of Langerhans
   d. Both exocrine and endocrine glands are ductless
   e. The circadian rhythm that occurs for many hormones produced in the body is important evidence for neuroendocrine control of the adenohypophysis

2. The following statements describe hormones:
   a. TRH (thyrotrophin-releasing hormone) is synthesised from a large precursor that contains multiple copies of TRH
   b. ACTH is derived from pro-opiomelanocortin (POMC)
   c. Oestrogen treatment of a normal adult will lead to large increases in free T_4 and free cortisol levels in blood
   d. The beta subunits of TSH, LH and FSH are homologous
   e. α-MSH is part of ACTH

3. The following statements describe transport of hormones:
   a. Thyroid hormones have receptors on the plasma membrane of target cells
   b. Peptide hormones are transported in blood bound to carrier proteins
   c. High concentrations of steroid hormones are stored in tissues such as the adrenal cortex and gonads
   d. Peptide hormones are not usually subjected to extraglandular activation
   e. Steroid hormones and thyroid hormones are very water soluble

4. The following statements describe thyroid function:
   a. Thyroglobulin is the plasma protein that transports T_4 and T_3 to their target tissues
   b. Reverse T_3 is (more or less) biologically inactive
   c. The thyroid gland is capable of taking up iodide from blood by an active process and then iodinating tyrosyl residues in thyroglobulin
   d. T_3 is the major thyroid hormone found in thyroglobulin

   e. Only a very small percentage of circulating T_3 and T_4 is not protein bound

5. As a result of direct feedback control:
   a. In patients with hyperthyroidism caused by a circulating antibody that binds to the TSH receptor, circulating levels of TSH will be significantly below normal levels
   b. A large dose of cortisol will suppress both CRH and ACTH in a normal subject
   c. Infusion of large amounts of glucose into a normal subject will result in decreased secretion of insulin
   d. Progesterone and testosterone both directly stimulate the secretion of LH
   e. Growth hormone levels are not reduced by negative feedback

6. In the adrenal cortex:
   a. Aldosterone secretion is decreased indirectly by hypernatraemia
   b. The zona reticularis is the principal source of adrenal cortisol production
   c. The zona glomerulosa lacks steroid 17α-hydroxylase and, therefore, cannot make cortisol or androgens
   d. Corticosteroid-binding globulin (CBG) levels are suppressed by androgen treatment
   e. Steroids must have an 11β-hydroxyl group to be active as glucocorticoids

7. In the endocrine control of plasma calcium ion levels:
   a. A falling plasma concentration of calcium ions raises the secretion of PTH from the parathyroids
   b. PTH increases the rate of calcium reabsorption by the kidneys
   c. PTH decreases the production of calcitriol
   d. PTH increases the rate at which calcium is exchanged from bone into plasma
   e. PTH receptors are present on the plasma membranes of kidney tubule cells and osteocytes

8. Upon binding of glucagon, the glucagon receptor affects its target cell metabolism by:
   a. Causing autophosphorylation of some of its own tyrosyl residues
   b. Interacting directly with the cell's transcriptional machinery
   c. Causing the alpha subunit of the membrane-bound complex G_s to be dissociated
   d. Causing the membrane-bound complex G_i to be dissociated

e. Interacting directly with adenylate cyclase to increase cyclic AMP levels in the cell

9. Steroid hormone receptors:
   a. Have structural features in common with receptors for thyroid hormones
   b. Have a molecular domain that can recognise specific nucleotide sequences in control genes
   c. Are located in the plasma membrane of their target cells
   d. Are relatively specific in their ability to bind only steroid hormones of a particular class (e.g. oestrogens, glucocorticoids, etc.)

True/false questions

Are the following statements true or false?

1. Destruction of the adrenal cortex in a subject (leading to primary hypoadrenocorticism) will result in pigmentation, which is a useful clinical sign.
2. LH and FSH are controlled by the same hypothalamic releasing hormone.
3. In normal subjects, aldosterone secretion is increased by either sodium depletion or potassium loading.
4. Inositol 1,4,5-trisphosphate (IP_3) and diacylglycerol are hormonal second messengers produced when phospholipase C acts upon the membrane phosphatidyl inositol 4,5-bisphosphate (PIP_2).
5. An early consequence of the binding of insulin to its receptor is the phosphorylation of tyrosine residues in the receptor, which enables specific enzymes to bind to the receptor and become activated.

6. Erythropoietin production by the kidney is increased by a low pO_2 in the blood supply to the kidney.
7. Cholera toxin interferes with the function of both G_s and G_i.
8. ADH secretion is inhibited in normal subjects by water loading.
9. Pregnenolone is the precursor of aldosterone, cortisol and cholecalciferol.
10. Oestrogen production from androgen in Sertoli cells involves the formation of an aromatic ring.
11. Cortisol inhibits the expression of the PNMT (phenylethanolamine N-methyl transferase) gene in the adrenal medulla.
12. The insulin receptor and the adrenaline β-adrenoceptor have similar structures and employ similar signal transduction mechanisms.
13. Atrial natriuretic factor (ANF) stimulates aldosterone secretion.

Short essay questions

1. Give an outline of how steroid hormones are synthesised in the body.
2. Describe possible causes for a newborn child having elevated levels of thyroid-stimulating hormone (TSH) in its blood.
3. Write short notes on each of the following
   a. pertussis toxin
   b. diacylglycerol (DAG)
   c. phosphodiesterase
   d. hormone-response element.
4. Outline the role of the skin, kidney and lung in the endocrine system.

Self-assessment: answers

Multiple choice answers

1. a. **False.** Cortisol and T_4 have limited water solubility and are classified as lipophilic hormones.
    b. **False.** Calcitriol is made in the kidney and calcitonin in the thyroid gland.
    c. **True.** These are insulin and glucagon.
    d. **False.** The exocrine glands are ducted.
    e. **True.** Clearly, a circadian rhythm in a hormone such as ACTH cannot be explained on the basis of negative feedback control and the hypothalamus and higher centres in the brain are involved.

2. a. **True.** Normal protein synthetic machinery is involved, coupled with post-translational modification.
    b. **True.** β-Endorphin is another product of POMC processing.
    c. **False.** Total T_4 and cortisol will increase as a result of an increase in plasma globulins binding these hormones (TBG and CBG) brought about by high oestrogen. However, free hormone levels are normal.
    d. **False.** It is the alpha subunits that are homologous. Variations between the beta subunits confers hormone specificity.
    e. **True.** α-MSH is the first 13 residues of ACTH.

3. a. **False.** Since they are lipid-soluble, thyroid hormones enter cells and react with nuclear receptors.
    b. **False.** Since they are water-soluble, carrier proteins are not required.
    c. **False.** Steroid hormones are made 'on demand'.
    d. **True.** Their extraglandular metabolism usually results in inactivation.
    e. **False.** They are poorly water soluble.

4. a. **False.** Thyroglobulin is involved in thyroid hormone synthesis. TBG is the transport protein.
    b. **True.** It is produced at the expense of T_3 when it is necessary to lower the BMR (e.g. in starvation).
    c. **True.** It is the only tissue in the body where iodination occurs.
    d. **False.** T_4 is the major thyroid hormone in thyroglobulin. Most T_3 is made extrathyroidally.
    e. **True.** Most of T_4 (99.97%) and T_3 (99.7%) is protein bound.

5. a. **True.** The high levels of T_4 and T_3 will suppress TRH and TSH.
    b. **True.** This is classic negative feedback control.
    c. **False.** Insulin secretion will increase to stimulate glucose uptake and storage.
    d. **False.** Both hormones inhibit LH; again this is negative feedback.
    e. **False.** Growth hormone increases IGF-1 production and it feeds back to inhibit GH secretion by stimulating somatostatin and inhibiting GHRH secretion.

6. a. **True.** Hypernatraemia will inhibit renin secretion leading to decreased angiotensin II levels and, therefore, lower aldosterone secretion.
    b. **False.** The zona fasciculata is the principal source of cortisol. The ZR makes mainly DHEA or DHEA sulphate.
    c. **True.** ZG cells do lack 17-hydroxylase but have aldosterone synthase allowing them to make aldosterone.
    d. **True.** This is the opposite effect to that seen with oestrogens.
    e. **True.** Because of that, cortisone per se is inactive as a glucocorticoid while cortisol is active. The inactivation of cortisol in the kidney (by conversion to cortisone) is vital to the action of aldosterone to control sodium balance.

7. a. **True.** The system is quite sensitive and the response prevents hypocalcaemia.
    b. **True.** This assists in returning blood calcium levels to normal if they have been low and PTH secretion has increased.
    c. **False.** Calcitriol production increases and it stimulates calcium absorption in the gut.
    d. **True.** By so doing, this increases blood calcium (and phosphate).
    e. **True.** Obviously, PTH receptors will be present in kidney tubules. In bone, it is the osteocytes where they are located rather than osteoclasts (despite the observation that osteoclastic activity is increased by PTH).

8. a. **False.** That describes insulin mechanism of action.
    b. **False.** All actions are via a second messenger.
    c. **True.** This leads to activation of adenylate cyclase and an increase in cyclic AMP.
    d. **False.** It acts through G_s.
    e. **False.** It acts via a G protein system (G_s).

9. a. **True.** The homology is especially high in the DNA-binding domain of the receptor.
    b. **True.** This is the DNA-binding domain.

c. **False.** They are in the cytosol or nucleus of target cells.

d. **True.** Their specificity resides in the hormone-binding domains, which have much reduced homologies.

True/false answers

1. **True.** The inability to synthesise cortisol leads to high secretion of ACTH and it has MSH activity.
2. **True.** Despite a long search for unique separate releasing hormones for LH and FSH, GnRH appears to function for both.
3. **True.** Aldosterone action is critical to the fine control of both electrolytes.
4. **True.** Calcium plays a vital role in the mechanism of action of hormones that work through DAG and IP_3.
5. **True.** This is termed 'autophosphorylation'.
6. **True.** This is an attempt to compensate for low pO_2 by increasing red cell production.
7. **False.** Cholera toxin acts through preventing the inactivation of $G_{s\alpha}$.
8. **True.** This enables water to be excreted in greater amounts to compensate.
9. **False.** Pregnenolone is the precursor of aldosterone and cortisol but it is 7-dehydrocholesterol which is the precursor of cholecalciferol (vitamin D).
10. **True.** Oestrogens are the only steroid hormones with aromatic A rings.
11. **False.** Cortisol induces PNMT by increasing transcription of the PNMT gene.
12. **False.** Both receptors are in plasma membranes but are quite distinct structurally.
13. **False.** ANF is part of the system that opposes aldosterone.

Short essay answers

1. The key points are:
   a. cholesterol (C_{27}) is the precursor of all steroid hormones
   b. steroid hormone-producing tissues receive the cholesterol from plasma LDL through receptor-mediated endocytosis
   c. the initial and rate-controlling reaction is the cleavage of six carbons from the side chain of cholesterol to give pregnenolone. The enzyme involved is cholesterol side-chain cleavage cytochrome P-450 (P-450$_{scc}$), a member of a large gene family
   d. the steroid hormone pathways from pregnenolone then vary according to tissue and cell type
   e. in order for cortisol and androgen to be made, 17α-hydroxylase has to be present. In the *adrenal cortex* that activity is restricted to the zonae fasciculata and reticularis, with the former making cortisol, the chief glucocorticoid in the

body, and the latter making mainly dehydroepiandrosterone (DHEA) and its sulphate
   f. 17-hydroxypregnenolone is the precursor of DHEA, which can be converted to testosterone and other androgens; testosterone is made in the *granulosa cells* of the ovary and *Leydig cells* of the testes
   g. in the *Sertoli cells* of the testes and the granulosa cells of the ovary, androgens such as testosterone are aromatised to give oestrogens
   h. in the *zona glomerulosa* of the adrenal cortex, 17-hydroxylase is absent but there is another cytochrome P-450 – aldosterone synthase – that accounts for that zone's ability to make aldosterone, the principal mineralocorticoid in the body
   i. in the *corpus luteum* and in the placenta, pregnenolone is converted to progesterone, which has important effects upon the uterus and is necessary for the maintenance of pregnancy
   j. the rate-controlling cholesterol side-chain cleavage step is controlled by different hormones in different tissues: ACTH controls it in the zonae fasciculata and reticularis of the adrenal; angiotensin II controls it in the zona glomerulosa of the adrenal; LH controls it in ovarian thecal cells and Leydig cells of the testes
   k. the cytochromes P-450 that catalyse the hydroxylation reactions involved in steroidogenesis use molecular oxygen and have a requirement for NADPH.

2. The very high levels of TSH are diagnostic of primary hypothyroidism. The thyroid is defective in its ability to make T_4. The molecular basis can be defects in any of the steps of thyroid hormone biosynthesis. The consequence is that TRH and TSH from the hypothalamus and pituitary, respectively, are secreted in increased amounts. Given the fact that these infants have low thyroid hormone levels and the role that T_4 plays in growth and development, it becomes important for them to start therapy with replacement T_4 as soon as possible. For that reason, and given the fact that they are normal at birth because of the T_4 they have obtained from their mothers, all newborn children should be screened for hypothyroidism by having their TSH measured.

3. a. **Pertussis toxin.** This is the toxin produced by the *Bordetella pertussis*, the bacterium that causes whooping cough. It alters the $G_{i\alpha}$ subunit of the G_1 regulatory protein by a process known as ADP-ribosylation. The altered $G_{1\alpha}$ cannot exchange GTP for GDP and adenylate cyclase is not inhibited in normal fashion. The end result is enhanced secretion of mucus in various parts of the lung.

b. **Diacylglycerol (DAG).** This is one of the products of phospholipase A_2 action in the plasma membrane on phosphatidyl inositol 4,5-bisphosphate. This hydrolysis participates in the response to several hormones. DAG activates protein kinase C, which, in turn, catalyses the phosphorylation of multiple proteins in target tissues for hormones operating by this mechanism.

c. **Phosphodiesterase (PDE).** This enzyme is critical to terminating the response to a hormone whose action is mediated by cyclic 3',5'-AMP. It does so by hydrolysing cyclic AMP to 5'-AMP and inorganic phosphate. Clearly cyclic AMP levels in cells are influenced by the relative activities of PDE and adenylate cyclase. The mechanism of action of many hormones involves cyclic AMP and PDE can be considered to be involved in 'switching off' the response of the cell to the hormone in question. Caffeine and related compounds are inhibitors of PDE.

d. **Hormone-response element (HRE).** HREs are part of the regulatory DNA region involved in the action of steroid and thyroid hormones (and others) on the transcription of genes in target tissues. This element binds a hormone–receptor complex and is usually located a few hundred nucleotides upstream from the transcription initiation site.

4. **Skin.** Vitamin D (cholecalciferol) is synthesised in skin by the action of ultraviolet light on 7-dehydrocholesterol. Cholecalciferol is the precursor of 25-hydroxycholecalciferol (made in the liver), which in turn is converted to the hormone calcitriol in the kidney as part of the defence against hypocalcaemia.

Kidney. The kidney produces several endocrine factors:

- *erythropoietin* (EP) is synthesised in the kidney in response to low oxygen tension in blood. The increased red cell synthesis that occurs, stimulated by EP, accounts for the polycythaemia observed in individuals who live at high altitude.
- *calcitriol* is synthesised in the kidney from 25-hydroxycholecalciferol, stimulated by parathyroid hormone (PTH). PTH is secreted in increased amounts in response to hypocalcaemia. Calcitriol contributes to restoring calcium in blood by increasing calcium absorption in the gut.
- *renin* is produced in the kidney in response to decreased pulsing pressure through the renal artery and/or reduced filtered sodium. Its role is to produce angiotensin I from angiotensinogen in blood; the angiotensin I is converted to angiotensin II, which by increasing aldosterone production causes increased sodium reabsorption.

The kidney is also the target for several hormones and responds by altering its activity.

The kidney is a target for *PTH*, with the response being increased calcitriol formation, increased calcium reabsorption and increased phosphate excretion.

The kidney is also a target for *antidiuretic hormone* (ADH), where the response is to increase water reabsorption.

The kidney is the site of action of *aldosterone*, the response being increased sodium reabsorption and increased potassium excretion.

Atrial natriuretic factor (ANF) is part of the system that responds to increased blood pressure and volume. It inhibits renin release from the kidney, reducing aldosterone production and sodium reabsorption in the kidney.

Lungs. Converting enzyme, which catalyses the conversion of angiotensin I to angiotensin II, is localised to the lung. ACE inhibitors are effective in the treatment of various forms of hypertension where angiotensin II levels should be lowered.

Nutrition

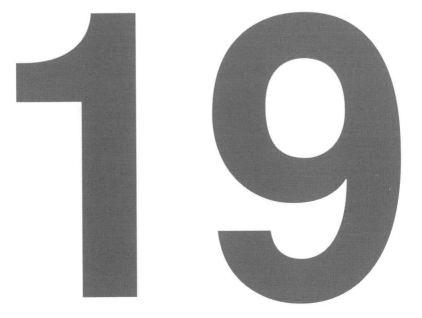

19

19.1 General aspects

It is essential that you have a knowledge of functional nutrition and this should include knowing the nutrients in the food that we eat and how they contribute to our well-being, growth and health. Important nutrition issues relate to (a) growth and development (b) the relationship between excess fat and coronary heart disease and diabetes mellitus (c) pregnancy (d) malnutrition.

A major impetus for the study of body composition in the population as a whole is the relationship between it and mortality. Body weight and height are the most commonly used parameters related to body composition and the term *body mass index* (BMI) is weight in kilograms divided by square of the height in metres. Normal ranges have been established for adult males (20–25) and women (18–24) and it is clear that values about 20% above or below this range are associated with increased relative mortality. Of particular concern in developed countries is the increased mortality seen in those who are obese, i.e. have a very large amount of body fat. The following are some of the principal facts and questions related to body composition.

- It is important to be able to determine how much fat a subject has. Lean body mass is calculated by methods that measure the gamma rays emitted by the naturally occurring potassium isotope (^{40}K) or by measuring neutron-activated ^{15}N. Total body water is measured by administering deuterium-labelled water and measuring it in body fluids.
- Given the fact that fat tissue ($0.9 \, \text{g/cm}^3$) is less dense than lean tissue ($1.1 \, \text{g/cm}^3$), a measure of body fat can be obtained by measuring body density. Weight is easy to measure and body volume is obtained by weighing a person in air and water with the differences in kilograms being the volume in litres (this is Archimedes' principle). Another way to gain information on the extent of body fat is to measure skinfold thickness at various sites in the body using skinfold callipers.
- Average data for a 70 kg man is 17% adipose tissue, 45% lean body mass, 25% extracellular water and 13% extracellular solids. However, if one calculates the energy stored in adipose tissue, it is about 100-fold greater than the energy stored in the lean body tissue. The values for fat, carbohydrate and protein are about 440, 4.3 and 34 MJ, respectively, in a 70 kg person.
- Changes occur during life: adults compared with newborn have a lower percentage of their body as brain, skin and abdominal viscera but show an increase in muscle and bone. The human fetus is quite lean and there are big increases in fat and protein late in fetal development: premature babies have many problems because of this late development, with the lower protein levels being especially critical. Less protein means fewer enzymes and less metabolic activity.

19.2 Nutrient requirements

There are six essential nutrients that must be included in our daily diet:

- carbohydrates
- proteins
- fats (lipids)
- water
- vitamins
- minerals.

Carbohydrates, fats and proteins are the major nutrients (fuels) in our diet and in the body. Carbohydrates and fats are the principal sources of energy but proteins can also be used and are especially important during fasting.

The dietary fuels

Carbohydrates

Carbohydrates should provide 50–60% of the energy in the typical Western diet. Most of the carbohydrates we eat should be in the form of *complex carbohydrates* such as starch. Dietary carbohydrate also has a protein-sparing action that is significant especially in undeveloped countries. Other complex carbohydrate known as dietary fibre is also present in our diet and there is evidence that it is beneficial in reducing the incidence of diverticular disease of the colon, cancer of the colon and coronary heart disease. Another major dietary carbohydrate is *sucrose*. Overindulgence in sucrose can cause dental caries, probably because bacteria living in the mouth efficiently use the glucose moiety to make dextrans, sticky polysaccharides that adhere to the teeth, building up dental plaque. High sucrose intake is also implicated in heart disease. Lactose, the disaccharide sugar found in milk, is the third significant dietary carbohydrate. Although it is very well handled in infants and young children, many people in Asia, Africa and South America have the tendency to develop lactose intolerance owing to falling levels of lactase in the gut (Box 7.1, p. 74).

Fat

Fat contributes 35–40% of the total calorie intake in a typical Western diet but the long-term public health aim is to reduce that towards 30%. Fat has high energy value and when in our food has satiety value. It is the source of the essential fatty acids *linoleate* and *linolenate*, which are precursors of compounds such as prosta-glandins, thromboxanes, leukotrienes and prostacyclin (p. 130). Dietary fat consists mainly of triacylglycerol, but there can also be significant amounts of cholesterol as cholesteryl esters.

It is recognised that a high fat intake in Western society is correlated with an increased incidence of cardiovascular disease. Cholesterol is especially important (p. 128) but total fat is also a concern. Although smoking is the greatest risk factor in terms of cardiovascular disease, excess fat intake and excess weight (as fat tissue) are also significant risk factors, but not as problematic as presented in the popular press.

Table 32 The fat-soluble vitamins

Symbol	Name	Human disease	Intake (μg)	Source
A	Retinol	Blindness, abortion, defects in epithelium	750	Fish oils, liver, dairy products
D	Calciferol	Rickets	25	Fish oil, milk, eggs, action of sunlight on skin
E	Tocopherol	Infertility		Vegetable oils, milk, wheat germ
K	Phylloquinone	Bleeding (infants)		Gut flora, vegetable oils

Protein

Dietary proteins vary with diet. From a nutritional point of view it is vital that they contain an adequate complement of essential amino acids (p. 110) and that they are available in sufficient quantity to meet the protein synthesis requirements of the body. If a person's diet does not contain enough of each essential amino acid then that person will go into *negative nitrogen balance*, where more nitrogen is excreted than is ingested. Protein quality is an important concept describing whether or not a particular dietary protein provides all of the essential amino acids. Egg and milk proteins are very rich in essential amino acids. Meat proteins also have the full complement of essential amino acids. Plants contain less protein and one has to eat a lot of cereal if one is to satisfy the requirement for essential amino acids. Clearly, one should eat a mixed diet and avoid 'food fads'.

19.3 Micronutrient requirements

Human diseases are caused by vitamin deficiencies and even in developed countries vitamin deficiencies occur in vulnerable groups. Vulnerable groups need to receive special consideration in their diets (e.g. women for iron and calcium; children, pregnant women and lactating women for many vitamins and minerals; the elderly; post-surgical patients).

Vitamins

Vitamins are required to be present in our diet. There has been a long history describing disorders related to diets deficient in vitamins including reports from China around 2000 BC (beri-beri), Greece around 500 BC (night blindness).

Vitamins are divided into two categories depending upon their water solubility.

The fat-soluble vitamins (Table 32)

The absorption of the fat-soluble vitamins from the gut follows the same path as fat. They are stored mostly in the liver, although vitamin E is also stored in adipose tissue. Significant quantities are stored so that the manifestation of deficiencies is slower than for the water-soluble group of vitamins. Another consequence of storage is that excess intake can be toxic; this is well established for both vitamins A and D. The vitamin activity of each is not confined to a single substance. They are mainly heat stable.

Vitamin A

Vitamin A (retinol) is the most important of the fat-soluble vitamins (Fig. 167). It was the first to be discovered. We derive most of our vitamin A from β-carotene, which is present in carrots, spinach, broccoli and apricots. The other source is retinol (vitamin A), which is present in liver, fish oil, eggs, kidney and dairy products.

Transport and metabolism. Dietary retinoids are transported from the intestine as retinol esters in chylomicrons for storage in the liver. Transport from the liver is with the retinol bound to retinol-binding protein (RBP). RBP binds to transthyretin. In retinoid-dependent epithelial tissues, retinol binds to cellular retinol-binding protein (CRBP) and is converted to retinoic acid. As shown in Figure 167, retinol exists in three oxidation states: as an alcohol (retinol), an aldehyde (retinal) and as an acid (retinoic acid). Retinal is formed from retinol by a dehydrogenation reaction that is reversible. Retinoic acid is produced from retinal by oxidation and that reaction is irreversible.

Function. The best defined function of vitamin A is in the visual process (Fig. 168). Retinoic acid behaves like a steroid hormone. The retinoic acid receptor (RAR) is a member of the thyroid hormone/steroid hormone receptor super family (p. 232). Effects include roles in growth and differentiation of epithelial tissue. There are effects on steroid hormone biosynthesis, synthesis of glycosaminoglycans, gametogenesis and differentiation of keratinocytes.

Hypervitaminosis A. Excess intake of vitamin A causes loss of appetite, abnormal skin pigmentation, loss of hair and dryness of skin, pain in the long bones

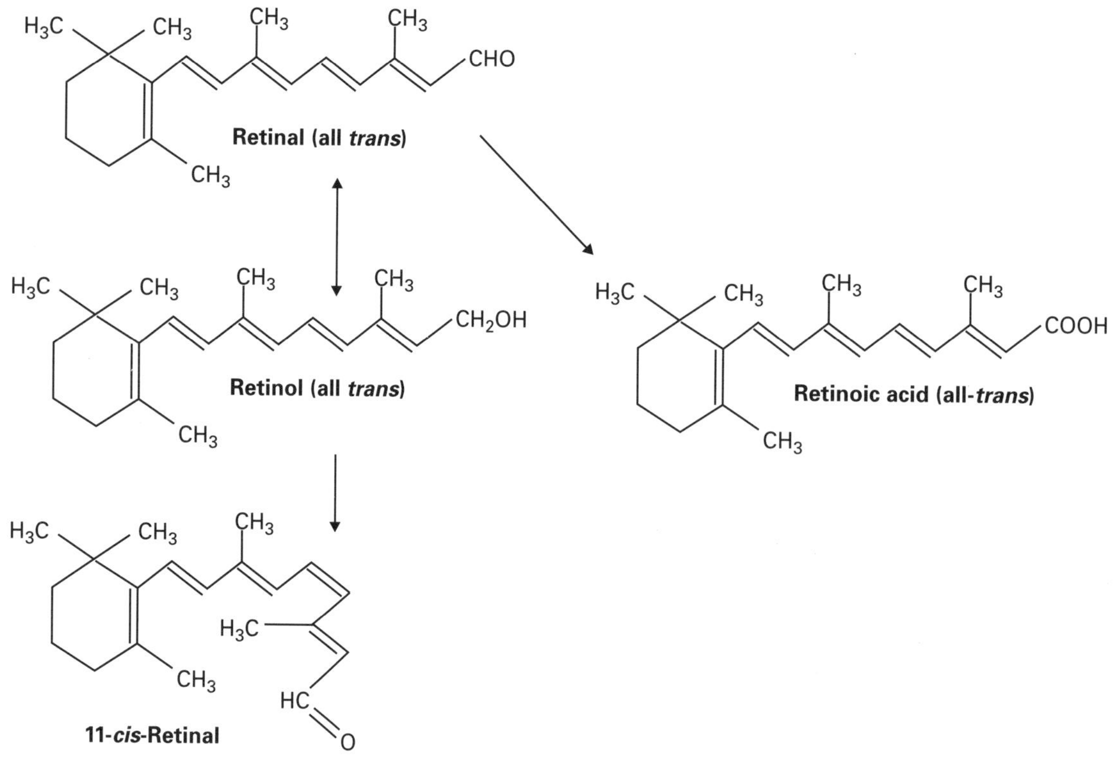

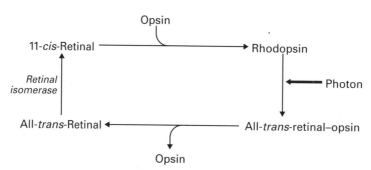

Fig. 167 Vitamin A forms. 11-*cis*-Retinal is the chromophore of rhodopsin, the photoreceptor of the rod outer segments in the eye.

Fig. 168 Retinal and the visual cycle.

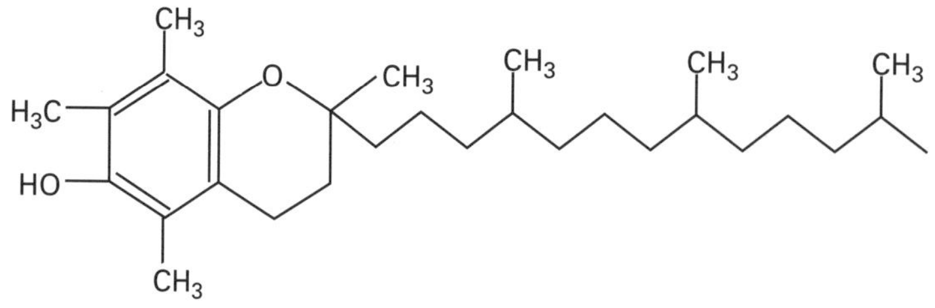

Fig. 169 The structure of α-tocopherol (vitamin E).

and bone fragility and very high doses (as found in polar bear liver) are lethal.

Vitamin E

The chief role of vitamin E (α-tocopherol, Fig. 169) is to participate in the protection of cells against oxygen free radicals. It is an anti-oxidant and functions in a complex system that includes the trace element selenium and the tripeptide glutathione. If our diet contains lots of polyunsaturated fatty acids (PUFA), then there is an increased demand for vitamin E. Under these conditions, a vitamin E deficiency results in haemolysis of red blood cells.

Vitamin K

Vitamin K is an anti-haemorrhagic factor (p. 256) since it is required as a coenzyme for the production of several of the blood coagulation factors, specifically prothrombin and factors VII, IX and X. Vitamin K is manufactured by colonic bacteria. A deficiency of vitamin K can occur

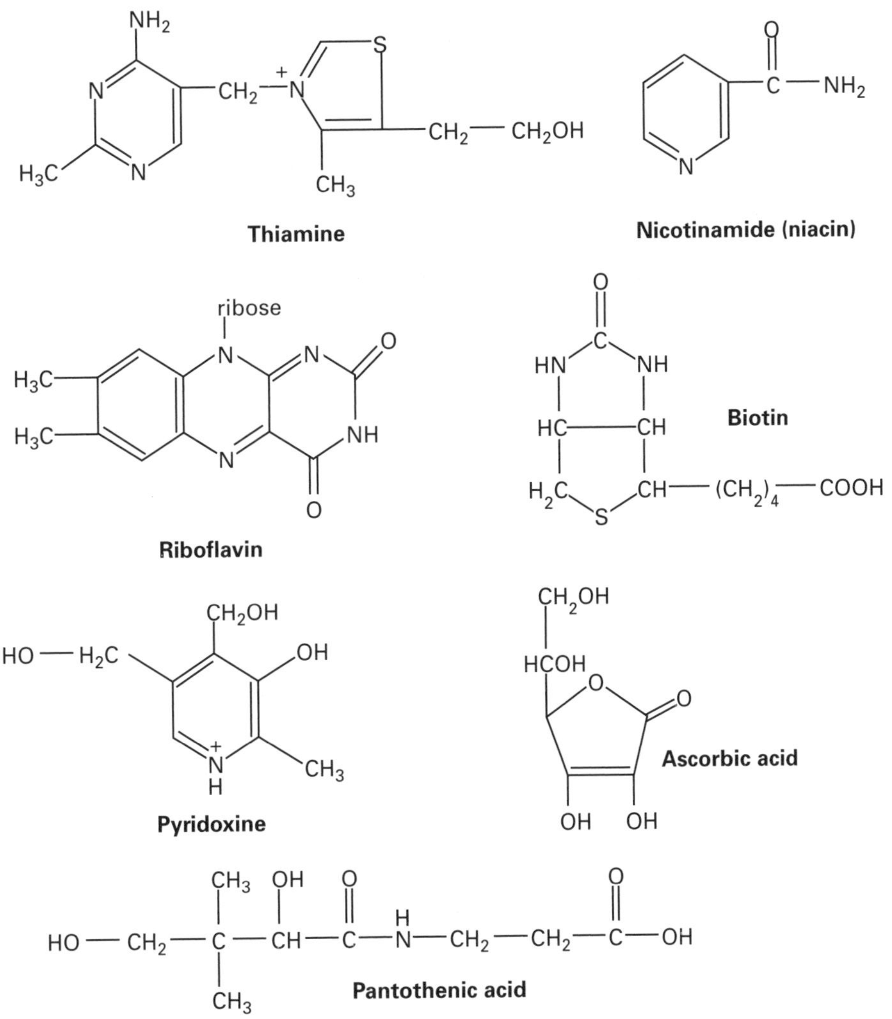

Fig. 170 The structure of some water-soluble vitamins.

in neonates, leading to haemorrhagic disease of the newborn. All newborn babies receive vitamin K as a preventive measure.

Vitamin D

Vitamin D is involved in the control of calcium metabolism in the body (pp. 226–227). It can be formed in skin that is exposed to UV light and is a pro-hormone, being the precursor of calcitriol.

The water-soluble vitamins

Many of the water-soluble vitamins are components of coenzymes or prosthetic groups for important enzymes in metabolism (Table 4, p. 72). Knowledge of the participation of specific vitamins in metabolism has practical (clinical) significance when one is treating subjects with inherited defects in critical pathways. Megadose vitamin therapy is a feature of many inborn errors of amino acid catabolism.

Thiamine, riboflavin, nicotinamide, pyridoxine, pantothenic acid and biotin are B vitamins and are widely distributed in foodstuffs. Folic acid is found in green leaves, vitamin B_{12} in liver and ascorbic acid (vitamin C) in fruits and vegetables. Structures of

several of the water-soluble vitamins are shown in Figure 170. Here is key information about the water-soluble vitamins:

Thiamine

Its coenzyme form is thiamine pyrophosphate (TPP), which is involved in several oxidative decarboxylation reactions including:

- the conversion of pyruvate to acetyl-CoA by the PDC
- the conversion of α-ketoglutarate to succinyl-CoA in the TCA cycle
- the metabolism of keto-acids derived from the three branched-chain amino acids
- it is also the coenzyme for transketolase in the pentose phosphate pathway
- because of its integral involvement in the metabolism of glucose and fatty acids, the daily requirements are linked to the total energy expenditure of any individual
- **deficiency** of thiamine leads to beri-beri.

The impairment of oxidative metabolism of glucose leads to altered nervous system and cardiac muscle function. Thiamine deficiency is not uncommon in alcoholics.

Nicotinamide (niacin)

Nicotinamide is found in the key coenzymes NAD^+, $NADP^+$, NADH and NADPH and, therefore:

- it is vital for oxidation-reduction reactions in metabolism catalysed by dehydrogenases
- the daily requirements are also linked to the total energy expenditure of any individual
- **deficiency** of nicotinamide (or nicotinic acid) leads to pellagra, where there are obvious skin lesions as well as cheilosis (cracked lips) and glossitis (inflamed tongue)
- **sources** of niacin are the diet but it is also formed from the amino acid tryptophan by a pathway that has several steps which are dependent upon adequate pyridoxine being present. Pellagra-like symptoms are occasionally seen in *Hartnup's disease*, an inherited disorder where tryptophan (and other neutral amino acids) absorption is impaired.

Vitamin B_2: riboflavin

Riboflavin is found in the prosthetic groups FAD and FMN, nucleotides which are:

- present in flavoprotein enzymes involved in oxidation–reduction reactions of intermediary metabolism
- involved in pyruvate and α-ketoglutarate dehydrogenase complexes, succinate dehydrogenase, fatty acyl-CoA dehydrogenase, the glycerol 3-phosphate shuttle and electron transport chain (FMN)
- **deficiency** of riboflavin affects epithelial tissues leading to cheilosis, angular stomatitis, glossitis and photophobia.

Vitamin B_6: pyridoxine

Pyridoxine exists in three oxidation states: pyridoxine (an alcohol), pyridoxal (an aldehyde) and pyridoxamine (an amine); all three are equally potent. It is as pyridoxal phosphate (PLP) that this vitamin participates in:

- essential enzymatic reactions of amino acid catabolism (Chapter 9) including transamination and decarboxylation
- glycogen phosphorylase where PLP is linked to it through the ε-amino group of a lysine.

Pantothenic acid

The importance of pantothenic acid becomes clear when one recognises the role of acetyl-CoA in intermediary metabolism. Pantothenate is also part of acyl carrier protein (ACP) involved in fatty acid synthesis (p. 123). Pantothenate contains a thiol group (derived from cysteine) through which acyl groups are bonded in both coenzyme A and ACP. Coenzyme A is involved in:

- pyruvate and α-ketoglutarate dehydrogenase complexes
- fatty acid beta-oxidation and fatty acid synthesis
- the catabolism of branched-chain amino acids
- **deficiency** of pantothenate is very rare.

Biotin

Biotin is the prosthetic group for four carboxylases that participate in critical pathways of intermediary metabolism, including:

- gluconeogenesis (pyruvate carboxylase)
- fatty acid synthesis (acetyl-CoA carboxylase)
- odd-numbered fatty acid oxidation (propionyl-CoA carboxylase)
- amino acid catabolism (propionyl-CoA carboxylase and β-methylcrotonyl-CoA carboxylase).

In these carboxylases, biotin is covalently attached through the ε-amino group of a lysine. Biotin is derived from the diet but is also made by gastrointestinal flora. Biotin deficiency in humans has been found only when diets included large amount of raw egg white. The latter contains a heat-labile glycoprotein, avidin, that binds biotin tightly. Rare disorders have been reported in enzymes of the biotin cycle, including failure to synthesise the biotinylated holocarboxylases.

Vitamin C: ascorbic acid

Vitamin C exists in two forms, ascorbic acid and dehydroascorbic acid.

Ascorbic acid is a donor of reducing equivalents and is critical for:

- the biosynthesis of collagen, where it is the coenzyme for both proline and lysyl hydroxylase
- wound healing and bone formation
- iron absorption in the gut since it is a reducing agent that can reduce ferric (Fe^{III}) iron in the diet to the absorbable ferrous iron (Fe^{II})
- the reaction catalysed by dopamine-β-hydroxylase in the catecholamine biosynthetic pathway.
- High concentrations are present in the adrenal cortex, where it may be important in preserving the cytochromes P-450 involved in steroid hormone biosynthesis.
- **Deficiency** leads to scurvy, an early sign of which is swollen bleeding gums.
- Diets that include fruits, fruit juice and vegetables provide the high levels that are consistent with good health.

Folic acid

Folate is a complex compound comprising a pteridine ring, *p*-aminobenzoic acid and one or more glutamic

---

BOX 19.2
Clinical note: Spina bifida

Evidence is accumulating that adequate folate intake by pregnant women can prevent spina bifida. The folate is required early in pregnancy to prevent neural tube defects. Adequate folate also may be beneficial in heart disease by lowering homocysteine levels.

acid residues. Tetrahydrofolate (FH_4) is the coenzyme derived from folate.

- The role of FH_4 is in one carbon metabolism (Chapter 9).
- **Deficiency** of folic acid results in megaloblastic anaemia owing to defects in stem cells.
- Folate is intimately involved with vitamin B_{12} (see later).
- Sulphonamide antibiotics work by inhibiting the incorporation of p-aminobenzoic acid (part of the folate structure) during bacterial folate synthesis.

Vitamin B_{12}: cobalamin

Vitamin B_{12} is the anti-pernicious anaemia factor. It has a complex structure that includes a haem-like corrin ring with four pyrroles; the pyrrole nitrogen atoms are bound to a central cobalt atom (hence the name cobalamin) and a side chain consisting of a phosphoribo-5,6-dimethylbenzimadozolyl group.

- It is synthesised by microorganisms and is found in meats, animal products and seafoods. It is not present in plants or yeasts and strict vegans may develop B_{12} deficiency and, therefore, anaemia.
- This anaemia is characterised by a macrocytic anaemia and is most commonly the result of defective absorption of vitamin B_{12} from the gut.
- B_{12} absorption requires the presence of a gastric secretory mucoprotein called *intrinsic factor*. This factor is secreted from the stomach where it binds vitamin B_{12} and then facilitates its absorption in the ileum.

Vitamin B_{12} is involved in only two reactions in the body:

- methyl-cobalamin is the coenzyme for homocysteine-methyltetrahydrofolate transferase. If vitamin B_{12} is deficient (or ineffective), then all of the folate taken in from the diet becomes trapped as methyl-tetrahydrofolate and is then unavailable for one-carbon metabolism and this impairs nucleotide synthesis
- adenosyl-cobalamin is the coenzyme for a mutase in the pathway from propionyl-CoA to succinyl-CoA. That pathway is involved in the catabolism of odd-numbered fatty acids and of the amino acids methionine, threonine, valine and isoleucine.

Folate is of use in the treatment of some of the symptoms of pernicious anaemia but it has no effect on the neurological symptoms. Indeed, its overuse by someone with pernicious anaemia may mask the neurological symptoms of that disorder.

Minerals

As well as energy, protein and vitamins, we require some other nutrients. The most obvious, apart from water, are the major structural elements: calcium, phosphorus, sodium, potassium and magnesium. Some of these elements are essential in structural components such as bones and teeth. Some are important in osmotic phenomena of fluids. Others are important in acid–base equilibrium. In addition, we require trace amounts of other elements, which are found as prosthetic groups in enzymes and carriers. The most important are iron, selenium, zinc, copper and iodine. In developed societies, mineral deficiencies are rare, although they do exist. Only iron and calcium (and possibly iodine) are likely to be deficient in the developed world, but deficiencies can also be common in certain types of patient.

Calcium

Most (99%) of body calcium is present in the skeleton (hydroxyapatite in bone). Calcium is needed by all cells. It is involved in almost all processes in the body and the plasma concentration of ionic calcium is subjected to exquisite control (p. 226).

Daily requirements. We need about 1 g per day in our diet but pregnant and lactating women require more. Sources of calcium include milk (cow's milk contains four times that of human milk), cheese and other dairy products. There are low levels in vegetables. Hard water is an important source.

Absorption. Dietary calcium is absorbed by an active process requiring transport proteins whose synthesis is controlled by calcitriol; about 70–80% is still excreted in faeces. Several compounds present in our food complex calcium and hinder its absorption. These include phytic acid (found in cereals), fatty acids (significant in fat malabsorption states) and oxalic acid (found in rhubarb).

Deficiency of calcium results in osteomalacia (rickets). It is caused by lack of vitamin D in the diet or insufficient production in the skin (owing to lack of sunlight).

Phosphorus

Phosphorus is required by all cells and its many functions have been described in Chapter 18.

Daily requirements. The average daily intake of dietary phosphorus is about 1.5 g.

Absorption. Phosphorus absorption is controlled by calcitriol action in the gut.

Defective phosphate metabolism (hypophosphataemia) can also lead to rickets. The clearest example is in X-linked hypophosphataemia, where renal reabsorption of phosphate is impaired.

Magnesium

The whole body contains about 25 g magnesium. It is essential in neuromuscular transmission and serves as a cofactor for many key enzymes, for example the kinases involved in phosphate group transfer in several reactions of glycolysis, acyl-CoA synthetase of fatty acid oxidation and glutamine synthase of amino acid metabolism.

Magnesium is found in bones and teeth and deficiency occurs in starvation and alcoholism.

Sodium and potassium

Sodium is the principal cation of the extracellular fluid while potassium is the principal cation of intracellular fluid. This ion gradient is maintained by the sodium pump (Na^+/K^+ ATPase) present in all cells and a major user of ATP. Sodium is involved primarily with the maintenance of osmotic equilibrium and body fluid volume while potassium is involved primarily with cellular enzyme function. Sodium/potassium balance in the body is under the fine control of aldosterone.

Sodium is present in most foods and sodium chloride is added during food processing. Requirements increase in hot weather, fever and during heavy work. Potassium is also widely distributed in foods.

Chlorine, as chloride

Chloride is required to maintain fluid and electrolyte balance and HCl production in the stomach. The chloride shift is important in carbon dioxide transport in blood (p. 62). It is supplied by many foods and also common salt.

Trace elements

Iron

The major requirement for iron is in haemoglobin and cytochrome synthesis, thus, this element has to be discussed in the context of anaemia. Iron deficiency results in deficiency of haemoglobin and is one of the most common forms of anaemia. Liver is a very good source of iron. Meat sources are absorbed much more efficiently than plant sources of iron. Milk and milk products are low in iron. Iron is not the only nutrient involved in red blood cell production; also required are folic acid, vitamin B_{12}, protein, pyridoxine, ascorbic acid and copper.

Absorption. Since iron is not actively excreted, iron balance in the body has to be controlled at the level of the intestinal mucosal cell; the assumption is that the level of iron-containing proteins such as ferritin in mucosal cells determines the rate and extent of iron absorption. It is Fe^{II} that is absorbed; efficient iron absorption depends upon reduction of dietary ferric to ferrous iron aided by reducing agents such as ascorbic acid. Iron is transported in blood in the form of transferrin.

Deficiency. Iron deficiency is common. In adults, deficiency can be caused by occult blood loss from the gastrointestinal tract. In children and adolescents, deficiency mainly results from poor nutrition.

Iodine

Forty per cent of the total body iodine is concentrated in the thyroid, where it can be used to iodinate a protein (thyroglobulin) leading to the production of the thyroid hormones (pp. 220–221). Some geographic locations have low iodine in the water supply and in plant products produced there. Iodine supplementation of common salt (76 µg/g salt) helps prevent iodine-deficiency goitre.

Copper and zinc

These metals are important components of enzyme systems; e.g. zinc is the prosthetic group of carbonic anhydrase and copper is a prosthetic group of cytochrome oxidase. As with iodine, seafoods are good sources of these metals as are liver and kidney.

Selenium

Selenium is the prosthetic group in glutathione reductase and is critical for overall anti-oxidant activity in cells.

Fluorine as fluoride

Although not an essential element, it appears beneficial to have fluoride in the diet since it reduces the incidence of dental caries by making teeth more resistant to acid (formed by bacteria in the mouth) by substituting for hydroxyl groups in hydroxyapatite.

Self-assessment: questions

Multiple choice questions

1. The following trace element is an integral part of the vitamin B_{12} molecule:
   a. Zinc
   b. Iron
   c. Copper
   d. Cobalt
   e. Molybdenum

2. In human nutrition:
   a. Fish and egg protein are of 'low quality'
   b. Linoleate is an essential fatty acid
   c. Phytate, present in most cereals, inhibits the absorption of dietary calcium
   d. Selenium acts as a cofactor for glutathione peroxidase
   e. Ferric iron (Fe^{III}) is absorbed more readily than ferrous iron (Fe^{II})

3. The following pairs link vitamins to deficiency states or to their role in the body:
   a. Nicotinamide and pellagra
   b. Pantothenate and fatty acid oxidation
   c. Riboflavin and energy metabolism
   d. Thiamine and beri-beri
   e. Pyridoxine and the pyruvate dehydrogenase complex

4. The following vitamins are synthesised in the liver by a pathway that involves pyridoxal phosphate and an aromatic amino acid:
   a. Vitamin K
   b. Vitamin D
   c. Thiamine
   d. Niacin (nicotinamide)
   e. Folate

5. The following statements describe nutrition:
   a. There is a long-term plan by nutritionalists to reduce the fat intake of the general population
   b. Vitamin C is required for the formation of both hydroxyprolyl and hydroxylysyl residues critical for collagen synthesis
   c. Iodine deficiency leads to the development of hyperthyroidism

   d. Fluoride intake makes teeth more resistant to acid and reduces the incidence of dental caries
   e. Chronic obstruction to bile flow can lead to hypocalcaemia in a subject

6. In the intestine:
   a. Vitamin B_{12} absorption requires ascorbic acid
   b. Iron is absorbed in the ferrous (Fe^{II}) form
   c. Fat-soluble vitamins are absorbed along with glucose
   d. Ferritin levels are involved in controlling the rate of iron absorption

True/false questions

Are the following statements true or false?

1. Biotin excretion in faeces plus urinary biotin equals the dietary biotin intake.
2. The Reference Nutrient Intake for thiamine, niacin and riboflavin is based upon the age and sex of individuals.
3. Increased intake of folate by pregnant women reduces the incidence of spina bifida.
4. Iron in vegetables is more readily absorbed than iron in liver.
5. Retinoic acid is the precursor of the all-*trans* retinal required for vision.
6. It is only the protein intake of an individual that determines whether or not they will be in positive nitrogen balance.
7. Tyrosine is an essential amino acid in normal subjects.
8. A deficiency in an essential amino acid in the diet of a subject leads to a positive nitrogen balance.
9. Fat-soluble vitamins tend to be stored in the body and high intake can lead to toxicity.

Short essay questions

1. Discuss the role of vitamins in
   a. carbohydrate metabolism
   b. fatty acid metabolism
   c. amino acid metabolism.
2. Prepare a table that highlights the roles of the various fat-soluble vitamins in the body and their active forms.

Self-assessment: answers

Multiple choice answers

1. a. **False.** Zinc is found in carbonic anhydrase.
   b. **False.** Iron is found in cytochromes and other haem proteins.
   c. **False.** Copper is found in cytochrome oxidase and tyrosinase.
   d. **True.** It is present in the corrin ring of B_{12}.
   e. **False.** Molybdenum is found in xanthine oxidase.

2. a. **False.** They are high quality, being of animal origin.
   b. **True.** It cannot be synthesised in the body and is needed as the precursor of arachidonate.
   c. **True.** It forms an insoluble complex with calcium and other metals.
   d. **True.** It is an important component of the anti-oxidant system in the body.
   e. **False.** It is ferrous iron which is absorbed. Ferric iron in the diet has to be reduced in the gut prior to absorption.

3. a. **True.** Nicotinamide is needed for NAD^+ and $NADP^+$.
   b. **True.** Pantothenate is needed for coenzyme A, which, in turn, is involved in fatty acid oxidation (and synthesis).
   c. **True.** Found in FAD and FMN, both involved in oxidative metabolism of fuels.
   d. **True.** In beri-beri, there is impaired oxidative metabolism of glucose owing to a lack of thiamine pyrophosphate, which has a role in the pyruvate dehydrogenase complex.
   e. **False.** It is not in any of the coenzymes/prosthetic groups in PDC. It is involved in amino acid catabolism.

4. a. **False.** Vitamin K can be made by colonic bacteria but not by the mammalian cell.
   b. **False.** Vitamin D can be made in the skin but only ultraviolet light is required.
   c. **False.** We get all of the required thiamine in our diet.
   d. **True.** Niacin can be synthesised starting from tryptophan.
   e. **False.** We derive all of the folate we require from folate polyglutamates in our diet.

5. a. **True.** The aim is to reduce the incidence of heart disease.
   b. **True.** It functions as a coenzyme in hydroxylation reactions.
   c. **False.** Iodine-deficiency hypothyroidism exists in areas of the world with low iodide in the water supply.

   d. **True.** Fluoride replaces hydroxyl groups in hydroxyapatite in teeth. Fluoroapatite is more resistant to acid.
   e. **True.** Vitamin D absorption is decreased and that can lower calcium levels through impaired calcium uptake.

6. a. **False.** It requires 'intrinsic factor' from the parietal cells of the stomach.
   b. **True.** Ascorbate aids in the reduction of ferric to ferrous iron.
   c. **False.** They are absorbed in phospholipid–bile salt micelles along with other fats.
   d. **True.** If they are high, this is a signal to decrease iron absorption.

True/false answers

1. **False.** Colonic bacteria synthesise biotin so excretion exceeds intake.
2. **False.** The recommended intakes depend on the total energy expenditure of the individual, i.e. we need more if we are using more fuel to support more energy expenditure. A middle-aged female who is very active in sport will need more of these vitamins than a young male 'couch potato'.
3. **True.** It may also help in reducing the incidence of cleft palate.
4. **False.** The efficiency is greatest from meat, especially liver, and the low efficiency from vegetables explains why some vegans develop iron-deficiency anaemia.
5. **False.** Retinol is the precursor of retinal. Retinal to retinoic acid is an irreversible step.
6. **False.** The quality of the protein is important but also whether or not the individual is receiving enough calories (from carbohydrate and fat). If not, they use protein as a fuel and may be in negative nitrogen balance.
7. **False.** Normal individuals are able to make tyrosine from phenylalanine.
8. **False.** A deficiency of any of the essential amino acids leads to negative nitrogen balance.
9. **True.** Hypervitaminosis A and D are potential problems for those taking large doses of these fat-soluble vitamins. Water-soluble vitamins, in contrast, are not toxic; many people take grams of vitamin C daily.

Short essay answers

1. **Carbohydrate metabolism.** *Nicotinamide* (niacin) is part of the cofactors NAD^+, NADH, $NADP^+$ and NADPH. NAD^+ is the cofactor for dehydrogenases involved in glycolysis, pyruvate dehydrogenase

complex (PDC) and the TCA cycle. *Lipoate* is also required by PDC as is *pantothenate* (part of coenzyme A). NADH is required for gluconeogenesis from pyruvate as is *biotin*. $NADP^+$ is required by both dehydrogenases in the pentose phosphate pathway and NADPH is a product of that pathway. *Thiamine* is part of a coenzyme, thiamine pyrophosphate, which is involved in PDC and also α-ketoglutarate dehydrogenase of the TCA cycle. It also functions in the pentose phosphate cycle where it is the coenzyme for transketolase. *Riboflavin* is part of the cofactors FAD and FMN. FAD is a cofactor in the PDC and is also the coenzyme for succinate dehydrogenase of the TCA cycle. FMN is a component of the electron transport chain. *Pyridoxal* is part of the coenzyme pyridoxal phosphate, which is an integral part of glycogen phosphorylase.

Fatty acid metabolism. *Pantothenate* is critical for fatty acid oxidation and synthesis because of its contribution to coenzyme A and acyl carrier protein. *Nicotinamide* and *riboflavin* are involved in fatty acid oxidation through the participation of NAD^+ and FAD in the beta-oxidation of fatty acids and the TCA cycle. Also, NADPH is required for fatty acid synthesis. *Vitamin B_{12}* participates in the metabolism of the propionyl-CoA, formed from odd-numbered fatty acids.

Amino acid metabolism. The most important vitamin related to amino acid catabolism is *pyridoxal*, given the role of pyridoxal phosphate in amino acid transamination and decarboxylation. It is also required for other reactions of amino acid metabolism. *Nicotinamide* and *riboflavin* are also important because of their role in branched-chain keto acid dehydrogenase and enzymes of the TCA cycle. *Folate* and *vitamin B_{12}* function in one-carbon metabolism, especially with the amino acids serine and histidine.

2. Table 33 describes the roles of the fat-soluble vitamins.

Table 33 The role of the fat-soluble vitamins

Vitamin	Active form	Function
A	Retinal, retinoic acid	Vision, growth and development
D	Calcitriol	Calcium absorption in gut
E	Hydroquinone	Anti-oxidant
K	Dihydrovitamin K	Coenzyme for γ-carboxylation of blood coagulation factors

Biochemical functions of blood

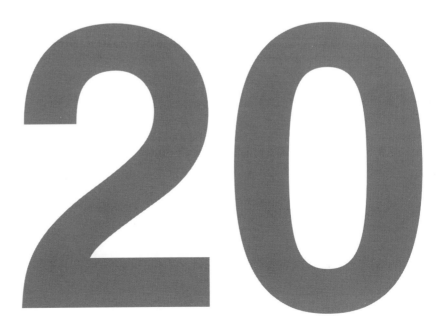

20.1 Plasma proteins

The plasma proteins have several critical functions:

- maintenance of oncotic pressure
- transport
- buffering
- immunity
- enzymatic
- blood clotting.

Many of the plasma proteins are synthesised in the liver, including albumin, α- and β-globulins, lipo-proteins and the proteins of blood coagulation. Their breadth of function is illustrated in Table 34. Immuno-globulins function as antibodies and are made in B lymphocytes (see below). The plasma proteins involved in hormone transport have been discussed in Chapter 18, those involved in lipid transport in Chapter 10 and those involved in blood coagulation are described in detail later in this chapter.

Clinical biochemists obtain measurements of the major classes of plasma protein in a patient's serum by carrying out protein electrophoresis on cellulose acetate or agarose gel. The major classes are pre-albumin, albumin, α_1- and α_2-globulins, β-globulins, and γ-globulins, as shown in Figure 171. Plasma protein electrophoretic analysis is of particular use in the diagnosis of nephrotic syndrome, hypogamma-

1. Apply mixture of proteins (e.g. plasma)

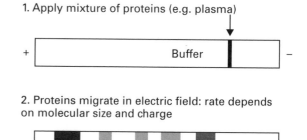

2. Proteins migrate in electric field: rate depends on molecular size and charge

3. After electrophoresis, proteins can be detected optically to produce an electrophoretogram

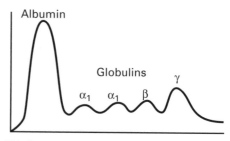

Fig. 171 Separation of plasma proteins by electrophoresis. Peaks indicate relative amounts of the different classes of protein; globulin peaks contain large mixtures of proteins.

globulinaemia, cirrhosis, α_1-antitrypsin deficiency and paraproteinaemia (high levels of an immunoglobulin made by a single clone of B lymphocytes).

Albumin

Albumin, a 66 kDa protein, is the most abundant plasma protein, being present at a concentration of about 4.5 g/dl in normal adults. About 14 g/day are made in the liver; its synthesis is stimulated by insulin. Serum albumin levels are low in liver disease. Normal serum albumin levels are an indication of good nutrition in patients. The most important functions of albumin are:

- to provide about 80% of the plasma oncotic pressure, which prevents loss of vascular fluid into tissues. It draws back into the venous ends of capillaries water that was forced through the arterial capillary walls by the hydrostatic pressure exerted by heart function
- to bind hydrophobic molecules. It has low affinity but, because of its high concentration in plasma, it has high capacity. Examples of ligands bound by albumin include fatty acids, bilirubin, calcium, thyroid hormones and many drugs including aspirin.

Haptoglobulin

Haptoglobulin is an α_2-globulin, molecular weight 90 000. Its chief role is to bind any free haemoglobin in the circulation, thus preventing it appearing in the glomerular filtrate in the kidney. The haptoglobin–

Table 34 The functions of plasma proteins

Role	Plasma protein
Maintenance of plasma oncotic pressure	Albumin
Protease inhibitor	Alpha-1 antitrypsin
Complexes extra-corpuscular haemoglobin	Haptoglobulin
Buffering	All plasma proteins
	Transport proteins
Hydrophobic compounds and Ca^{2+}	Albumin
Copper	Ceruloplasmin
Iron	Transferrin
Fat	Beta-lipoproteins
Cortisol	Corticosteroid-binding globulin (CBG)
Thyroid hormones (T_4 and T_3)	Thyroxine-binding globulin (TBG), transerythretin (pre-albumin)
	Hormone-related activity
Angiotensin I precursor	Angiotensinogen
Mediator of growth hormone action	Insulin-like growth factor I
	Blood coagulation
Non-vitamin K dependent	Fibrinogen, factors V, VIII, XI, XII
Vitamin K dependent	Prothrombin, factors VII, IX, X
	Immunity
Antibodies	Gamma-globulins, especially IgG and IgA

haemoglobin complex is then cleared by cells of the reticuloendothelial system.

Alpha-1 antitrypsin

Alpha-1 antitrypsin has a molecular weight of 52 000. Various serine proteases are inhibited by being complexed with α_1-antitrypsin. It is especially important as an inhibitor of leucocyte elastase in the lower respiratory tract. Low levels of α_1-antitrypsin are found in about 5% of cases of *emphysema*.

Enzymes in blood

Enzymes which function in blood include those required for blood coagulation (see below). Low concentrations of other enzymes are present in plasma arising from cell breakdown with release into blood of cellular contents. When tissues are damaged by a disease process, large amounts of tissue enzymes are released and their measurement is used to aid diagnosis, e.g. creatine kinase and LDH for heart disease; amylase for pancreatitis, alanine aminotransferase in liver disease.

20.2 Immunoglobulins

Immunoglobulins (antibodies) belong to one of the systems that combat invasion of the body by foreign, potentially toxic, organisms present in the environment. Antibodies have the ability to bind to antigens on pathogens and this facilitates their removal by phagocytes.

Classes of antibodies

Immunoglobulins are a family of proteins and are divided into five classes, with each class having a distinct set of functions. They are all glycoproteins with variable proportions of carbohydrate in each class.

IgG

- major antibody of the secondary immune response
- can cross the placenta.

IgM

- this antibody is made by the fetus in utero
- the predominant early antibody in response to an antigen.

IgA

- predominant immunoglobulin in secretions such as saliva, colostrum, human milk, tears, and GI and respiratory secretions.

IgD

- occurs on cell surfaces: precise function unknown.

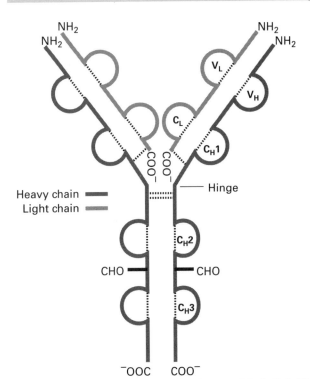

Fig. 172 Schematic representation of an immunoglobulin G (IgG) molecule. Light (L) and heavy (H) chains are shown with their constant (C) and variable (V) regions. The dashed lines represent disulphide bonds.

IgE

- found on mucosal surfaces
- triggers histamine release when antigen binds to it
- is a defence against worm parasites.

Antibody structure

IgG (γ-globulin) has a typical antibody structure (Fig. 172). There are pairs of larger ('heavy'; H) and smaller ('light'; L) chains. Each L chain has a molecular weight of 25 000 and is common to all classes of immunoglobulin. The H chains vary for each class and each has a molecular weight of 50 000–70 000. The chains are linked by disulphide bonds that are both intra- and interchain. Important aspects of immunoglobulins include:

- each L chain has one variable (V) and one constant (C) domain
- each H chain has one variable and three constant domains in IgG
- the two H chains are linked to each other through two interchain disulphide bonds at the 'hinge' region. The hinge allows for flexibility and thus there are two antigen-binding sites per IgG molecule
- variable regions of both L and H chains are at the N-terminal end of IgG. This is the site for antigen to bind to antibody
- located within the variable domains of the L and H chains are *hypervariable regions* through which the paired H_V and L_V contribute to the antigen-binding site of the IgG.

Antibody diversity

Antibodies are made by B lymphocytes and it is important to recognise that all of the antigen-binding specificities are present in the various clones of B cells *before* they encounter the antigen. There are tens of millions of antigen specificities, which exceeds the number of genes in the human genome. Gene shuffling allows a limited number of genes to give rise to the vast number of antigen-binding specificities.

1. A gene coding for the variable region of an L chain is made by shuffling 300 V_L genes so that one of them can finish attached to any one of four joining genes (J_L) which link the variable construct to the single gene coding for the constant region of the L chain. There will be at least 1200 possible V_L/J_L constructs.

2. Similar shuffling occurs for H chain variable region but there is an extra class of genes involved. Therefore, any one of about 200 V_H genes can be attached to any one of 12 D (diversity) genes, which in turn can be next to any one of four J_H genes, which join the variable region construct of the H chain to the constant region. As a result, there can be at least $200 \times 12 \times 4$ V_H gene constructs, i.e. 9600.

3. Since an antigen-binding site will be composed of the L chain variable region and the H chain variable region, there will be at least $1200 \times 9600 = 11.52$ million antigen-binding specificities.

20.3 Blood coagulation

Blood coagulation is a process that results in the formation of a fibrin clot, which seals a damaged or injured blood vessel. Blood coagulation must be:

(a) on demand, initiated by injury to a blood vessel
(b) rapid and controlled
(c) localised at the site of injury to the vessel
(d) temporary.

The following series of events occur after injury to a vessel.

1. Local vasoconstriction occurs within a few seconds to limit blood loss, with endothelin being secreted by endothelial cells.

2. Next there is platelet plug formation. Disruption of the endothelium exposes collagen and subendothelial elements to which platelets adhere. The platelet plug formed temporarily stops the flow of blood. For the platelets to aggregate and form the plug, a plasma protein known as von Willebrand's factor (vWF) is required. It forms a bridge between the platelet and the subendothelium. This is accomplished by binding of vWF to specific receptors – Glycoprotein Ib/Glycoprotein IX – on the surface of the activated platelets as well as to the subendothelium.

3. The coagulation cascade and fibrin formation are

BOX 20.1
Clinical note: Von Willebrand's disease

Patients with a deficiency of vWF will have defective platelet plug formation; this can be measured by assaying 'bleeding time'. In that test a very small cut is made and the time taken for blood flow to stop is measured. Bleeding time should not be confused with clotting time. In the latter it is the efficiency of clot formation that is assayed.

---

initiated by exposure of negatively charged phospholipids such as phosphatidylserine on the surface of activated platelets or damaged cell membranes. A series of events is triggered at the site with control being achieved by a multiple enzyme cascade that amplifies the early events. The critical step occurs when insoluble fibrin is made from soluble fibrinogen, and the fibrin molecules are crosslinked to increase the tensile strength of the clot.

4. The transient nature of the clot is attested to by the early elaboration of platelet-derived growth factor (PDGF) for permanent tissue repair and the initiation of fibrinolysis.

The blood coagulation cascade

The key feature of blood coagulation is that inactive coagulation factors are present in blood and that they are activated in a stepwise fashion (Fig. 173). By international agreement, Roman numerals are used for each well-characterised clotting factor (Table 35) and a lower case letter a is added to the numeral to indicate the active form of a coagulation factor, e.g. Xa. Blood coagulation schemes always appear rather complex but we will dissect the system shown in Figure 173 by starting from the end-product – a tough fibrin clot – and work backwards to describe the entire system.

Thrombin acts on fibrinogen to produce fibrin

Fibrinogen consists of two pairs of three non-identical polypeptide chains (α, β and γ) joined by disulphide bonds. The subunit structure is usually denoted as $(A\alpha B\beta\gamma)2$. The presence of many negative charges in the A and B portions of the α and β chains prevents aggregation of fibrinogen. However, when these are removed by the action of the protease *thrombin*, the fibrin molecules formed can aggregate, become insoluble and form a clot of weak tensile strength as they surround the platelet plug.

Covalent bonds stabilise the clot

Bonds are formed between lysine and glutamine residues in α and γ chains in adjacent fibrin molecules, catalysed by the active form of factor XIII (XIIIa), which is a *fibrin transamidase*. Another action of thrombin is to convert factor XIII to XIIIa.

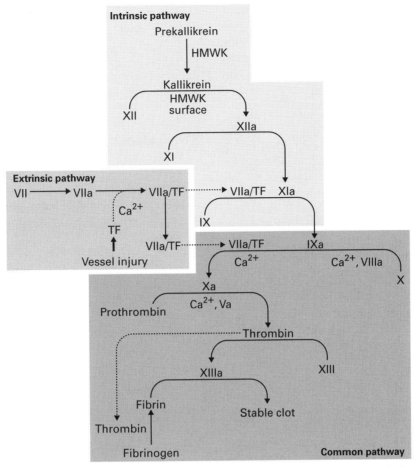

Fig. 173 The traditional blood coagulation scheme showing the reactions of the intrinsic and extrinsic pathways. TF, tissue factor; HMWK, High-Molecular-Weight Kininogen.

Table 35 Nomenclature for coagulation factors

Number	Factor
I	Fibrinogen
II	Prothrombin[a]
III	Tissue factor
IV	Calcium
V	Proaccelerin
VII	Proconvertin[a]
VIII	Antihaemophilic factor
IX	Christmas factor[a]
X	Stuart factor[a]
XI	Plasma thromoplastin antecedent
XII	Hageman factor

[a]Vitamin K-dependent factor.

Thrombin is made from prothrombin; Factor Xa is required

The above scheme would cause clotting to occur whenever fibrinogen, thrombin and factor XIII were present and this would be disastrous. Since fibrinogen is always present in normal individuals then the enzymes must not be active under normal conditions. They exist as proenzymes (zymogens) that must be modified to become active when a clot is required to plug up a damaged vessel. Thrombin is generated in the process of coagulation from its precursor in plasma, prothrombin. Thrombin is produced from prothrombin by the action of factor Xa and everything must now hinge on the formation of Xa.

Factor X is activated by extrinsic and intrinsic pathways

Two principal pathways have been defined:

- the *intrinsic pathway* in which all of the components are found in plasma (Fig. 173)
- the extrinsic pathway, which is activated by Tissue Factor, a transmembrane protein that is not present in plasma and is contributed by tissue at the site of vessel injury (Fig. 173)
- these two pathways are followed by a *common pathway*, which is the reactions occurring following the activation of factor X.

Both pathways are required because of Tissue Factor Pathway Inhibitor

A defect in one pathway will give a bleeding disorder even if the other pathway is unaffected, e.g. a defect in factor VII, a component of the extrinsic pathway causes a bleeding disorder despite all of the factors of the intrinsic pathway being present. The extrinsic pathway appears to be very active when assayed in vitro and it has always been difficult to understand why the intrinsic pathway plays any role under normal circumstances. That is now understood better since a factor has been identified that after a short period of time inhibits the extrinsic pathway – Tissue Factor Pathway Inhibitor (TFPI) – making it necessary for the intrinsic pathway to function.

The current model links the extrinsic and intrinsic pathways

When a vessel is damaged it is the factor VIIa/Tissue Factor that activates both factor X to Xa and IX to IXa. Also, thrombin produced through the action of Xa can activate factors IX and VIII, thus continuing the process after TFPI inhibits the action of VIIa/TF. With this model, factor XII, High Molecular Weight Kininogen (HMWK) and prekallikrein play only a minor role. However, when blood is placed in a test tube it will clot through the complete intrinsic pathway.

Two non-enzymic factors are required

These are factors V and VIII, so-called 'positioning factors'. Thrombin action on them gives the more active forms Va and VIIIa. Factor VIII in plasma is stabilised by vWF. The low levels of vWF found in von Willebrand's disease lead to low factor VIII levels and the potential for bleeding (this is secondary factor VIII deficiency). Thrombin also activates *Protein C* which digests the active forms of factors Va and VIIIa in the presence of *Protein S*. This latter action of thrombin is important in achieving balance and limiting blood clotting to the site of the damaged vessel. Both Protein C and Protein S contain Gla residues and are vitamin K-dependent factors (see below).

The vitamin K-dependent factors

Vitamin K (Fig. 174) deficiency leads to defects in blood coagulation. Dihydrovitamin K is the coenzyme for a carboxylase that brings about post-translational modification of prothrombin and factors VII, IX and X (Fig. 175) An extra carboxyl group is added to several glutamates in these factors forming γ-carboxyglutamate (Gla) residues. The regeneration of dihydrovitamin K from the 2,3-epoxide involves two reductions catalysed by enzymes that are inhibited by coumarin anti-coagulants such as warfarin. Factors with Gla residues bind calcium at least 10 times more effectively than the same factors with glutamate residues. The binding of these factors to phospholipid surfaces through calcium localises them at the site of injury to a blood vessel where platelet plug formation has occurred and an active phospholipid surface has been made available.

Haemophilias

Haemophilia A results from deficiency of factor VIII. Inheritance is X-linked so females are carriers and male descendants of these carriers can be affected.

Haemophilia B (Christmas disease) results from factor IX deficiency. Inheritance is also X-linked.

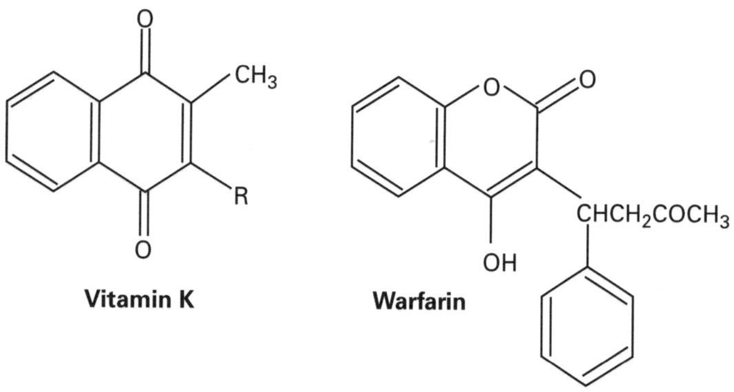

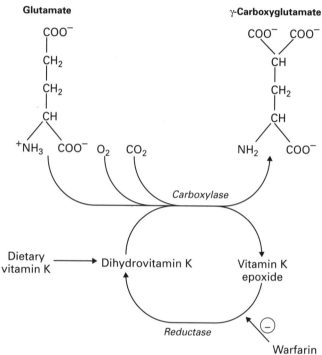

Fig. 174 The structure of vitamin K (R is an alkyl side chain that varies in different vitamin K derivatives) and warfarin.

Fig. 175 The role of dihydrovitamin K in the formation of γ-carboxyglutamate residues in prothrombin and factors VII, IX and X and the site of action of warfarin, an anti-coagulate.

Anti-coagulants

Calcium chelators. Citrate, EDTA and oxalate act by complexing ionic calcium, which is required in several steps in the blood coagulation cascade. Citrated blood is used in blood transfusions. Calcium chelators are added to blood to prepare plasma to carry out tests for blood clotting activity. Following centrifugation to sediment all the cells, the clear plasma remains on the top layer. After the plasma is prepared it can be recalcified and the rate of formation of clots can be measured following activation of the system. Serum is prepared by letting blood clot in a tube and then centrifuging at high speed to sediment down all the cells leaving the serum as the top layer. Serum is depleted in fibrinogen and coagulation factors relative to plasma.

Heparin. This sulphated glycosamino-glycan is made in mast cells and inhibits clotting at several points by increasing several hundred-fold the activity of antithrombin III. Antithrombin III is a serum proteinase inhibitor that inhibits thrombin and also IXa and Xa (but not VIIa). Heparin is used clinically as an acute anti-coagulant.

Warfarin. This coumarin-related compound is an inhibitor of dihydrovitamin K regeneration (Fig. 175) and is used for chronic anti-coagulation of patients. In contrast to heparin, it has no effect when added to a blood sample (a person and his/her liver is needed for warfarin to be effective). Also, warfarin is a rat poison.

Fibrinolysis

In order for a damaged blood vessel to undergo repair the clot must be dissolved and this is accomplished by fibrinolysis. Tissue type plasminogen activator (tPA) is in vascular tissues and binds to fibrin clots. It brings about the activation of plasminogen (also bound to clots) to *plasmin*, a serine protease that dissolves the clot. Recently, tPA has been used successfully to treat patients who have suffered a stroke or a heart attack because of the formation of a clot in a cerebral or coronary artery.

20.4 Red cell metabolism

The red cell is notorious for having limited biochemical

apparatus. One critical difference between erythrocytes and their precursors, erythroblasts and reticulocytes, is the absence of mitochondria, which are lost within 24 hours of reticulocytes entering the circulation. The consequence of this is that ATP synthesis has to occur via an anaerobic pathway: glycolysis. The other limitation applies to pathways for the generation of NADPH, with only the pentose phosphate pathway being available. Clearly, glucose is the key fuel in the mature red cell.

Roles of glucose metabolism in erythrocytes

The glucose metabolic pathways in red cells are reviewed in Figure 176. The importance of other metabolic intermediates has been discussed in other chapters:

- ATP is required for ion pumps (p. 141)
- NADH is required to maintain the iron in haemoglobin as Fe^{II} (interaction with oxygen can form methaemoglobin (Fe^{III}_+), which cannot bind oxygen; *methaemoglobin reductase* requires reduced cytochrome b_5, the level of which is dependent upon adequate NADH)
- 2,3-bisphosphoglycerate (2,3-BPG) is the most important negative modulator of oxygen – haemoglobin association (p. 60)

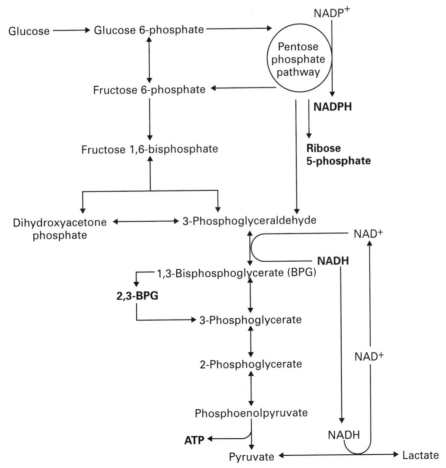

Fig. 176 Glucose metabolism in red blood cells.

- NADPH is required to maintain adequate levels of reduced glutathione, which protects against oxygen free radicals
- ribose 5-phosphate contributes to the maintenance of AMP (ATP) levels.

Enzyme deficiencies in red cells

Glucose 6-phosphate dehydrogenase deficiency (Favism) is estimated to affect 400 million people worldwide. Highest frequencies are found in tropical Africa, in the Middle East, in tropical and subtropical Asia, in some areas of the Mediterranean and in Papua New Guinea. It leads to impaired generation of NADPH in affected tissues. Since catalase and glutathione (via glutathione peroxidase) are essential for the detoxification of hydrogen peroxide, the defence of the cell against this compound depends ultimately and heavily on glucose 6-phosphate dehydrogenase. The commonest clinical manifestations are jaundice and acute haemolytic anaemia. The acute haemolytic anaemia can be triggered by drugs, by infections, or by the ingestion of fava beans (hence, favism). Epidemiological data indicate strongly that absence or low activity of the enzyme can confer relative resistance against *Plasmodium falciparum* malaria.

Self-assessment: questions

Multiple choice questions

1. Factor VIII:
   a. Has proteolytic activity similar to thrombin
   b. Is a participant in the extrinsic pathway
   c. Binds calcium in a similar fashion to factor IX
   d. Is a positioning factor that participates in the activation of factor X by factor IXa
   e. Levels in blood are low in von Willebrand's disease

2. Vitamin K:
   a. Participates directly in the formation of the fibrin clot
   b. Absorption from the gut would be impaired when fat absorption is defective
   c. Is an activator of the translation of the prothrombin mRNA in the liver
   d. Deficiency can lead to haemorrhagic disease of the newborn
   e. Dependent factors include prothrombin and factors VII, IX and X

3. The formation of a fibrin clot:
   a. Is dependent upon the presence of calcium ions
   b. Requires platelet-derived phospholipid
   c. Requires the participation of several non-enzymic glycoprotein factors
   d. Can be blocked in vitro by the addition of heparin to blood
   e. Will not occur in blood from which red cells have been removed

4. The following plasma constituents have the accompanying roles:
   a. Albumin — transports hydrophilic molecules
   b. Haptoglobulin — binds extracorpuscular haemoglobin
   c. Transerythretin — binds cortisol
   d. VLDL — is a major transporter of cholesterol
   e. Albumin — is elevated in plasma in nephrotic syndrome

5. The following statements describe immunoglobulin structure as exemplified by IgG:
   a. The heavy chains make major contributions to antigen-binding sites
   b. The light chains make major contributions to antigen-binding sites
   c. The light chains are linked to heavy chains by disulphide bonds, which in turn are the only disulphide bonds in the immunoglobulin molecule
   d. IgG has two specific antigen-binding sites
   e. Light chains and heavy chains have the same number of variable domains

6. Antibodies:
   a. Of the IgG class are the major immunoglobulins in plasma
   b. Of the IgM class are smaller than IgG
   c. Of the IgA class are found in significant quantities in human secretions
   d. Of the IgG class can cross the placenta
   e. Of the IgE class are found on mucosal surfaces

7. The liver is the chief site in the body for the synthesis of:
   a. The principal plasma protein
   b. Immunoglobulins
   c. Factor VIII
   d. Insulin-like growth factor I
   e. Angiotensinogen

True/false questions

Are the following statements true or false?

1. You would expect to find many aspartate or glutamate residues in the A and B portions of the Aα and Bβ chains of fibrinogen.
2. The concentration of fibrinogen would be identical in plasma and serum samples prepared from the same subject.
3. All of the plasma proteins are made in the liver.
4. There are identical numbers of constant domains in the heavy chains and light chains of IgG.
5. Gene shuffling results in there being a small number of antigen specificities in B lymphocytes.

Short essay questions

1. Write an account of the changes that occur when fibrinogen is converted to fibrin.
2. Explain the ability of warfarin to serve as an anti-coagulant.
3. Describe how you would prepare plasma and serum and any differences that exist between them.
4. Discuss the findings you would expect in a subject with pyruvate kinase (PK) deficiency.
5. Explain the biochemical consequences to a patient of having a defect in erythrocite glucose 6-phosphate dehydrogenase.
6. List three plasma proteins synthesised in the liver that have a role in transporting compounds in blood and in each case write a few sentences that explain the significance of the role.

Self-assessment: answers

Multiple choice answers

1. a. **False.** Factor VIII is not an enzyme.
   b. **False.** It is part of the intrinsic pathway.
   c. **False.** It is not one of the vitamin K-dependent factors with γ-carboxyglutamate residues
   d. **True.** This is an accurate description of its action. Factor V has a similar role in the activation of prothrombin to thrombin, catalysed by factor Xa.
   e. **True.** This explains why subjects with vWF deficiency bleed. vWF binds factor VIII, thus maintaining a higher level of it in plasma.

2. a. **False.** Its action is indirect at the level of post-translational modification of specific blood coagulation factors.
   b. **True.** It is a fat-soluble vitamin.
   c. **False.** It acts as a coenzyme in a reaction that occurs post-translationally.
   d. **True.** Newborns have low level of vitamin K since they do not have enough colonic bacteria to synthesis the vitamin K.
   e. **True.** These are the blood coagulation factors with several γ-carboxyglutomate residues replacing glutamate.

3. a. **True.** Removal of calcium ions prevents blood clotting.
   b. **True.** Phospholipid vesicles provide a platform for efficient activation of the clotting cascade.
   c. **True.** These are factors V and VIII.
   d. **True.** Heparin activates antithrombin III, which inhibits the action of thrombin and other serine proteases of the coagulation cascade.
   e. **False.** Red cells play no part in the formation of a clot: plasma plus platelets are all that is required.

4. a. **False.** It is the major transporter of hydrophobic molecules.
   b. **True.** This allows for any haemoglobin released from erythrocytes by haemolysis to be cleared in the reticuloendothelial system after binding to haptoglobulin.
   c. **False.** It is involved in thyroid hormone transport and also binds retinol-binding globulin.
   d. **False.** LDL is the major transporter of cholesterol (receptor-mediated endocytosis).
   e. **False.** Its levels are low in nephrotic syndrome owing to unusually high excretion in urine.

5. a. **True.** These are found at the N-terminal region of the heavy chains.
   b. **True.** These are found at the N-terminal region of the light chains.
   c. **False.** The light and heavy chains are linked by disulphide bonds but there are also disulphide bonds at the 'hinge' and also intrachain disulphide bonds creating the loops.
   d. **True.** Where there are 'paired' H_v and L_v domains.
   e. **True.** Each chain has one variable domain.

6. a. **True.** They can be readily seen in plasma electrophoretograms.
   b. **False.** They are fives times larger.
   c. **True.** These secretions include saliva, human milk, tears and gastrointestinal secretions.
   d. **True.** This gives the fetus some protection from antigens to which the mother has been exposed.
   e. **True.** Levels of IgE are especially high in persons who are hyperallergic.

7. a. **True.** It is albumin.
   b. **False.** These are made in lymphocytes.
   c. **True.** Basically, all the blood coagulation factors are made in the liver.
   d. **True.** This is its chief site of formation and it is stimulated by growth hormone.
   e. **True.** It is secreted into blood and is converted to angiotensin I by the action of renin.

True/false answers

1. **True.** Glutamate and aspartate are dicarboxylic acids and it is the concentration of negative charges in the A and B fibrinopeptides that prevent fibrinogen from aggregating to form a clot.
2. **False.** Serum is prepared by letting a blood sample clot and this means that the serum has low concentrations of fibrinogen compared with plasma prepared by centrifuging blood that is prevented from clotting by the addition of heparin or the removal of calcium ions.
3. **False.** Whereas most are made in the liver, including the most abundant one albumin, many are not, including the immunoglobulins and enzymes released as a result of normal cell turnover throughout the body.
4. **False.** The heavy chains have three and the light chains have one.
5. **False.** On the contrary, gene shuffling accounts for the enormous diversity of antibodies that can be generated in response to antigens.

Short essay answers

1. Fibrinogen is present in plasma at relatively high concentrations (*c.* 350 mg/dl) and is very water soluble. It consists of three non-identical pairs of polypeptide chains (α, β and γ) that are linked by

disulphide bonds. The critical structural feature is that the N-terminal portions of the α and β chains have many negative charges provided by aspartate and glutamate. When these are removed in the form of fibrinopeptides A and B by the action of thrombin, the fibrin monomers that remain have binding sites exposed that allow them to aggregate to form a low-tensile-strength clot. The aggregated fibrin is held together by non-covalent bonds. Isopeptide bonds are formed between ε-amino groups of lysines and amide groups of glutamines in neighbouring fibrin molecules to give a stable fibrin clot with high tensile strength. This reaction is catalysed by activated factor XIII (formed from XIII by thrombin action).

2. Several blood coagulation factors – prothrombin, factors VII, IX and X – are modified in the liver by having several of their glutamate (Glu) residues carboxylated to form γ-carboxyglutamate (Gla) residues. This gives these proteins a greatly increased ability to bind calcium. The coenzyme for the carboxylase involved in Gla formation is dihydrovitamin K. In the reaction, dihydrovitamin K is converted to a 2,3-epoxide and the latter has to be converted back to dihydrovitamin K if there is to be efficient formation of the Gla-containing factors. The reductases involved in the conversion are inhibited by coumarins such as warfarin. Warfarin is used for chronic anti-coagulation of patients. It is frequently described as a 'blood thinner'.

3. To prepare plasma one has to prevent clotting of the blood sample. This can be done by adding heparin to inhibit multiple steps in the blood coagulation cascade or by complexing calcium ions by use of compounds such as oxalate, citrate or EDTA. The treated blood sample is then subjected to centrifugation at sufficient speed (g) to sediment down all formed elements in blood, including red cells, leucocytes, neutrophils, etc. Lying above the cell layer is *plasma*. It is plasma that is used for PT and aPTT assays that are used to evaluate the extrinsic and intrinsic pathways, respectively.

To prepare serum a blood sample is allowed to clot, usually in a tube standing on ice. The sample is then centrifuged and serum will appear as a clear liquid phase above the formed elements plus clot, which centrifuge to the foot of the tube. Serum will have low levels of fibrinogen and other clotting factors compared with plasma.

4. Red cell metabolism is much impaired in subjects with PK deficiency since red cells are dependent upon glycolysis for ATP synthesis and PK catalyses the step in glycolysis in which net ATP formation is achieved. Red cell lysis will occur and the subject will be anaemic. Increased red cell turnover will lead to increased bilirubin synthesis, which, if it overwhelms the liver's capacity to handle it, will

lead to hyperbilirubinaemia (jaundice). Since PK activity is low, glycolytic intermediates that precede it will accumulate, including 2,3-BPG. An increase in the red cell ratio of 2,3-BPG to ATP will help establish the diagnosis.

5. Glucose 6-phosphate dehydrogenase (G-6-PDH) catalyses the first step in the pentose phosphate pathway, which has a principal role of generating NADPH and ribose 5-phosphate. In subjects with a G-6-PDH deficiency, it is red blood cells (RBCs) that are especially at risk since they have a limited number of metabolic pathways available to them (they lack mitochondria) and have no other source of NADPH. A principal role of NADPH in RBCs is to maintain levels of glutathione which plays a key role in the response of cells to oxidative stress. RBCs in someone with G-6-PDH deficiency will tend to haemolyse, especially when the person takes drugs or foodstuffs (e.g. fava beans) that generate lots of oxygen radicals. In these circumstances, RBC turnover is enhanced because of increased lysis. Oxygen delivery to tissues will be less efficient. In addition, the ability of the body to deal with bile pigments, metabolites of the haem part of haem proteins, is exceeded, leading to jaundice.

6. Three plasma proteins could be albumin, thyroxine-binding globulin (TBG) and transferrin.

Albumin. This major plasma protein is the most prominent transporter of hydrophobic molecules in plasma. Examples of such molecules are free fatty acids, unconjugated bilirubin, aspirin and aldosterone. Fatty acids are important fuels for muscles, especially cardiac muscle, and they have to be transported from their storage site in adipose tissue through an aqueous medium. Albumin also binds calcium: this is of clinical importance as the total calcium in blood will be altered if albumin concentrations are altered.

TBG. The major plasma protein binding thyroxine and triiodothyronine, the thyroid hormones, is TBG. The extent of binding is very high and, clearly, if the level of TBG changes then the total amount of these hormones will change. Knowledge of this is important when one is examining thyroid hormone levels in patients. The level of TBG is increased by oestrogen and this will happen if one treats a subject with oestrogen or if the patient is pregnant.

Transferrin. This protein is responsible for transporting ferric iron in the body. All cells with mitochondria require iron for their cytochromes. Iron is required for haemoglobin synthesis and for cell division and growth. Clearly, iron has to be delivered to cells and this is the function of transferrin. Other proteins are involved in controlling the actual uptake of iron from transferrin into cells.

Biochemical genetics and inborn errors of metabolism

21

21.1 Introduction

Over 3000 diseases probably have a genetic basis. Many chronic diseases have a genetic component and genetic predispositions to at least some forms of cancer have been found. Rapid progress has been made recently in understanding the molecular basis of many inherited diseases. Modern techniques of molecular genetics can be used to find the genes involved and to follow these genes from one generation to another. Biochemistry can link a genetic condition and its associated disease. It may then provide the basis for rational treatment. These advances have put diagnosis of genetic disease and genetic counselling on a secure footing and may ultimately enable 'gene therapy'.

The concept of inherited disease was first recognised by Garrod from his studies of four families in which 11 individuals had the relatively harmless disorder, alkaptonuria. In this condition the subject's urine turns black on standing and there is arthritis in later life. The biochemical basis was accumulation and excretion of homogentisic acid resulting from lack of an enzyme which breaks down a metabolic product of the aromatic amino acids, phenylalanine and tyrosine.

Human genetic makeup and mutation

Genes are arranged on chromosomes at loci, sites where each particular gene is to be found. If the loci on maternal and paternal chromosomes carry identical versions of a gene, the individual is said to be homozygous. If the genes are different, the individual is heterozygous.

In the human body most cells are diploid, containing 23 pairs of chromosomes (22 autosomes plus XX or XY sex chromosomes). In each pair of chromosomes one is of maternal and the other of paternal origin. Maternal and paternal germ cells are haploid (only one copy of each chromosome per cell, i.e. 22 autosomes plus X or Y). Females have two X chromosomes but the X chromosome is unpaired in males.

The role of genes in controlling protein structure and function is discussed in Chapters 13 and 15. Table 36 lists the patterns of inherited diseases. New mutations in germ cells are passed on to succeeding generations. New somatic cell mutations are not, but may be important, e.g. in the development of cancer.

21.2 Patterns of inheritance

Knowledge of Mendelian inheritance is important in investigating inherited disease. Different patterns of inheritance will be seen depending upon whether the mutant gene is dominant or recessive and whether it is on an autosome or a sex chromosome.

Autosomal recessive disorders:

- mutant gene must be one of the 22 autosomes
- only in the homozygous state will the clinical condition be apparent
- pedigree shows horizontal pattern
- both sexes equally affected
- affected person's offspring are all unaffected unless the other parent is a carrier
- examples include alkaptonuria, cystic fibrosis, Tay–Sachs disease and phenylketonuria.

Autosomal dominant disorders:

- heterozygotes will manifest the disease, i.e. the subject has one abnormal and one normal gene
- pedigree shows vertical pattern
- both sexes equally affected and able to pass the defective gene on
- examples include familial hypercholesterolaemia and Huntington's disease
- lack of penetrance may be an indication that exogenous or environmental factors are involved in the expression of phenotype, e.g. acute intermittent porphyria.

Table 36 Gene changes that can cause disease

Type	Change	Example
Chromosome duplication	Three copies instead of two for one chromosome	Chromosome 21 in Down's syndrome
Amplification	Duplication of a section of DNA, particularly triplet repeats	Myotonic dystrophy
Translocation	Movement of a section of DNA within a chromosome or between chromosomes	Burkitt's lymphoma
Point mutations	Single base change, may or may not affect function (p. 191)	Beta-thalassaemia
Deletions/insertions	Will result in a frameshift (p. 191)	Alpha-thalassaemia
Mitochondrial DNA changes	Affects mitochondrially coded proteins	Familial mitochondrial encephalomyopathy
Multifactorial polygenic changes	A clear genetic change which may affect several genes but in addition an environmental factor is involved	Diabetes mellitus
Disorders of the mechanism protecting against genome damage	Gene changes have an indirect effect in that the body cannot repair somatic gene damage	Hereditary non-polyposis colon cancer

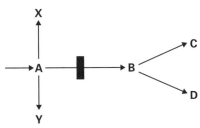

Fig. 177 A defect in a pathway enzyme will have several effects: A↑, X, Y (minor metabolites) ↑, B, C and D↓. In addition changing levels of components of the pathway may influence other systems.

X-linked recessive disorders:

- abnormal gene is on the X chromosome
- the disorder is almost completely confined to males
- the pattern is oblique
- males have unaffected parents but do have affected uncles
- transmitted only by female carriers
- examples include haemophilia A and B, and Duchenne's muscular dystrophy.

21.3 Inborn errors of metabolism

Mutations can affect biochemical pathways

Figure 177 shows the possible consequences of a deficiency in an enzyme involved in a metabolic pathway. Given that there are thousands of inborn errors of metabolism it will only be possible to discuss a few of them here. Those which are presented illustrate important aspects of diagnosis and therapy.

Amino acid metabolism

There are many disorders in amino acid metabolism some of which are summarised in Table 37. PKU is presented in some detail since it has had great significance in terms of testing procedures and therapy.

Phenylketonuria

PKU is an example of an autosomal recessive disorder. If it is not diagnosed at birth, the phenotype includes mental retardation, neurological seizures and diluted pigmentation of hair and skin.

Biochemical basis. The deficiency of phenylalanine catabolism occurs because phenylalanine 4-hydroxylase is absent or greatly reduced. The enzyme converts phenylalanine into tyrosine, the precursor of dopamine, noradrenaline, adrenaline and thyroid hormones (Fig. 178). Phenylalanine 4-hydroxylase is a mixed-function oxidase with a requirement for reducing power, so that the complete system is rather complex (Fig. 179). Clearly, low rates of conversion of phenylalanine to tyrosine can also occur if the tetrahydrobiopterin (THBP) coenzyme is not regenerated owing to defective *dihydropteridine reductase*. THBP is also required in the biosynthesis of the neurotransmitters, dopamine, noradrenaline, adrenaline and serotonin. Treatment of PKU caused by defective THBP metabolism involves the addition of DOPA and 5-hydroxytryptophan to the diet in addition to restriction of phenylalanine.

Genetic basis. In the classic form of PKU, most mutations are point mutations in either a splice site (40%) or the coding region (single amino acid change: 20%).

Clinical effects. Although the phenylalanine 4-hydroxylase enzyme is present in the liver, the effects are far more wide-ranging, i.e. a defect in one tissue may give clinical symptoms in another tissue. The block in conversion of phenylalanine causes elevated levels of this amino acid in blood and urine. It is the resultant hyperphenylalaninaemia that impairs brain development leading to mental retardation. The term phenylketonuria was coined because a minor catabolic pathway was increased in PKU resulting in the excretion of large quantities of phenylpyruvic acid (a phenylketone). Phenylpyruvic acid is *not* the cause for the clinical abnormalities, merely a symptom of their occurrence. Since phenylalanine is a competitive inhibitor of tyrosinase in melanocytes, there is reduced melanin formation in these subjects.

Table 37 Inborn errors of amino acid metabolism

Amino acid	Name of disorder	Enzyme affected
Phenylalanine	Phenylketonuria (PKU)	Phenylalanine hydroxylase Dihydropteridine reductase
Tyrosine	Tyrosinaemia I Tyrosinaemia II	Fumarylacetoacetate hydrolase Tyrosine aminotransferase
Methionine	Homocystinuria	Cystathionine synthase in the methionine salvage pathway
Branched amino acids	Maple syrup urine disease	Branched-chain keto acid dehydrogenase
Phenylalanine and tyrosine	Alkaptonuria	Homogentisic acid oxidase
Tyrosine	Albinism	Tyrosinase
All amino acids	Hyperammonaemia	Urea cycle defect, e.g. ornithine transcarbamylase

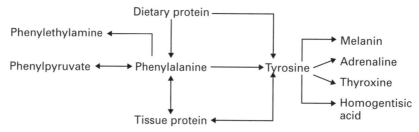

Fig. 178 Phenylalanine and tyrosine metabolism.

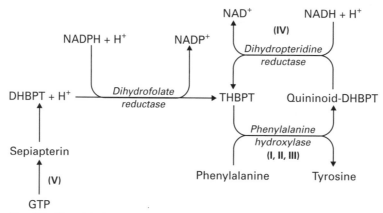

Fig. 179 Phenylalanine hydroxylase and its coenzyme requirement. Defects in phenylalanine hydroxylase itself resulting in types I, II and III PKU; defects in regeneration of the tetrahydrobiopterin (THBPT) coenzyme result in type IV PKU, and deficient production of the THBPT precursor causes type V PKU.

The diagnosis of PKU is made in neonates. Children with PKU cannot be recognised at birth by physical examination since they have been protected from defective phenylalanine metabolism by their mothers. However, when they consume and metabolise protein they will develop hyperphenylalaninaemia and only a few months' exposure to this will cause reduced mentation (5IQ points lost per month). Every newborn in the UK is screened for hyperphenylalaninaemia by the Guthrie test, which is a microbiological assay carried out on a dried spot of blood taken (ideally) after the baby is about 5 days old and has had several meals containing protein. The aim is to identify newborn children with the defect in order that dietary therapy can be instituted, by restricting phenylalanine intake in the diet. However, enough phenylalanine must be included since it is one of the essential amino acids.

Carbohydrate metabolism

Glycogen storage diseases

There are several glycogen storage diseases (GSDs) (Table 38): in each case there are excessive levels of glycogen in liver or muscle. In several of these it is easy to predict the outcome from a knowledge of the significance of the metabolic pathway that becomes impaired:

- hepatic glucose 6-phosphatase deficiency will lead to hypoglycaemia, given the critical role of G-6-Pase in glucose production by either glycogenolysis or gluconeogenesis
- muscle phosphorylase deficiency will affect the ability to support a high level of muscular contraction given the key role that glycogen serves as the fuel supporting such work.

Table 38 The glycogen storage diseases

Type	Enzyme affected	Tissues affected	Symptoms
I	Glucose 6-phosphatase	Liver, kidney, intestine	Large liver and kidney, stunted growth, acidosis, hypoglycemia, hyperlipidaemia
II	Lysosomal glucosidase	All organs	Cardiomegaly, hepatomegaly
III	Debrancher system	Liver, muscle, heart	Hepatomegaly, normal lipids and glucose
IV	Brancher enzyme	Generalised	Hepatosplenomegaly, ascites, cirrhosis, liver failure
V	Muscle phosphorylase	Skeletal muscle only	Weakness and cramping of skeletal muscle on exercise, no rise of blood lactate
VI	Liver phosphorylase	Liver	Hepatomegaly, normal spleen, no hypoglycemia, lipaemia or acidosis
VII	Phosphofructokinase-1	Skeletal muscle, red blood cells	Weakness and cramping of skeletal muscle on exercise

Table 39 Disorders in carbohydrate metabolism

Disorder	Defective enzyme
Essential fructosuria	Fructokinase
Hereditary fructose intolerance	Fructose 1-phosphate aldolase
Galactosaemia	Galactokinase or galactose 1-phosphate uridyl transferase
Haemolytic anaemia	Pyruvate kinase, glucose 6-phosphate dehydrogenase

Other disorders

Other disorders in carbohydrate metabolism are listed in Table 39. Because of the severity of the form of galactosaemia involving defective galactose 1-phosphate uridyl transferase, blood samples from newborn infants are screened for high levels of galactose. The condition is treated by withdrawing lactose (and galactose) from the diet.

Lipid metabolism

Familial hypercholesterolaemia (FH) and sphingolipi-doses are discussed in Chapter 10.

Management of genetic diseases

Biochemical approaches

Understanding the biochemical nature of the defect can greatly aid the management of genetic diseases. Here are some successful strategies:

- **control of metabolite levels,** e.g. limit uptake of precursors which might undergo toxic accumulation (used in phenylketonuria)
- **supply the missing metabolite,** e.g. give thyroxine to treat thyroid insufficiency caused by defects in thyroid hormone synthesis
- **use drugs to alter metabolite levels,** e.g. to assist in clearance of an accumulating metabolite (use of cholestyramine complexes to increase cholesterol excretion in FH) or to modulate an enzyme activity (inhibition of cytosolic HMG-CoA reductase (control step of cholesterol biosynthesis) in FH)
- **replace affected organ(s)** by transplant, e.g. cystic fibrosis could be treated by a lung or heart/lung transplant; FH homozygotes need a liver transplant to survive; and adult polycystic kidney disease is treatable by kidney transplant
- **supply the missing protein,** this is easy if blood is the tissue affected (factor VIII injections in haemophilia A).

Gene therapy: potential and problems

The aim of gene therapy is to replace the mutated gene with a good copy of the cloned sequence. In practice, there are many problems and certain conditions to be met. It may be almost impossible to physically replace the mutated copy in a precise way and it may be necess-ary to use viral vectors to introduce the gene. Again, there is the problem of targeting the gene to the correct tissue. Also, it is difficult to arrange for the correct expression, even if the normal promoter is included in the construct (even small changes in the expression may be problematic). Also, there are ethical questions, e.g. germ line gene therapy.

The basis of gene therapy is the use of retroviral vectors carrying a base sequence or gene for the missing protein. It is used to 'infect' the affected tissue with essentially a genetically engineered virus that integrates into the DNA and can express the protein to correct the disease. Liposomes (small lipid vesicles) may be an alternative mode of delivery, e.g. for cystic fibrosis therapy.

21.4 **DNA analysis and inherited disease**

Diagnostic methods

Accurate and early diagnosis is needed for successful management and treatment of inherited disease. As well as carrying out diagnosis in existing individuals and making a prognosis for them, we also need to advise them on the prospects for any children they may have. In addition we need the ability to make antenatal diagnosis to advise parents of the likely prognosis for any baby they have conceived.

Diagnosis can be biochemical or DNA-based. While the latter is more modern, the former is still very useful for some conditions. Normally it is done at 12–16 weeks of gestation by amniocentesis, with a positive diagnosis being followed by counselling. Amniotic cells can be cultured for chromosome and biochemical tests. An enzyme assay carried out on amniotic cells for hexosaminidase A is used to screen for Tay–Sachs disease (p. 130), which causes cerebral degeneration/death at 3–4 years. Carriers for Tay–Sachs disease have been screened for in Jewish populations and this allows for appropriate counselling for couples who are both heterozygotes for this autosomal recessive disorder. Amniocentesis is risky and it is done at a relatively late stage of development of fetus. Chorionic villus sampling to obtain fetal cells can be done as early as 6–8 weeks. DNA is extracted from the samples for DNA analyses.

Genetic approaches to inherited disease

Human molecular genetics has revolutionised the detection and monitoring of the mutant genes that cause inherited diseases. The major advantage of DNA analysis for antenatal testing is that the technique is not limited to proteins that the amniocytes express. It is the DNA of the fetal cell which is analysed and that reflects the DNA in every other cell in the body.

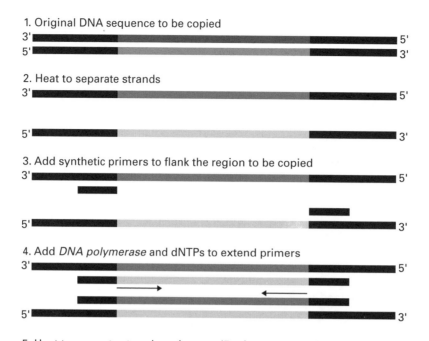

1. Original DNA sequence to be copied

2. Heat to separate strands

3. Add synthetic primers to flank the region to be copied

4. Add *DNA polymerase* and dNTPs to extend primers

5. Heat to separate strands and repeat (5 minutes per cycle)

Fig. 180 The polymerase chain reaction for amplification of specific DNA sequences.

Molecular genetics has provided routine techniques:

- for extracting DNA from samples
- for amplifying parts of its sequence to produce enough DNA for other techniques
- for cleaving it at sites where specific short sequences occur
- for determining the length of cleavage fragments
- for determining the sequence of DNA chains hundreds of nucleotide units in length
- for isolating fragments containing sequences of interest
- for locating the positions of sequences of interest on specific chromosomes
- for detecting differences between almost identical sequences
- for expressing sequences which specify the amino acid sequences of proteins.

The following is a summary of biochemical methods now common in medical genetics.

Cloning. Amplification of DNA can be carried out by cloning. The DNA to be amplified is cleaved into fragments, typically thousands of base pairs in length, which are inserted into the DNA of a suitable bacteriophage or other vector that is used to infect bacteria growing in a dish of solid medium. Each phage particle, carrying its unique inserted sequence, produces a plaque on the dish which contains thousands of new phage, all identical to the original. Phage from each plaque is then propagated in a bacterial culture and harvested.

Polymerase chain reaction. Amplification of DNA sequences may also be achieved by means of the polymerase chain reaction (PCR). In this technique samples of DNA are used as a template for the in vitro synthesis of new chains (Fig. 180). The whole process is made more convenient by the availability of purified DNA polymerase from thermophilic bacteria which is not destroyed by the high temperatures needed to separate the DNA strands. Repeated cycles of duplication can be performed with a single reaction mixture by programmed temperature changes between the temperatures needed for separation of the DNA chains, for annealing the primers, which are added in excess at the start, and for DNA synthesis.

Restriction enzymes. Specific cleavage of DNA molecules is carried out using restriction endonucleases or restriction enzymes (Fig. 181). These enzymes, which are part of a bacterial system for preventing phage infection, recognise specific short, typically six, but sometimes four or eight, base-pair sequences within a DNA double helix and cleave both chains at this site. The cleavage sequences are often palindromic, reading the same from left to right or from right to left. Both

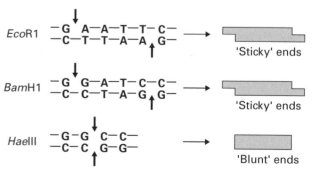

Fig. 181 Examples of restriction endonucleases.

chains may be cut between neighbouring base pairs to produce blunt ends or the cuts to the two chains may be offset producing sticky ends. Since 4^6 or 4096 different six base sequences are possible, an enzyme which recognises such a sequence will cleave DNA into fragments with an average length of 4096 base pairs. Many such enzymes, each specific for its own cleavage sequence, have been identified and isolated. The enzymes are named after the strain of bacteria in which they occur, e.g. *Eco*R1 from *E. coli*, *Bam*H1 from *Bacillus amyloliquefaciens*. The polynucleotides produced from DNA by treatment with restriction enzymes are known as restriction fragments.

Fragment separation by gel electrophoresis. Restriction fragments may be separated from one another and their lengths measured by electrophoresis on agarose gels. All polynucleotides are negatively charged, carrying one negative charge on the phosphate of each nucleotide unit. Their electrophoretic migration rate towards the positive electrode depends only on their length and not on their base composition or sequence. Because of the sieving action of the gel, short fragments migrate faster than long fragments. A mixture of fragments can thus be separated and the lengths of individual fragments determined by running the mixture on a gel together with marker fragments of known length.

Restriction mapping. Regions of DNA can be mapped by a combination of cleavage with restriction enzymes and measurement of fragment lengths. The restriction map produced in this way is a physical map of the DNA showing the distances between the various restriction sites. Such a map is the basis for a complete base sequence determination of the region.

Restriction fragment length polymorphisms, (RFLPs). Mutations occasionally lead to creation of a new cleavage site or removal of a former one. A mutation may thus alter the lengths of restriction fragments produced from a particular region of the DNA. Two fragments may no longer be separated and thus appear as a single fragment with a length of the two combined. Alternatively, a single fragment may have a new site created within it and appear as two shorter fragments. These fragment patterns, which are known as restriction length polymorphisms or RFLPs, behave like Mendelian genes and can be traced from parents to offspring. More importantly they can be mapped on the chromosomes and provide much more useful markers than conventional genes.

RFLPs in the diagnosis of inherited disease. Mapping restriction sites and locating genes on chromosomes provide powerful and incisive tools for studying the inheritance of mutant genes responsible for inherited diseases. Because crossing-over events are rare between sites or genes that are close together on a chromosome, following the inheritance of an RFLP gives very strong evidence about whether a neighbouring gene, perhaps one involved in an inherited disease, has been passed on or not.

DNA sequencing. DNA fragments up to several hundred base pairs long can be sequenced directly by the Sanger 2,3 dideoxy method.

Southern blotting. DNA fragments containing known sequences can be located after gel electrophoresis by the process of Southern blotting. After electrophoretic separation, the fragments are converted to single chain form by treatment with alkali and transferred, or blotted, from the gel to a sheet of nitrocellulose. If the sheet is then probed with short lengths of DNA of known sequence, the probes, which are usually radio-actively labelled for easy detection, will anneal with those separated fragments that have a complementary sequence. After excess probes have been washed away, only probes that have annealed will remain on the sheet. Detection of their radioactivity reveals the positions of the required fragments.

Locations of genes on chromosomes can be revealed using a similar technique. Probes, short lengths of DNA carrying either a radioactive or fluorescent marker, can be annealed with suitable chromosome preparations thus showing on which chromosome and where within the chromosome, sequences complementary to the probe are located. This provides a much more powerful method than conventional genetics for finding gene loci on chromosomes.

Production of proteins of therapeutic value by recombinant DNA technology. A fragment of DNA which codes for a protein can be inserted into a suitable vector that has a promoter sequence near the point of insertion. Expression of the DNA sequence, i.e. transcription to mRNA and translation to protein, may then be achieved by introducing the vector into a host cell. Notice that direct transfer of eukaryotic DNA fragments into bacteria will not work since bacteria cannot deal with any introns the DNA may contain. Better to isolate the relevant RNA from eukaryotic tissue and make so-called cDNA by copying this RNA sequence into DNA using reverse transcriptase. Another problem is that bacteria are incapable of carrying out any post-translational modification the manufactured protein may require. Expression vectors that can use eukaryotic hosts have been developed. Examples of the use of this methodology are:

* preparation of **factor VIII** for treatment of haemophilia A. Previously haemophiliacs were treated with blood products enriched with this factor. However, some blood used for the preparation was HIV-contaminated and many treated haemophiliacs developed AIDS
* preparation of **growth hormone** which is used to treat children who are deficient in this hormone. Several growth hormone preparations proved to be contaminated and Creutzfeldt–Jakob disease (CJD), a fatal encephalopathy, developed in some treated subjects. Human growth hormone is now manufactured by recombinant DNA technology. This eliminates the risk of CJD and also produces

growth hormone in much larger quantities than were previously available

- **insulin** which had previously been prepared from the pancreas of animals, is now produced by recombinant DNA technology; the product is not antigenic.

The Human Genome Project

The Human Genome Project aims to characterise the complete human genome, including its 50 000–100 000 genes. It is enabling technology for molecular medicine.

Molecular medicine will enable the early detection of diseases, gene therapy and powerful analytical approaches to determine the biochemical nature of diseases. The ultimate aim is to determine the complete DNA sequence, an enormous task given that the human genome is 3×10^9 bp (i.e. equivalent to a DNA molecule 5 feet long). Most of the DNA (>90%) is non-coding (introns/intergenic sequence/junk DNA) and only 10% is coding. There is a need to identify the exon/intron boundaries in the DNA sequence.

Self-assessment: questions

Multiple choice questions

1. The following are characteristics of sphingolipidoses:
   a. Autosomal recessive inheritance
   b. The defective enzymes are hydrolases
   c. Significant pathology in heterozygotes
   d. Diagnosis is possible using enzyme assays
   e. The defective enzymes are in catabolic rather than anabolic pathways

2. The following pairs link cause and disease:
   a. Glucose 6-phosphate dehydrogenase deficiency and favism
   b. Homocystinuria and methionine metabolism
   c. Niemann–Pick disease and sphingomyelin accumulation
   d. Defective tetrahydrobiopterin biosynthesis and PKU type I
   e. Hyperammoninaemia and urea cycle defect

3. The following tests for inborn errors of amino acid catabolism instituted by Guthrie are recommended:
   a. Retesting as soon as possible after a positive test result is obtained for an aminoacidopathy
   b. Carrying out the assay for the offending amino acid in blood rather than for a metabolite of the amino acid in urine
   c. Ensuring that blood samples (dried spots of blood) are withdrawn after the child has had several protein-containing meals
   d. Carrying out the test when the child reaches 5 years of age
   e. Recognising that there can be multiple causes leading to the same phenotype

4. In inheritance of disease:
   a. In autosomal recessive disorders the mutated gene must be on one of the autosomes
   b. Lack of penetrance in autosomal dominant inheritance indicates that external factors are not involved in the expression of phenotype
   c. In autosomal dominant inheritance both sexes are equally affected
   d. An X-linked recessive inheritance pedigree shows sons and mothers with the disorder
   e. In autosomal recessive disorders heterozygotes are usually normal

True/false questions

Are the following statements true or false?

1. The mutation that results in the formation of HbS (sickle cell haemoglobin) rather than HbA is a single base change in the DNA coding for β chains of haemoglobin.
2. Albinism results from a defect in melanin biosynthesis.
3. PCR stands for polymerase chain reductase.
4. Familial hypercholesterolaemia is an example of a disease where the inheritance is autosomal recessive.
5. Restriction enzymes recognise sequences in DNA that are often palindromic.
6. Differential clinical symptoms may result from different mutations in a given gene.
7. Prenatal diagnosis of an inherited disease requires that the biochemical nature of the defect is understood.
8. Linked polymorphisms (RFLPs or AFLPs) are of greater value in disease diagnosis than mapping conventional genes.
9. DNA probes can be used to identify the chromosomal location of genes.
10. Recombinant methods always employ bacteria as the host cell for producing proteins to be subsequently used in therapy.
11. Southern blotting cannot be carried out at the North pole.
12. A cDNA library prepared from a tissue, e.g. liver, would be much smaller than a genomic library prepared from liver.

Short essay question

Contrast the testing procedures used in the diagnosis of phenylketonuria (PKU) with those used in Tay–Sachs disease (TSD).

Self-assessment: answers

Multiple choice answers

1. a. **True.** The only exception is Fabry's disease.
   b. **True.** These are lysosomal enzymes involved in sphingolipid breakdown.
   c. **False.** The enzyme produced from one allele is sufficient.
   d. **True.** Heterozygotes can be found upon screening, where the enzyme activity is measured and found to be half of normal.
   e. **True.** There is no evidence for increased synthesis.

2. a. **True.** Favism is a condition where subjects develop sever haemolytic anaemia when they eat fava beans; it is caused by glucose 6-phosphate dehydrogenase deficiency.
   b. **True.** The methionine salvage pathway is defective.
   c. **True.** Sphingomyelin accumulates because of a defect in sphingomyelinase.
   d. **False.** The classic type I form of PKU results from defective phenylalanine hydroxylase. Defective synthesis of its coenzyme is type V.
   e. **True.** The urea cycle defect results in inadequate clearance of ammonia produced in deamination reactions.

3. a. **True.** Two things are accomplished. It finds out if the defect was 'transient'; and confirms the diagnosis so therapy can be started promptly and with confidence.
   b. **True.** This eliminates problems related to kidney malfunction.
   c. **True.** If the child is not challenged with amino acids (protein), then the defect could be missed. Therefore, testing must not occur too soon.
   d. **False.** In many cases the untreated affected child will have an achievable IQ of about 50 by aged 5 years.
   e. **True.** The best example is PKU, where there are several potential causes for increased phenylalanine in blood. In types IV and V, the child needs additional therapy.

4. a. **True.** This must be obvious.
   b. **False.** It is the external (exogenous) factors contributing to the phenotype that results in the abnormal phenotype not being expressed in their absence.
   c. **True.** Only one bad copy of the gene is needed so there is no sex preference.
   d. **False.** The mothers are not affected since they have good copy of the X chromosome.
   e. **True.** This makes it important to find these carriers by enzyme assay or DNA analysis.

True/false answers

1. **True.** Codon 6 of the β chain changes from GAG in HbA to GUG in HbS. Valine substitutes for glutamate.
2. **True.** Tyrosinase is defective and this enzyme is required for melanin synthesis.
3. **False.** It stands for polymerase chain reaction.
4. **False.** Inheritance is autosomal dominant.
5. **True.** The palindromic sequence occurs in four to eight base pairs of DNA.
6. **True.**
7. **False.** Duchenne's muscular dystrophy is an example of a disorder where prenatal diagnosis was available before dystrophin was identified as the affected protein.
8. **True.** It is the linkage that is critical in terms of their utility in disease diagnosis.
9. **True.** The DNA probes contain radioactive or fluorescent markers.
10. **False.** Bacteria cannot deal with introns nor can they carry out post-translational modifications of the required protein.
11. **False.** Southern was the name of the scientist who developed the technique.
12. **True.** It corresponds to the exons whereas the genomic library would include exons and introns.

Short essay answer

Both disorders are autosomal recessive. However, a key difference between them is that at this time there is no treatment for TSD whereas for PKU adoption of a strict dietary regimen prevents the development of the major symptom, mental retardation. TSD homozygotes die within 3 years of birth after a life that features blindness and mental retardation.

In TSD the important testing that has been introduced is to find heterozygotes in the population. This is done by measuring the defective enzyme, hexosaminidase A, in blood samples from susceptible populations. Heterozygotes have half the normal amount of the enzyme. Heterozygotes who are married and wish to have children are offered amniocentesis carried out around week 13 during any pregnancy. Amniocytes are cultured and hexosaminidase A measured. The absence of activity indicates that the fetus is a homozygote for the disorder. Heterozygotes will have half normal activity but that ensures them a normal life.

In PKU it is the newborn baby who is evaluated. The baby's phenylalanine hydroxylase activity is determined by measuring their blood phenylalanine. PKU infants will have highly elevated blood phenylalanine levels, which appear after the baby has had several meals containing protein. The finding of elevated phenylalanine in a dried spot of blood leads to a follow-up test for confirmation of the finding. Since PKU babies are normal (because their mother prevented phenylalanine accumulating), the testing (Guthrie test) is carried out on all newborn babies.

Since PKU can also be caused by defects in the biopterin coenzyme for phenylalanine hydroxylase, dihydropteridine reductase is measured in babies who have hyperphenylalaninaemia since the therapy for this form of PKU is more complicated.

Index

Copper, 246, 247Q/248A
  in metalloenzymes, 28
Core biochemistry courses, 1
Co-repressors, bacterial DNA
    transcription, 181, 186Q/188A
Cori cycle, 97–98, 100Q/102A
Coronary artery disease, plasma enzymes,
    31 (Box)
Corpus luteum, 225, 236
Corticosteroid-binding globulin,
    233Q/235A, 252 (Table)
Corticotrophin (adrenocorticotrophic
    hormone), **140**, 223, 224,
    233Q/235A
Corticotrophin-releasing hormone, 140,
    223 (Table), 224
Cortisol, 140, 222 (Fig.), 224, 233Q/235A,
    234Q/236A
  binding to renal mineralocorticoid
    receptor, 232
Cotransport, 50–51, 74–75
Coumarin anticoagulants, 256, 257
Counter-regulatory hormones, 139–140,
    149Q/151A
Coupled assays, 30–31, 40Q/43A
Covalent bonds
  cleavage, 36, 41Q/44A
  enzyme inhibition, 34, 41Q/44A
  peptides, 13 see also Disulphide bonds
Covalent control, glycogen metabolism,
    95, 104
Covalent modification
  gluconeogenesis enzymes, 96
  irreversible, 39
  reversible, 38, 41Q/44A
C-peptide, 220
Creatine, synthesis, transmethylation, 113,
    116Q/118A
Creatine kinase, heart, 144, 146 (Box)
Creatine phosphate, muscle, 147,
    148Q/150A
Creatine phosphokinase, coronary artery
    disease, 31 (Box)
Creatinine, 148Q/150A
CREB (cyclic AMP response element
    binding protein), 229
Cretinism, 225
Creutzfeldt–Jakob disease, risk in growth
    hormone therapy, 269
Crigler–Najjar disease, 215
Cristae, mitochondria, 85
C-terminal ends, 13, 15
CTP
  inhibition of pyrimidine nucleotide
    synthesis, 156
  phospholipid synthesis, 129,
    160Q/161A
Cyanide, on cytochrome oxidase, 85,
    88Q/91A
Cyclic AMP
  catabolism, 229, 230, 234Q/237A
  DNA transcription control, E. coli, 181,
    186Q/188A
  on glycogen metabolism, 95,
    100Q/102A–103A
  hormone signal transduction, 228–230
Cyclic AMP response element binding
    protein, 229
Cyclic GMP, nitric oxide action, 232
Cyclooxygenase pathway, 130
Cysteine, 14 (Fig.), 22Q/24A, 111, **120**
  disulphide bonds, 13, 19
Cystic fibrosis
  gene therapy, 209
  organ transplantation, 267
  pancreatic enzyme therapy, 32 (Box)
Cytochrome b-c₁ complex, mitochondrial
    electron transport, 85

Cytochrome oxidase, 60, 88Q/91A, 114
  mitochondrial electron transport, 85
Cytochromes, P450, 114, 116Q/119A
  drug metabolism, 213
  ethanol-oxidising system, 212
  haem catabolism, 213
  induction, 213 (Box)
  steroid synthesis, 221
Cytoplasm, oxidation of NADH, 84–85
Cytosine, 154 (Table)
  nucleic acids, 167, 172Q/174A
Cytoskeleton, 48
Cytosol, 48 (Table)

D
DAG (diacylglycerol), 124, 133Q/135A,
    230, 234Q/236A:237A
dATP, 157, 168, 173Q/174A
dCTP, 168, 173Q/174A
Deacylase see Thioesterase
Deamination, 109
Death rates, body mass index, 240
Debranching enzymes, glycogenolysis, 94,
    101Q/103A
  defects, 266 (Table)
Decarboxylation, 112, 116Q/118A
  oxidative
    α-ketoglutarate, 83
    coenzymes, 72 (Table)
DeCase (orotidine 5′-monophosphate
    decarboxylase), 156
Degeneracy, genetic code, 190, 198Q/200A
Dehalogenase, thyroidal, 221
7–Dehydrocholesterol, 227 (Fig.)
  vitamin D from, 128, 132Q/134A, 237
Dehydroepiandrosterone, 222 (Fig.)
Dehydrogenases, 29
Deletions, genetic, 264 (Table)
δ-aminolaevulinic acid, 111, 114
δ-aminolaevulinic acid dehydratase, 114
δ-aminolaevulinic acid synthase, 114, 115,
    116Q/119A
Delta cells, 227
ΔG⁰′, 71
Denaturation, 16, 17, **20**, 22Q/24A:25A,
    23Q/25A
  of enzymes, 31–32
De novo pathways
  purine nucleotide synthesis, 154, 155
  pyrimidine nucleotide synthesis, 156,
    160Q/161A
Dental caries, 240
  fluoride, 246, 247Q/248A
Deoxycorticosterone, 222 (Fig.)
Deoxyribonucleotides, synthesis, 157–158
Deoxyribose, 165
Deoxyribose backbones, DNA, 167
Deoxythymidine, synthesis, 157–158,
    160Q/161A
Depilatories, 19
Desaturation, fatty acids, 123,
    132Q/134A:135A
  see also Unsaturated fatty acids
dGTP, 168
Diabetes mellitus, 138
  ketoacidosis, 83 (Box), 138
  from steroid treatment, 140
Diacylglycerol, 124, 133Q/135A, **230**,
    234Q/236A:237A
Diarrhoea, salt/glucose solutions, 75 (Box)
Dielectric constant, water, 7, 9Q/10A
Dietary nutrients
  amino acid requirements, 110
  carbohydrates, 72–75, 240
  cholesterol, 126
  fats, 75–76, 240–241
  fibre, 72, 145, 240
  proteins, **106**, 241, 247Q/248A

    intake rate, 107
    vitamins, 241–245
Diffusion across cell membranes, 50
Digestion
  carbohydrates, 73–74
  fats, 75–76
  proteins, 106–107
Digestive enzymes
  covalent modification, 39
  protein turnover in production, 107
  therapeutic use, 32 (Box)
Dihydrofolate reductase, 157, 162
  inhibitors, 157 (Box)
Dihydroorotase, 156
Dihydropteridine reductase, 265
5α-Dihydrotestosterone, 223, 224
Dihydrovitamin K, 256, 261
Dihydroxyacetone phosphate, 96, 124
24,25-Dihydroxycholecalciferol, 226
1,25-Dihydroxycholecalciferol (calcitriol),
    212, 217, **226–227**, 235, 237
Dihydroxyphenylalanine, 221 (Fig.)
Di-iodotyrosine, 220
Diisopropylfluorophosphate, 38
Dimethylallyl pyrophosphate, 126 (Fig.)
2,4-Dinitrophenol, 86, 88Q/91A
Dipalmitoyl phosphatidyl choline,
    48 (Box), 133Q/135A
Dipeptidases, 106
Dipeptides, 13
Diphosphatidylglycerol (cardiolipin), 129,
    132Q/134A
Diploidy, 264
Disaccharides, 73, 88Q/90A
Dissociation
  acids, 7, 9Q/10A
  oxygen and haemoglobin, 59–61
Distal histidine residues, haem groups, 59
Disulphide bonds, 13, 14 (Fig.), **19**,
    23Q/25A
  immunoglobulins, 253, 259Q/260A
Diurnal variation, 233Q/235A
  growth hormone secretion, 140
  HMG-CoA reductase, 127
DNA, 12–13, **164–175**, 172Q/174A
  analysis, 267–270, 271Q/272A
  hormone-responsive elements, 232,
    234Q/237A
  repair, 170
  sequencing, 269
  sterol response element, 127
  see also Replication, genetic
DNA-binding proteins, 181, 186Q/188A
DNA ligase, 169, 170, 173Q/175A
DNA polymerases, **168**, 169, 170,
    173Q/174A:175A
DNA viruses, 204, 208Q/209A
  replication, 205
dNTP, deoxyribonucleotide synthesis, 157
Domains, proteins, 21, 23Q/25A
  immunoglobulins, 253, 259Q/260A
Dominant genes, 264–265, 271Q/272A
DOPA, for phenylketonuria, 265
Dopamine β-hydroxylase, 221 (Fig.)
Double helix, nucleic acids, 165–167,
    172Q/174A
Double sieve mechanism, protein
    synthesis errors, 191
Double-stranded DNA, RNA viruses, 204,
    208Q/209A
Downstream direction, nucleic acids, 166,
    179
Drugs
  anticancer drugs, 157, 160Q/161–162A
  enzyme inhibitors, 35 (Box), 41Q/44A
  induction of cytochromes P450, 213 (Box)
  metabolism in liver, 213, 216Q/217A
  see also Antibiotics; named drugs

Haemoglobin (*contd*)
  oxygen affinity, 12, 59–60
  quaternary structure, 20
  tertiary structure, 19
Haemoglobinopathies, 63
  see also Sickle cell disease; Thalassaemias
Haemolytic anaemia *see* Glucose
      6-phosphate dehydrogenase
      deficiency; Pyruvate kinase,
      deficiency
Haemolytic jaundice, 215
Haemophilias, 256
  recombinant factor VIII therapy, 269
Haem oxygenase, 213
Hair, keratin, 19
Haploidy, 264
Haptoglobin, 252–253, 259Q/260A
Hartnup's disease, 244
HDL, 124 (Table)
Heart
  fuel metabolism, 143–144,
      148Q/150A:151A, 149Q/151A
    fatty acids, 88Q/90A, 144,
      148Q/151A
  insulin, 231
Heart disease
  dietary fats, 241 (Box), 247Q/248A
  fibrinolysis for, 257
  folate, 244
  low-dose aspirin, 130
  plasma enzymes, 31 (Box), 146 (Box)
Heavy chains, immunoglobulins, 21, **253**,
      259Q/260A
Heavy metals, 34, 41Q/44A
Helicases, bacteria, 171
Heparin, 256–257, 259Q/260A
Hereditary fructose intolerance, 267
      (Table)
Herpes viruses, 204 (Table)
Heterotrophs, 70
Heterotropic allosteric binding,
      haemoglobin, 59, 60
Heterozygosity, 264
Hexokinase, 29, 35 (Table), 40Q/43A, 77,
      88Q/90A
  Cori cycle, 100Q/102A
  coupled assay, 30–31
  EC number, 29
  isoenzyme kinetics, 33–34, 77
  sampled assay, 30
  specificity, 28
  substrate enfolding, 36
Hexosaminidase A deficiency, 130, 267
Hexose monophosphate shunt *see* Pentose
      phosphate pathway
HGPRTase *see* Hypoxanthine–guanine
      phosphoribosyltransferase
High molecular weight kininogen, blood
      coagulation, 256
Hinges, immunoglobulins, 253
Histamine, 111
Histidine, 14 (Fig.), 22Q/24A, 111, 120
  haemoglobin, 16, 59, 62
Histones, 12, 164, **170**, 173Q/175A,
      186Q/188A
HIV *see* Human immunodeficiency virus
HMG-CoA, 82, 88Q/90A
  in cholesterol synthesis, 126,
      132Q/134A
HMG-CoA reductase, 127, 132Q/134A
  inhibitors, 127 (Box), 132Q/134A
Homeostasis, 220
Homocysteine-N^5-methyl-FH$_4$ transferase,
      113, 245
Homocystinuria, 265 (Table), 271Q/272A
Homogentisic acid, 264
Homotropic allosteric binding,
      haemoglobin, 59–60

Homozygosity, 264
Hormone-responsive elements, DNA, 232,
      234Q/237A
Hormones, 12, 220–237
  counter-regulatory, 139–140, 149Q/151A
  gastrointestinal tract, 76, 220 (Table)
  inactivation in liver, 213
  mechanisms, 228–232
  receptors, **52**, 53Q/54A, 228
  steroids *see* Cortisol; Glucocorticoids;
      Steroid hormones
Hormone-sensitive lipase (HSL), 80,
      133Q/135A
  ACTH on, 140
  adipose tissue, 142, 148Q/150A
Human genome, 164 (Table), 172Q/174A
Human Genome Project, 270
Human growth hormone *see* Growth
      hormone
Human immunodeficiency virus, 204
      (Table)
  drugs against, 35 (Box), 208Q/209A
  infection mechanism, 205
Hyaline membrane disease (respiratory
      distress syndrome), 48 (Box)
Hydration of ions, 7, 9Q/10A
Hydrochloric acid, 106
Hydrocortisone *see* Cortisol
Hydroeicosatetranoic acids, 130
Hydrogen, metabolism reactions, 70
Hydrogen bonds, 6–7, 9Q/10A
  enzyme action, 35–36
  peptides, 13
Hydrogen ions, 7, 9Q/10A
  acid catalysis, 37
  haemoglobin binding, 59, 60
  phosphofructokinase-1 regulation, 79,
      87Q/89A
  see also pH; Proton gradients
Hydrogen peroxide, glucose 6-phosphate
      dehydrogenase, 258
Hydrolases, 29, 271Q/272A
  and aminoacyl-tRNA synthetases,
      191–192, 199Q/200A
Hydrolysis, 8, 9Q/10A
  carbohydrates, 73–74
  fats, 75
  proteins, 16, 23Q/25A
Hydroperoxyeicosatetranoic acids, 130
Hydrophilia (molecular), 7, 9Q/10A,
      48–49
Hydrophilic hormones *see* Water-soluble
      hormones
Hydrophobia (molecular), 7, 9Q/10A,
      48–49
  protein side chains, 19, 22Q/24A
Hydroxy amino acids
  threonine, 14 (Fig.), 22Q/24A, 108, 111
  see also Serine
β-Hydroxybutyrate dehydrogenase, 82
  heart, 144
β-Hydroxybutyric acid, 82, 88Q/90A
25-Hydroxycholecalciferol, 226, 227 (Fig.)
1-Hydroxylase, calcium metabolism, 226,
      227
17α-Hydroxylase, 236
17-Hydroxypregnenolone, 236
11β-Hydroxysteroid dehydrogenase type
      II, 232
5-Hydroxytryptophan, for
      phenylketonuria, 265
25-Hydroxy-vitamin D, 212, 216Q/217A
Hypercholesterolaemia, 128 (Box),
      132Q/134A, 133Q/135A
HMG-CoA reductase inhibitors, 127
Hyperthyroidism, 225
Hypervariable regions, immunoglobulins,
      253

Hypophosphataemia, 245
Hypothalamic–pituitary–adrenal cortical
      axis, 224
Hypothalamic–pituitary–gonadal axis,
      224–225
Hypothalamic–pituitary–thyroid axis,
      225–226
Hypothalamus, 223–226
Hypothyroidism, primary, 225–226, 236
Hypoxanthine, 155
  catabolism, 158
Hypoxanthine–guanine
      phosphoribosyltransferase
      (HGPRTase), 160Q/161A
  absence, 155, 158 (Box)

I
Ice, 6
I-cell disease, 197 (Box)
Icosahedral viruses, 205
IDL (intermediate density lipoproteins),
      125, 132Q/134A
IgG (immunoglobulin G), 21, **253**,
      259Q/260A
IgM, IgA, IgD, IgE antibodies, 253,
      259Q/260A
Imidazole group, histidine, 14 (Fig.)
Immune system, self *vs* non-self, cell
      surface carbohydrates, 50
Immunoglobulins, 253–254, 259Q/260A
  G *see* IgG
IMP, 160Q/161A
  catabolism, 158
Inborn errors of metabolism, 265–267
Indoles
  metabolism of, 213
  tryptophan, 14 (Fig.)
Induced fit, enzyme action, 36
Inducers, bacterial DNA transcription,
      186Q/188A
Inducible proteins, 180, 186Q/188A
Induction, cytochromes P450, 213 (Box)
Infection, viral, 205
Influenza viruses, 204 (Table)
Inheritance, Mendelian, 264–265,
      271Q/272A
Inhibitors, of enzymes, **34–35**, 38,
      41Q/44A
Initial rates (v), enzyme reactions, 30
Initiation
  polypeptide synthesis, 192
  RNA synthesis, 179, 186Q/188A
Initiation complexes, 193, 199Q/201A
Inosine, catabolism, 158
Inosine monophosphate, 154 (Fig.), 155
Inositol trisphosphate, 95, **230**,
      234Q/236A
Insertions, genetic, 264 (Table)
Insulin, 12, **138**, 139, 148Q/150A
  on adipose tissue, 139 (Table), 142,
      148Q/150A
  adrenaline on release, 140
  on gluconeogenesis, 96, 97
  on glycogen metabolism, 95,
      100Q/102A
  on glycogen phosphorylase, 38
  on lipoprotein lipase, 125, 132Q/134A
  liver, 139 (Table), 141, 148Q/150A
  inactivation, 213
  lysosomal protein catabolism, 108
  marathon running, 147
  on pyruvate metabolism, 80
  receptors, 21, 111, 234Q/236A
  tyrosine kinase, 231
  recombinant, 270
  secretion, 138, 148Q/150A
  synthesis, 199Q/201A, 220

281

Plasmin, 257
Plasmodium falciparum, glucose
    6-phosphate dehydrogenase, 258
Platelet-derived growth factor, 231, 254
Platelets
    aspirin on, 130
    function, 254, 259Q/260A
Ploidy, 264
Point mutations, 191, 201
Polar bear liver, 241
Polarity, nucleic acids, 165–166
Polar molecules
    impermeability of cell membranes, 49
    water, 6, 7
Polio virus, 204 (Table)
Poly A tails, messenger RNA, 184
Polycistronic messengers, bacteria,
    186Q/188A
Polymerase chain reaction, 268
Polymerisation, biochemical, **8**, 10
Polypeptides, 13, 22Q/24A
    hormones, 223
Polysaccharides, 72–73, 88Q/90A
Polysomes, 192
Polyunsaturated fatty acids, 75
    and vitamin E, 242
P/O ratios, ATP yield, 86
Porphobilinogen, 114
Porphyrias, 115 (Box)
Porphyrin rings, 114
Positioning factors, blood coagulation,
    256, 259Q/260A
Positive-strand RNA, viruses, 206,
    208Q/209A
Post-translational modification
    hormones, 220
    proteins, 195–197, 199Q/201A
Potassium, 246
    on aldosterone secretion, 224,
      234Q/236A
Potency, enzymes, 28
Potential gradients, electrical, 51,
    53Q/54A
PP cells, 227
Precipitation, proteins, 15–16,
    22Q/24A:25A
Precursor proteins, side chains, 13
Pregnancy
    calcitonin, 227
    hormones, 220, 224
Pregnenolone, 221, 234Q/236A
Prekallikrein, blood coagulation, 256
Premature babies
    body composition, 240
    neonatal jaundice, 215
Prenatal diagnosis, 272
    amniocentesis, 267
    chorionic villus sampling, Tay–Sachs
      disease, 267
Preprocollagen, 197
Preproinsulin, 220
Primary hypothyroidism, 225–226, 236
Primary structure, proteins, 17
Primary transcript, RNA splicing, 184–185
Primases, 169
Primers, DNA replication, 169,
    173Q/174A:175A, 178 (Table)
Probes, DNA, 269, 271Q/272A
Procollagen, 197
Product inhibition, nucleotide synthesis,
    155, 156, 160Q/161A
Progesterone, 222, **224–225**, 236
Progress curves, enzyme reactions, 30,
    40Q/43A
Prohormones, 220, 224
Proinsulin, 220
Prokaryotes
    DNA replication, 168

DNA transcription control, 180–181
initiation of protein synthesis, **192**, 195,
    199Q/201A
mRNA, 190
see also Bacteria
Prolactin, 223 (Table)
Proline, 14 (Fig.), 22Q/24A, 23Q/25A
    collagen, 16
    collagen biosynthesis, 197, 199Q/201A
Promoters, 179, 186Q/188A
    eukaryotes, 181
    lac, E. coli, 181
    see also Start codons
Proof-reading
    DNA replication, 169–170
    protein synthesis, 191
Pro-opiomelanocortin, 140, 223,
    233Q/235A
Propionyl-CoA, 123
    metabolism, 82, 245
Prostacyclin, 130
Prostaglandins, 130–131
Prosthetic groups, enzymes, 28–29,
    40Q/43A, **72**
Proteases, 29
    digestive, 38, 106
    HIV, 35 (Box)
    peptidases, 106
    see also Carboxypeptidases
Protein(s), 12–25
    catabolism, 107–110
    cell membranes, 49–50, 53Q/54A
      transport function, 39, 50
    dietary, **106**, 241, 247Q/248A
    digestion, 106–107
    DNA transcription control, 180,
      186Q/188A
    energy content, 240
    metabolism, 106–120
    and nucleic acids, 172Q/174A
    post-translational modification and
      transport, 195–197, 199Q/201A
    purification, 15–16, 22Q/24A:25A
    storage as fuel, 138
    structure, 16–21
    synthesis, 12, 22Q/24A, **190–201**
    viral, 205
    see also Enzymes
Protein C, 256
Protein conservation phase, starvation,
    140
Protein kinase A, 228–229
    on glycogen metabolism, 95,
      100Q/102A, 104
Protein kinase C, activation, 230
Protein–lipid–enzyme complexes,
    mitochondrial electron transport,
    85
Protein S, 256
Prothrombin, 255
    vitamin K action, 256, 259Q/260A
Prothrombin time, 215, 216Q/217A
Proton donors, 37
Proton gradients, metabolism, 70, **85–86**,
    88Q/91A
Protoporphyrin III, 115
Proximal histidine residues, haem groups,
    59
PRPP (phosphoribosylpyrophosphate),
    155, 156, 160Q/161A
PRPP synthetase, on pyrimidine
    nucleotide synthesis, 156
Pseudoirreversible inhibitor, methotrexate
    as, 157 (Box)
Pumps *see* ATPases; Ion pumps; Sodium
    pump
Punctuation *see* Unpunctuated genetic
    code

Purification, proteins, 15–16, 22Q/24A:25A
Purine nucleotides, 154–156, 160Q/161A
    in nucleic acids, 165, **167**, 172Q/174A,
      198Q/200A
Purines, catabolism, 158
Pyridoxal phosphate, 116Q/118A, 244,
    247Q/248A, 249
    aminotransferases, 109
Pyridoxine, 243 (Fig.), 244, 247Q/248A
Pyrimidine nucleotides, 154
    metabolites, 159
    in nucleic acids, 165, **167**, 172Q/174A,
      198Q/200A
    synthesis, 155–156, 160Q/161A
Pyrimidine phosphoribosyltransferase,
    156, 160Q/161A
Pyrophosphatases, 168
Pyrophosphate
    from protein synthesis, 191
    from RNA synthesis, 179, 186Q/188A
Pyrophosphate bonds, ATP, 70, 87Q/90A
Pyruvate
    aerobic metabolism, 79–80
    gluconeogenesis pathway, 96–97,
      101Q/103A
    from glucose, 77
    see also PEP/pyruvate substrate cycle
Pyruvate carboxylase, 96,
    100Q/102A:103A
    acetyl-CoA, 101Q/103A
    Cori cycle, 100Q/102A
Pyruvate dehydrogenase complex, **79–80**,
    87Q/90A, 88Q/90A:91A,
    100Q/103A, 248–249
Pyruvate kinase, 77, 79, 88Q/91A,
    100Q/103A
    Cori cycle, 100Q/102A
    deficiency, red cells, 259Q/261A
    liver-type, 97, 101Q/103A

Q
Quaternary structure, 23Q/25A
    proteins, 17, 20–21

R
Radiation (ionising), 170
Radiochemistry, enzyme reactions, 30,
    42Q/44A
Reading frames, polypeptide synthesis,
    192
Receptor-mediated endocytosis, 51–52
    cholesterol, 127
Receptors
    of hormones, **52**, 53Q/54A, 228
    insulin *see* Insulin, receptors
    viral infection, 205
    see also Signal transduction systems
Recessive genes, 264, 265, 271Q/272A
Recombinant DNA technology, 269–270,
    271Q/272A
Red cells, 58
    glucose 6-phosphate dehydrogenase
      deficiency, 101Q/103A
    lactate production, 87Q/90A
    metabolism of, 257–258
    nutrients, 246
    see also Erythropoietin
5α-Reductase, 224
Reduction/oxidation, metabolism, 70
Reductive biosynthesis, coenzymes,
    72 (Table)
Regulation (signal proteins), 12
Rehydration solutions *see* Salt/glucose
    solutions
Release factors, protein synthesis
    termination, 194
Release of viruses, 206